Advances and Updates in Fetal and Neonatal Surgery

Editors

KUOJEN TSAO
HANMIN LEE

CLINICS IN PERINATOLOGY

www.perinatology.theclinics.com

Consulting Editor
LUCKY JAIN

December 2022 • Volume 49 • Number 4

ELSEVIER

1600 John F. Kennedy Boulevard • Suite 1800 • Philadelphia, Pennsylvania, 19103-2899

http://www.theclinics.com

CLINICS IN PERINATOLOGY Volume 49, Number 4
December 2022 ISSN 0095-5108, ISBN-13: 978-0-323-98757-8

Editor: Kerry Holland
Developmental Editor: Karen Solomon

Clinics in Perinatology (ISSN 0095-5108) is published quarterly by Elsevier Inc., 360 Park Avenue South, New York, NY 10010-1710. Months of issue are March, June, September, and December. Business and Editorial Offices: 1600 John F. Kennedy Blvd., Ste. 1800, Philadelphia, PA 19103-2899. Customer Service Office: 3251 Riverport Lane, Maryland Heights, MO 63043. Periodicals postage paid at New York, NY and additional mailing offices. Subscription prices are $331.00 per year (US individuals), $823.00 per year (US institutions), $376.00 per year (Canadian individuals), $860.00 per year (Canadian institutions), $448.00 per year (international individuals), $860.00 per year (international institutions), $100.00 per year (US and Canadian students), and $195.00 per year (International students). International air speed delivery is included in all Clinics subscription prices. All prices are subject to change without notice. **POSTMASTER:** Send address changes to *Clinics in Perinatology*, Elsevier Health Sciences Division, Subscription Customer Service, 3251 Riverport Lane, Maryland Heights, MO 63043. **Customer Service: Telephone: 1-800-654-2452** (U.S. and Canada); **1-314-447-8871** (outside U.S. and Canada). **Fax: 1-314-447-8029. E-mail: journalscustomerservice-usa@elsevier.com** (for print support); **journalsonlinesupport-usa@elsevier.com** (for online support).

Reprints. For copies of 100 or more, of articles in this publication, please contact the Commercial Reprints Department, Elsevier Inc., 360 Park Avenue South, New York, NY 10010-1710. Tel. 212-633-3874; Fax: 212-633-3820; E-mail: reprints@elsevier.com.

Clinics in Perinatology is also published in Spanish by McGraw-Hill Interamericana Editores S.A., P.O. Box 5-237, 06500 Mexico D.F., Mexico.

Clinics in Perinatology is covered in *MEDLINE/PubMed (Index Medicus) Current Contents, Excepta Medica, BIOSIS and ISI/BIOMED.*

Contributors

CONSULTING EDITOR

LUCKY JAIN, MD, MBA
George W. Brumley Jr Professor and Chairman, Emory University School of Medicine, Department of Pediatrics; Chief Academic Officer, Children's Healthcare of Atlanta; Executive Director, Emory + Children's Pediatric Institute, Atlanta, Georgia, USA

EDITORS

KUOJEN TSAO, MD
Professor of Pediatric Surgery, Obstetrics/Gynecology and Reproductive Medicine, Chief, Division of Pediatric Surgery, Department of Pediatric Surgery, McGovern Medical School at the University of Texas Health Science Center, Houston, Texas, USA

HANMIN LEE, MD
Surgeon-in-Chief, UCSF Benioff Children's Hospital; Chief, Division of Pediatric Surgery, University of California, San Francisco, San Francisco, California, USA

AUTHORS

MEREDITH A. ATKINSON, MD, MHS
Associate Professor, Division of Pediatric Nephrology, Johns Hopkins University School of Medicine, Baltimore, Maryland, USA

AHMET A. BASCHAT, MD
Professor, Department of Gynecology and Obstetrics, The Johns Hopkins Center for Fetal Therapy, Baltimore, Maryland, USA

CARA L. BERKOWITZ, MD
Division of Pediatric General, Thoracic and Fetal Surgery, Children's Hospital of Philadelphia, Philadelphia, Pennsylvania, USA

MARTIN L. BLAKELY, MD, MS
Professor of Pediatric Surgery and Pediatrics, Monroe Carell Jr. Children's Hospital at Vanderbilt Vanderbilt University Medical Center, Nashville, Tennessee, USA

CARESSA CHEN, MD
University of California San Francisco, San Francisco, California, USA

DANIEL A. DEUGARTE, MD
Department of Surgery, UCLA and Harbor-UCLA Medical Center, David Geffen School of Medicine at UCLA, UCLA Division of Pediatric Surgery, Westwood Clinic Location, Los Angeles, California, USA

LAUREN L. EVANS, MD
Cedars-Sinai Medical Center, Los Angeles, California, USA

DIANA FARMER, MD
Professor and Chair, Department of Surgery, University of California Davis Medical Center, Sacramento, California, USA

MARLA B. FERSCHL, MD
Professor of Pediatric Anesthesia, Department of Anesthesia and Perioperative Care, University of California San Francisco, San Francisco, California, USA

THOMAS E. HAMILTON, MD
Thoracic and Fetal Surgery, Esophageal and Airway Treatment (EAT) Endowed Chair in Pediatric General Surgery at CHOP, Attending Surgeon, Department of General, Children's Hospital of Philadelphia, The Hub for Clinical Collaboration, Philadelphia, Pennsylvania, USA

DAVID N. HANNA, MD
Vanderbilt University Medical Center, Nashville, Tennessee, USA

MICHAEL R. HARRISON, MD
University of California San Francisco, San Francisco, California, USA

MATTHEW T. HARTING, MD, MS
Associate Professor, Department of Pediatric Surgery, Children's Memorial Hermann Hospital, University of Texas McGovern Medical School, Houston, Texas, USA

BRITTANY N. HEGDE, MD
Pediatric Surgery Research Fellow, Department of Pediatric Surgery, McGovern Medical School at the University of Texas Health Science Center at Houston, Center for Surgical Trials and Evidence-Based Practice (C-STEP), McGovern Medical School at the University of Texas Health Science Center at Houston, Houston, Texas, USA

SHINJIRO HIROSE, MD
Professor and Chief, Division of Pediatric, Thoracic, and Fetal Surgery, University of California-Davis Medical Center, Sacramento, California, USA

RANU R. JAIN, MD
Professor, Assistant Division Chief of Pediatric Anesthesia, Program Director Pediatric Anesthesia Fellowship, Department of Anesthesiology, University of Texas HSC at Houston, Houston, Texas, USA

TIM JANCELEWICZ, MD, MA, MS
Associate Professor, Division of Pediatric Surgery, Le Bonheur Children's Hospital, University of Tennessee Health Science Center, Memphis, Tennessee, USA

SEBASTIAN K. KING, PhD, FRACS
Professor, Colorectal and Pelvic Reconstruction Service, Department of Paediatric Surgery, The Royal Children's Hospital; Department of Paediatrics, University of Melbourne; F. Douglas Stephens Surgical Research Group, Murdoch Children's Research Institute, Melbourne, Australia

HANMIN LEE, MD
Director, Fetal Treatment Center; Professor & Chief, Division of Pediatric Surgery, University of California San Francisco, Division of Pediatric Surgery, University of California San Francisco, San Francisco, California, USA

SU YEON LEE, MD
Pediatric and Fetal Surgery Research Fellow, Department of Surgery, Division of Pediatric, Thoracic and Fetal Surgery, University of California Davis Medical Center, Sacramento, California, USA

MARC A. LEVITT, MD, FACS
Professor, Division of Colorectal and Pelvic Reconstruction, Children's National Hospital, The George Washington School of Medicine, Washington, DC, USA

VALERIE L. LUKS, MD
Division of Pediatric General, Thoracic and Fetal Surgery, Children's Hospital of Philadelphia, Philadelphia, Pennsylvania, USA

JENA L. MILLER, MD
Assistant Professor, Department of Gynecology and Obstetrics, The Johns Hopkins Center for Fetal Therapy, Baltimore, Maryland, USA

SARAH MOHAMEDALY, MD, MPH
Division of Pediatric Surgery, Department of Surgery, University of California, San Francisco, California, USA

SOMALA MOHAMMED, MD, MPH
Assistant Professor of Surgery, Harvard Medical School, Attending Surgeon, Boston Children's Hospital, Boston, Massachusetts, USA

ALYSSA R. MOWRER, MD
Division of Pediatric Surgery, Department of Surgery, Medical College of Wisconsin, Children's Wisconsin, Milwaukee, Wisconsin, USA

GEORGE B. MYCHALISKA, MD
Section of Pediatric Surgery, Department of Surgery, Fetal Diagnosis and Treatment Center, University of Michigan Medical School, C.S. Mott Children's Hospital, Ann Arbor, Michigan, USA

AMAR NIJAGAL, MD
Division of Pediatric Surgery, Department of Surgery, University of California, San Francisco, The Liver Center, University of California, The Pediatric Liver Center at UCSF Benioff Children's Hospitals, San Francisco, California, USA

RAMESHA PAPANNA, MD, MPH
Associate Professor, Department of Obstetrics, Gynecology and Reproductive Sciences, UT Health Science Center at Houston, Houston, Texas, USA

ANURADHA PATEL, MD
Monroe Carell Jr. Children's Hospital at Vanderbilt, Vanderbilt University Medical Center, Nashville, Tennessee, USA

WILLIAM H. PERANTEAU, MD
Division of Pediatric General, Thoracic and Fetal Surgery, Children's Hospital of Philadelphia, Philadelphia, Pennsylvania, USA

MARCELINA PUC, BA
Division of Pediatric General, Thoracic and Fetal Surgery, Children's Hospital of Philadelphia, Philadelphia, Pennsylvania, USA

LAURA A. RAUSCH, MD, MPH, MA
Vanderbilt University Master of Public Health School, Geriatric Research Education and Clinical Center, Vanderbilt University Medical Center, Nashville, Tennessee, USA

MARISA E. SCHWAB, MD
General Surgery Chief Resident, University of California San Francisco, Division of
Pediatric Surgery, University of California San Francisco, San Francisco, California, USA

BRIANNA L. SPENCER, MD
Department of Surgery, University of Michigan, Michigan Medicine, Ann Arbor, Michigan,
USA

KUOJEN TSAO, MD
Professor of Pediatric Surgery, Obstetrics/Gynecology and Reproductive Medicine,
Chief, Division of General and Thoracic Surgery, Department of Pediatric Surgery,
McGovern Medical School at the University of Texas Health Science Center, Houston,
Texas, USA

AMY J. WAGNER, MD
Division of Pediatric Surgery, Department of Surgery, Medical College of Wisconsin,
Children's Wisconsin, Milwaukee, Wisconsin, USA

Contents

Maternal–fetal surgery is fraught with inherent controversy from within the medical community and general public. Despite these challenges, the field of maternal–fetal surgery evolved into an international enterprise. Carefully nurtured by pioneers with foresight and resilience, the field navigated ethical dilemmas with rigorous scientific methodology, collaboration, transparency, and accordance. These central pillars are consistent throughout the brief but momentous history of maternal–fetal surgery, serving as the catalyst for its success. The maturation of fetal intervention is an exemplar of technological innovation propelling clinical innovation, as well as a celebration of mastering the delicate balance between caution and optimism.

Significant advances in maternal–fetal medicine and gene sequencing technology have fostered a new frontier of in utero molecular and cellular therapeutics, including gene editing, enzyme replacement therapy, and stem cell transplantation to treat single-gene disorders with limited post-natal treatment strategies. In utero therapies take advantage of unique developmental properties of the fetus to allow for the correction of mono-genic disorders before irreversible disease pathology develops. While early preclinical studies in animal models are encouraging, more studies are needed to further evaluate their safety and efficacy prior to widespread clinical use.

Anesthesia for fetal and neonatal surgery requires subspecialized knowl-edge and expertise. Attention to important anatomic, physiologic, and metabolic differences seen in pregnancy and at birth are essential for the optimal care of these patients. Thorough preoperative evaluations tailored intraoperative strategies and careful postoperative management are critical when devising the anesthetic approach for each of these cases.

Myelomeningocele is the most common congenital neurologic defect, and the only nonlethal disease addressed by fetal surgery. A randomized control trial has established amelioration of the Arnold–Chiari II malformation, reduced ventriculoperitoneal shunt rate, and improvement in distal neurologic function in patients that receive in utero repair. Long-term follow-up of these school-age children demonstrates the persistence of these effects. The use of stem cells in fetal repair is being investigated to further improve distal motor function.

The most severe forms of congenital anomalies of the kidney and urinary tract present in fetal life with early pregnancy renal anhydramnios and are considered lethal due to pulmonary hypoplasia without fetal therapy. Due to the high rate of additional structural anomalies, genetic abnormalities, and associated syndromes, detailed anatomic survey and genetic testing are imperative when stratifying which pregnancies are appropriate for fetal intervention. Restoring amniotic fluid around the fetus is the principal goal of prenatal treatment. The ongoing multi-center Renal Anhydramnios Fetal Therapy (RAFT) trial is assessing the safety and efficacy of serial amnioinfusions to prevent pulmonary hypoplasia so that the underlying renal disease can be addressed.

Congenital diaphragmatic hernia is an anomaly that is often prenatally diagnosed and spans a wide spectrum of disease, with high morbidity and mortality associated with fetuses with severe defects. Congenital diaphragmatic hernia is thus an ideal target for fetal intervention. We review the literature on prenatal diagnosis, describe the history of fetal intervention for congenital diaphragmatic hernia, and discuss fetal endoscopic tracheal occlusion and the Tracheal Occlusion To Accelerate Lung growth trial results. Finally, we present preclinical studies for potential future directions.

Extracorporeal life support, initially performed in neonates, is now commonly used for both pediatric and adult patients requiring pulmonary and/or cardiac support. Data suggests the clinical feasibility of Extracorporeal Membrane Oxygenation for premature infants (29–33 weeks estimated gestational age [EGA]). For extremely premature infants less than 28 weeks EGA, an artificial placenta has been developed to recreate the fetal environment. This approach is investigational but clinical translation is promising. In this article, we discuss the current state and advances in neonatal and "preemie Extracorporeal Membrane Oxygenation" and the development of an artificial placenta and its potential use in extremely premature infants.

Congenital diaphragmatic hernia (CDH) is a challenging surgical disease that requires complex preoperative, perioperative, and postoperative care. Survival depends on successful reduction and repair of the defect, and numerous complex decisions must be made regarding timing and preparation for surgery. This review describes the challenges and controversies inherent to surgical CDH care and provides recommendations for management based on the most recent evidence.

Congenital lung malformations represent a spectrum of lesions, each with a distinct cause and tailored clinical approach. This article will focus on the following malformations: congenital pulmonary airway malformations, formally known as congenital cystic adenomatoid malformations, bronchopulmonary sequestration, congenital lobar emphysema, and bronchogenic cyst. Each of these malformations will be defined and examined from an embryologic, pathophysiologic, and clinical management perspective unique to that specific lesion. A review of current recommendations in both medical and surgical management of these lesions will be discussed as well as widely accepted treatment algorithms.

Esophageal atresia with or without tracheoesophageal fistula and tracheobronchomalacia encompass 2 of the most common complex congenital intrathoracic anomalies. Tailoring interventions to address the constellation of problems present in each patient is essential. Due to advances in neonatology, anesthesia, pulmonary, gastroenterology, nutrition and surgery care for patients with complex congenital tracheoesophageal disorders has improved dramatically. Treatment strategies tailored to the individual patient needs are best implimented under the aegis of a comprehensive longitudinal multidisciplinary care team.

The 2 most common congenital abdominal wall defects are gastroschisis and omphalocele. Gastroschisis is a defect in the abdominal wall with exposed abdominal contents. Mortality rates are low but lengths of stay are often prolonged by bowel dysmotility and other intestinal abnormalities in complicated cases. Omphalocele is a defect through the umbilical cord with herniated abdominal contents covered by a sac. It is associated with other genetic abnormalities and other anomalies that can lead to significant morbidity and mortality. Prenatal diagnosis in both conditions allows for improved prenatal consultation and coordinated perinatal care to improve clinical outcomes.

PROGRAM OBJECTIVE
The goal of *Clinics in Perinatology* is to keep practicing perinatologists, neonatologists, obstetricians, practicing physicians and residents up to date with current clinical practice in perinatology by providing timely articles reviewing the state of the art in patient care.

TARGET AUDIENCE
Perinatologists, neonatologists, obstetricians, practicing physicians, residents and healthcare professionals who provide patient care utilizing findings from *Clinics in Perinatology*.

LEARNING OBJECTIVES
Upon completion of this activity, participants will be able to:
1. Recognize that assessment, diagnosing, preoperative and postoperative planning, as well as postoperative management of fetal and neonatal surgeries and interventions to ensure safe and comprehensive care, demands a multidisciplinary and collaborative scientific approach.
2. Discuss the difficulties, controversies, and ethical and safety concerns which impact the development and application of fetal and neonatal surgical interventions and procedures.
3. Review best practice guidelines and recommendations for medical and surgical management of fetal and neonatal complications and disorders to ensure safe and ethical treatment that lowers the risk of morbidity and mortality.

ACCREDITATION
The Elsevier Office of Continuing Medical Education (EOCME) is accredited by the Accreditation Council for Continuing Medical Education (ACCME) to provide continuing medical education for physicians.

The EOCME designates this journal-based CME activity for a maximum of 14 *AMA PRA Category 1 Credit*(s)™. Physicians should claim only the credit commensurate with the extent of their participation in the activity.

All other health care professionals requesting continuing education credit for this enduring material will be issued a certificate of participation.

DISCLOSURE OF CONFLICTS OF INTEREST
The EOCME assesses conflict of interest with its instructors, faculty, planners, and other individuals who are in a position to control the content of CME activities. All relevant conflicts of interest that are identified are thoroughly vetted by EOCME for fair balance, scientific objectivity, and patient care recommendations. EOCME is committed to providing its learners with CME activities that promote improvements or quality in healthcare and not a specific proprietary business or a commercial interest.

The planning committee, staff, authors, and editors listed below have identified no financial relationships or relationships to products or devices they or their spouse/life partner have with commercial interest related to the content of this CME activity:
Meredith A. Atkinson, MD, MHS; Ahmet A. Baschat, MD; Cara L. Berkowitz, MD; Martin L. Blakely, MD; Caressa Chen, MD; Daniel A. DeUgarte, MD; Lauren L. Evans, MD; Diana Farmer, MD; Marla B. Ferschl, MD; Thomas E. Hamilton, MD; David N. Hanna, MD; Michael R. Harrison, MD; Matthew T. Harting, MD, MS; Brittany N. Hegde, MD; Shinjiro Hirose, MD; Ranu R. Jain, MD; Tim Jancelewicz, MD, MA, MS; Sebastian K. King, PhD, FRACS; Hanmin Lee, MD; Su Yeon Lee, MD; Marc A. Levitt, MD, FACS; Valerie L. Luks, MD; Jena L. Miller, MD; Sarah Mohamedaly, MD, MPH; Somala Mohammed, MD, MPH; Alyssa R. Mowrer, MD; George B. Mychaliska, MD; Amar Nijagal, MD; Ramesha Papanna, MD, MPH; Anuradha Patel, MD; William H. Peranteau, MD; Marcelina Puc; Laura A. Rausch, MD, MPH, MA; Marisa E. Schwab, MD; Brianna L. Spencer, MD; Jeyanthi Surendrakumar; Doreen Thomas-Payne, MSN, BSN, RN, PMHNP-BC; KuoJen Tsao, MD; Amy J. Wagner, MD

UNAPPROVED/OFF-LABEL USE DISCLOSURE
The EOCME requires CME faculty to disclose to the participants:
1. When products or procedures being discussed are off-label, unlabelled, experimental, and/or investigational (not US Food and Drug Administration [FDA] approved); and
2. Any limitations on the information presented, such as data that are preliminary or that represent ongoing research, interim analyses, and/or unsupported opinions. Faculty may discuss information about pharmaceutical agents that is outside of FDA-approved labelling. This information is intended solely for CME and is not intended to promote off-label use of these medications. If you have any questions, contact the medical affairs department of the manufacturer for the most recent prescribing information.

TO ENROLL

To enroll in the *Clinics in Perinatology* Continuing Medical Education program, call customer service at 1-800-654-2452 or sign up online at http://www.theclinics.com/home/cme. The CME program is available to subscribers for an additional annual fee of USD 265.00.

METHOD OF PARTICIPATION

In order to claim credit, participants must complete the following:

1. Complete enrolment as indicated above.
2. Read the activity.
3. Complete the CME Test and Evaluation. Participants must achieve a score of 70% on the test. All CME Tests and Evaluations must be completed online.

CME INQUIRIES/SPECIAL NEEDS

For all CME inquiries or special needs, please contact elsevierCME@elsevier.com.

CLINICS IN PERINATOLOGY

SERIES OF RELATED INTEREST

Obstetrics and Gynecology Clinics of North America
https://www.obgyn.theclinics.com

THE CLINICS ARE AVAILABLE ONLINE!
Access your subscription at:
www.theclinics.com

Foreword

Fetal and Neonatal Surgery: Then and Now

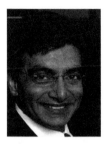

Lucky Jain, MD, MBA
Consulting Editor

Advances in fetal and neonatal surgery mirror the gains made in the entire field of neonatal-perinatal care. It is hard to believe that the first fetal surgical intervention was performed in 1963 without any ultrasound or other imaging modality when Dr Albert William Liley performed a fetal transfusion for severe erythroblastosis fetalis (**Fig. 1**).[1] The procedure was successful and paved the way for subsequent interventions in this malady that was associated with much morbidity and mortality. Advances in fetal imaging have not only improved our understanding of organ development and embryology but also allowed for entire teams of providers to accomplish interventions that were inconceivable in 1963. These teams include specialists in maternal-fetal medicine, neonatology, surgery, radiology, anesthesia, and more. As technology has advanced and the access to life-saving medical interventions has spread on a global scale, mothers and babies have experienced improved health outcomes.

While the list of procedures for fetal anomalies continues to grow, congenital diaphragmatic hernia (CDH) stands out as the most intriguing and challenging conditions to fix. While overall mortality for infants born with CDH has decreased over time, lung hypoplasia and pulmonary hypertension put a significant dent in survival. Fetal tracheal occlusion as a potential approach to prevent lung hypoplasia was pioneered by Dr Michael Harrison and colleagues and continues to evolve as a treatment modality (**Fig. 2**).[2]

In this issue of the *Clinics in Perinatology*, Drs Tsao and Lee have put together a series of articles on fetal and neonatal surgery written by global leaders in the field. These authors and their teams exemplify the spirit that has shaped the field and will most certainly continue to create innovation and hope in this complex field. As always, I am grateful to the publishing staff at Elsevier, including Kerry Holland and Karen

Clin Perinatol 49 (2022) xv–xvii
https://doi.org/10.1016/j.clp.2022.09.002
0095-5108/22/© 2022 Published by Elsevier Inc.

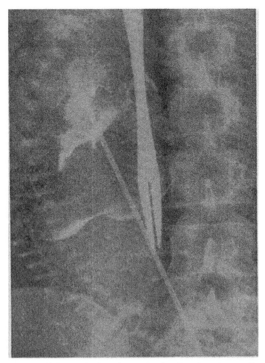

Fig. 1. Contrast medium and the coiled catheter in the fetal peritoneal cavity from the original case report by Dr Albert William Liley. The Tuohy needle has been withdrawn and lies on the mother's abdominal skin. (*From* LILEY AW. INTRAUTERINE TRANSFUSION OF FOETUS IN HAEMOLYTIC DISEASE. Br Med J. 1963 Nov 2;2(5365):1107-9.)

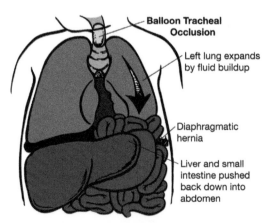

Fig. 2. The effects of tracheal occlusion in fetuses with CDH. Occluding the trachea of fetuses with CDH increases lung volume, decreases herniation of abdominal viscera, and improves postnatal lung function. (*From* Graves CE, Harrison MR, Padilla BE. Minimally Invasive Fetal Surgery. Clin Perinatol. 2017 Dec;44(4):729-751.)

Justine Solomon, for their support in allowing us to bring a broad range of clinically relevant topics to you.

Lucky Jain, MD, MBA
Emory University School of Medicine, and
Children's Healthcare of Atlanta
1760 Haygood Drive, W409
Atlanta, GA 30322, USA

E-mail address:
ljain@emory.edu

REFERENCES

1. Liley AW. Intrauterine transfusion of foetus in hemolytic disease. Br Med J 1963; 2(5365):1107–9. https://doi.org/10.1136/bmj.2.5365.1107.
2. Graves C, Harrison M, Padilla BE. The effects of tracheal occlusion in fetuses with congenital diaphragmatic hernia (CDH). Occluding the trachea of fetuses with CDH increases lung volume, decreases herniation of abdominal viscera, and improves postnatal lung function. Clin Perinatol 2017;44:1–29. https://doi.org/10.1016/j.clp.2017.08.001.

Preface

Advances and Updates in Fetal and Neonatal Surgery

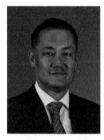 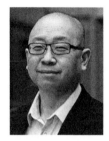

KuoJen Tsao, MD   Hanmin Lee, MD
Editors

We are delighted to focus on fetal and neonatal surgery in this issue of *Clinics in Perinatology*. Tremendous advances in fetal and neonatal treatment have been made in the last 10 years with the recognition that there is a continuum of care from fetal diagnosis and potential therapy through neonatal care. Both fetal surgical care and neonatal surgical care are multidisciplinary fields that rely on the expertise of perinatologists, neonatologists, pediatric surgeons, anesthesiologists, and many other maternal and pediatric specialists.

Fetal surgery has matured from a field of case reports and single-institution, small case series to national and international registries and prospective randomized trials with rigorous scientific methodology. These efforts have been largely driven by collaborative fetal care consortia, such as the International Fetal Medicine and Surgery Society, Eurofetus, and the North American Fetal Therapy Network. Only with such collaboration across multiple centers can the field of fetal intervention, encumbered by relatively small numbers of cases at each center, best share data and analyze results. Of course, balanced within fetal surgery is the need to provide excellent care for the fetus while maintaining a prioritization on maternal health and safety for the pregnant woman. Similar to fetal surgery, neonatal surgery has made great strides over the last decade. Advances in neonatal care and pediatric anesthesia have paralleled the technical advances in pediatric surgery, which has allowed effective treatment of neonates with complex surgical and medical conditions. The multidisciplinary collaboration among neonatologists, pediatric anesthesiologists, and pediatric surgeons is the foundation of advances in neonatal care as we strive for shorter hospital stays and less morbidity, as well as for survival. As this neonatal care evolves, more attention to long-term outcomes is needed to truly understand the impact of our fetal and neonatal surgical therapies.

Clin Perinatol 49 (2022) xix–xx
https://doi.org/10.1016/j.clp.2022.09.001
0095-5108/22/© 2022 Published by Elsevier Inc.

We are delighted to share the expertise of many of the world's leaders with their thoughtful review of the literature and their centers' experiences on the subjects covered in this issue of *Clinics in Perinatology*. We are incredibly grateful to the authors for their excellence in clinical care and their well-written articles. We hope that the following pages will help educate, inform, and inspire our colleagues around the world. We dedicate this effort to the many patients and their families who have been under our care and bravely and graciously allowed us to be a part of their lives. They educate, inform, and inspire us.

KuoJen Tsao, MD
Division of Pediatric Surgery
Department of Pediatric Surgery
University of Texas McGovern Medical School
Houston, TX 77030, USA

Hanmin Lee, MD
UCSF Benioff Children's Hospital
Division of Pediatric Surgery
University of California, San Francisco
San Francisco, CA 94158, USA

E-mail addresses:
KuoJen.Tsao@uth.tmc.edu (K. Tsao)
hanmin.lee@ucsf.edu (H. Lee)

The Rearing of Maternal–Fetal Surgery

The Maturation of a Field from Conception to Adulthood

Caressa Chen, MD[a], Lauren L. Evans, MD[b],
Michael R. Harrison, MD[a],*

KEYWORDS

- Fetal surgery • Fetal intervention • Fetal therapy • In utero therapy • Fetus as patient
- Maternal–fetal surgery

KEY POINTS

- The history of maternal–fetal surgery is brief but momentous.
- Fetal intervention involves many inherent challenges and ethical dilemmas.
- The field has made considerable advancements through rigorous scientific methodology, collaboration, transparency, and international accordance.

INTRODUCTION

In less than 60 years, the field of maternal–fetal surgery has evolved from mildly successful fetal transfusions to a flourishing international field, redefining first-line treatments for a range of disease processes. From its conception, the field has been characterized by 4 guiding principles: rigorous scientific methodology, collaboration, transparency, and international accordance. These central motifs have propelled the field forward, surmounting the challenges and ethical minefield inherent to maternal–fetal surgery.

The ethically charged issues surrounding the field were, and continue to be, the largest threats to success. Within the field of medicine, there was potential friction as this new specialty relied on cooperation between the many different specialties it spanned. Maternal–fetal intervention is unique as it necessitates care for 2 different

[a] University of California San Francisco, 1700 4th, Street BH204 Byers Hall, San Francisco, CA 94158, USA; [b] Cedars-Sinai Medical Center, 8700 Beverly Boulevard North Tower #8215, Los Angeles, CA 90048, USA
* Corresponding author. University of California San Francisco, 550 16th Street, 5th Floor Mission Hall, San Francisco, CA 94158.
E-mail address: michael.harrison@ucsf.edu

patients and consideration of both maternal and fetal health. Balancing potential risks conferred to the mother and potential benefits to the child were even more difficult initially as risks were not well-characterized and benefits were not well-established. The duality of the role of clinician and innovator likewise posed potential moral predicaments. Technology and innovation drove the field of fetal surgery forward but had to be implemented cautiously. Early adopters carefully navigated the continuum between research, innovation, and clinical practice.

Maternal–fetal intervention was subject to intense scrutiny as it raised fundamental questions about the fetus' right to life and the inevitable issue of abortion. Another challenge consistent throughout the field's history is appropriate patient selection. The first fetal surgeries were performed on women pregnant with fetuses with the worst prognosis, but often those were the ones too severe to benefit. Identifying the appropriate cases meant finding a balance between universality and selectivity.

The early creation and adoption of consensus guidelines allowed the field to proceed with ethical and scientific integrity. Led by pioneers with foresight and resilience, maternal–fetal surgery overcame the challenges described above and grew exponentially (**Fig. 1**). As ethical dilemmas surfaced, timely mechanisms of oversight and guidelines prevented potential pitfalls, allowing the field to reach rapid actualization despite its moral delicacy. This article focuses on the careful stewardship and concatenation of events that led to the successful maturation of a nascent field into an enterprise in less than 60 years. It is an overview but by no means a comprehensive review of the countless achievements in its brief but momentous history.

PLANNING AND PREPARATION: THE FIRST FETAL INTERVENTIONS AND ADVANCES IN FETAL DIAGNOSTICS

Innovation in fetal therapy began in the 1960s when Sir William Liley performed a percutaneous fetal transfusion for erythroblastosis fetalis.[1] Others soon reported modifications to techniques, surgical approaches, and equipment.[2–4] Ultimately, open hysterotomy was abandoned due to significant maternal mortality and morbidity[5] and percutaneous techniques were limited by rudimentary anesthesia and fetal imaging.[6] The earliest innovators were too early and adopted a pessimistic view of the future of fetal surgery.[7]

In the 1970s advancements in fetal diagnostics, with fetoscopy and ultrasound, offered new opportunities for understanding pathophysiology.[5,8] Image-guided interventions developed,[9–11] but fetoscopy was largely abandoned in favor of the noninvasive ultrasound.[12] The early lessons from fetal intervention and new era of diagnostics informed the ensuing articles of modern fetal surgery.

A FETUS IN RAPID DEVELOPMENT: DEVELOPING THE FOUNDATIONS OF MODERN FETAL THERAPY

No historical recounting of the field of maternal–fetal surgery is complete without mention of the visionary and pioneer Mike Harrison, whose singular achievements are eclipsed only by the legacy of trainees he created.[13] In 1978 Harrison joined the University of California San Francisco (UCSF), drawn by the opportunity to work with Al DeLorimier and his team on their fetal lamb model.

In the following decade, crucial work was conducted to refine large animal models, laying the groundwork for human fetal intervention. Harrison and his team executed extensive preclinical studies to recreate, understand, and develop techniques for the repair of a variety of fetal diseases, primarily congenital diaphragmatic hernia (CDH),[14,15] lower urinary tract obstruction (LUTO),[16] and hydrocephalus.[17] He

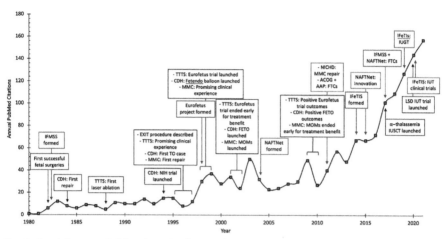

Fig. 1. Fetal Surgery Publication Timeline. PubMed was queried with keywords "fetal surgery," "prenatal surgery," "antenatal surgery," "*in utero* stem cell transplantation," and "*in utero* gene therapy," human results only. The publications per year demonstrate the exponential growth of modern fetal–maternal surgery. Landmark achievements (*black*) appear as inflection points, spurring increased activity in the field, which prompted oversight in the form of societies and consensus statements/guidelines (*red*).

continued his commitment to understanding and optimizing maternal outcomes through innovation. For example, after recognizing that metal staples rendered primates infertile, he and his team developed an absorbable stapling device.[18] Simultaneously, Maria Michejda and Gary Hodgen established preclinical models of hydrocephalus and spina bifida, demonstrating improved outcomes in fetuses who underwent surgical treatment.[19–21] Harrison set the precedent of establishing a robust animal model to understand the pathophysiology of the disease, followed by utilization of the model to test the feasibility, safety, and efficacy of intervention—this remains a cornerstone of maternal–fetal surgery.[22]

Shortly after Harrison's arrival, was the organic formation of the UCSF Fetal Treatment Program (FTP)—a group of obstetricians, geneticists, sonographers, surgeons, cardiologists, and other specialists. Harrison credits the diversity of expertise and collaborative weekly discussions as the impetus for the eventual launch of the fetal surgery enterprise.[22] Additionally, this was an early instance of coordination among a multidisciplinary clinical team—which would become a paradigm for patient care in maternal–fetal surgery.

A BOUNCING, THRIVING NEWBORN: EARLY CLINICAL SUCCESS AND FOUNDING THE INTERNATIONAL FETAL MEDICINE AND SURGERY SOCIETY

1982 was a milestone year for maternal–fetal surgery. Harrison and the FTP successfully performed the first human *in utero* placement of a vesicoamniotic shunt for a fetus with congenital hydronephrosis.[23] Weeks after this breakthrough event, another fetus presented that was not amenable to stent placement due to severe oligohydramnios.[24] Nearly 20 years after open hysterotomy was abandoned due to preterm premature rupture of membranes (PPROM) and fetal loss, Harrison performed the first open decompression of the urinary system. He used the tocolytic, anesthetic, and surgical techniques previously optimized in 25 nonhuman primate fetuses[25] to successfully create bilateral ureterostomies. There were no fetal or maternal complications, and the fetus developed until delivery. However, the baby had irreversibly damaged kidneys and lungs, dying shortly after birth from respiratory failure.[24] Similar to patients with early erythroblastosis, this patient's disease was too severe to be remedied at the time of intervention, highlighting the continued issue of optimal patient selection and timing.[6] Immediately after, Bill Clewell achieved another percutaneous shunt placement, placing the first ventriculoamniotic shunt for a case of fetal hydrocephalus.[26]

Aware of the precarious position of the fledgling field and anticipating negative public perception, Harrison organized early leaders of the field to engage in a frank discussion of the present and future of fetal intervention.[22,27] This meeting, entitled "Unborn: Management of the fetus with a correctable congenital defect," was held among 24 international experts who would (the following year) formally become the International Fetal Medicine and Surgery Society (IFMSS). Together, they wrote a consensus statement composed of self-imposed ethical guidelines for fetal intervention. Specifically, they defined criteria for intervenable diseases, emphasizing that surgery should only be conducted for structural defects with well-defined lethal natural histories, accurate diagnostic modalities, and no effective postnatal treatment. Additionally, interventions should be attempted after validation in preclinical animal models. The importance of coordinated care from a multidisciplinary team was highlighted, and initial standards of specialized fetal treatment centers (FTCs) were set. Lastly, they underscored the theme of transparency, through publications of all outcomes and by establishing a registry.[27] With this early formulation of guidelines, the field made a concerted and conscious effort to avoid the fate of other burgeoning surgical fields, which were nearly destroyed by negative media coverage and poor initial survival.[22,28] The framework established at this meeting continues to uphold the enterprise of maternal–fetal surgery today.

In 1986 early results from the International Fetal Surgery registry demonstrated discouraging results for shunting in hydrocephalus.[29] Despite initial success, cases that were technically successfully carried fetal mortality of 10%, and surviving babies remained severely handicapped.[6] Patients who underwent shunting prenatally had worse outcomes than those who underwent shunting postnatally. As a result, an international voluntary moratorium was placed on shunts for hydrocephalus.[12,22]

A TODDLER WITH A TALENT FOR TANTRUMS: THE FIRST CLINICAL TRIAL AND THE NEAR DEMISE OF FETAL SURGERY

By the early 1980s the pathophysiology of CDH was well-characterized, the poor natural history of severe CDH was established,[30,31] and feasibility of prenatal repair in animal models was demonstrated.[32,33] In 1984 Harrison and his team attempted the first human fetal repair of severe CDH but were unsuccessful, hampered by the unforeseen inability to reduce the herniated liver without kinking the umbilical vein.[22] He later reported successful repair in fetuses without liver herniation.[34] Considering his challenging experience Harrison admitted that fetal surgery was "at a crossroads." Despite convincing preclinical evidence and promising early clinical experience, the efficacy of new interventions was unclear. This led him to move beyond establishing feasibility with retrospective case studies and pursue a prospective controlled trial to truly assess the efficacy of CDH repair.[35]

After a lengthy approval process, in 1994 Harrison began the first National Institutes of Health (NIH)-funded phase 1 trial in maternal–fetal surgery, comparing prenatal open CDH repair to conventional postnatal repair.[22] The trial was momentous for many reasons. By conducting a prospective trial, Harrison and his team redefined the standard of clinical evaluation, bringing about a paradigm shift. After nitroglycerin demonstrated great promise in preventing preterm labor in animal models, nitroglycerin was used in mothers in the trial. Unfortunately, the nitroglycerin—specifically the solubilizing propylene glycol—led to reversible yet serious cases of maternal pulmonary edema. The trial was suspended and underwent intramural and NIH-initiated investigations. This was the first incidence of serious maternal injury, and it sowed dissension within the UCSF FTP, leading to internal discord. Obstetricians within the group viewed fetal surgery and the FTP as a threat to maternal health. Despite Harrison's 7-hour attempt to advocate for the FTP and the future of maternal–fetal surgery, the organization was dissolved. Determined to keep fetal surgery alive, Harrison reorganized his supporters to form the UCSF Fetal Treatment Center, which continues today.[22]

The trial resumed, proving prenatal repair safe and feasible, but with no survival improvement.[36] As a result, open fetal CDH repair was abandoned and Harrison returned to experimental animal work, paving the way for minimally invasive techniques of CDH repair.

FIRST DAY OF SCHOOL: THE REVIVAL OF FETOSCOPY AND THE FIRST RANDOMIZED CONTROLLED TRIALS

In the late 1980s, advanced ultrasonography led to a better diagnosis and understanding of twin–twin transfusion syndrome (TTTS). Julian De Lia and Kurt Benirschke developed a laser-directed vascular coagulation technique,[37] and in 1988 De Lia performed the first human fetoscopic laser ablation for severe TTTS.[38] Yves Ville and Kypros Nicolaides followed with the first endoscopic laser ablation under local anesthesia.[39] By 1995 De Lia had successfully performed 26 cases, noting an impressive 53% survival with 96% normal development.[40]

With the rising promise of TTTS, the European Commission formed the Eurofetus project to stimulate research and development. The project included a formal consortium between fetal medicine centers and an endoscopic instruments manufacturer (Karl Storz). This collaboration resulted in miniature endoscopes and instruments specifically for fetal surgery. The Eurofetus group also established a registry for all fetoscopic cases.[12,41]

Widespread adoption of fetoscopic laser therapy was prevented by lingering skepticism, likely due to concerns about maternal safety and efficacy.[12] In response, the Eurofetus group organized the first randomized controlled trial (RCT) in maternal–fetal surgery: a multi-center trial for severe TTTS, comparing fetoscopic-directed laser ablation and amnioreduction. The successful coordination and execution of this RCT was a tour de force for the group and a milestone for the field. The trial began in 1999 and concluded early due to clear superiority in laser-treated patients. Fetoscopic laser ablation remains a paragon, exemplifying the importance of collaboration and rigorous clinical trials; in less than 20 years, laser ablation progressed from an experimental first case to the first-line treatment for select stages of TTTS.

TESTING BOUNDARIES: EXPANDING BEYOND THE REPAIR OF STRUCTURAL DEFECTS

As the consequences of open fetal surgery—namely PPROM and preterm labor—became apparent, enthusiasm for minimally invasive fetoscopic interventions grew. Thorough preclinical studies established fetal and maternal safety,[42–45] setting the stage for modern fetal endoscopic surgery.

In 1993, 2 groups independently realized that fetal tracheal occlusion (TO) was the key to reversing pulmonary hypoplasia.[46,47] Coupled with the resurgence in fetoscopic surgery, this prompted a new minimally invasive approach to CDH. Groups globally began to optimize occlusion techniques with varying success, using foam plugs,[47] external clips,[48] endotracheal tubes with/without magnetic flow valves,[49] umbrellas,[50] and detachable balloons.[51] Notably, this represented a significant shift in fetal intervention: from repair of only anatomic defects to interventions designed to manipulate physiology.[22]

Harrison developed the *ex utero* intrapartum treatment (EXIT) procedure, to secure the airway while the fetus remained on placental support.[52] Originally designed to reverse TO, the technique has since widened its indications to causes of airway obstruction and thoracic abnormalities.[53] In 1997, Harrison's group published the first successful human fetoscopic TO,[54] quickly supported by a follow-up report of 8 fetuses.[55] These promising results inspired the first US fetal surgery RCT, evaluating the treatment of severe CDH with fetal endoscopic (Fetendo) intratracheal balloon placement and birth by EXIT procedure with balloon removal, compared with standard postnatal care. The trial ran from 1999 to 2001, with equivocal results. TO did not improve survival or morbidity rates, the benefit likely offset by the high rate of preterm delivery and an unexpected high control group survival rate.[56]

Using different severity criteria, a European fetal endoscopic tracheal occlusion (FETO) task force was formed to continue investigating TO.[12] In 2001 they launched the FETO trial– an international RCT for temporary TO in severe CDH.[57] TO was performed through endoscopic balloon placement and reversed weeks later, using a second endoscopic procedure developed by Jan Deprest.[57,58] FETO increased survival rates, although PPROM continued to be a challenge.[59]

COMING OF AGE: A NEW STANDARD FOR EVALUATING FETAL INTERVENTIONS

Building on promising preclinical studies and with the development of improved magnetic resonance imaging (MRI), interest in myelomeningocele (MMC) repair began rising in the early 1990s.[60] The focus on MMC represented another milestone in the field: shifting from intervention on only life-threatening anomalies, to a nonlethal, highly morbid condition. For the first time, the field was ready to improve morbidity alone and embrace the improving perioperative risks. After demonstrating feasibility in sheep,[61] in 1997 Joseph Brunauer published the first two human fetal endoscopic repairs of MMC.[62] Due to high perinatal mortality, minimally invasive approaches were abandoned. In 1998 N. Scott Adzick and Brunauer independently reported the first open fetal repairs for MMC[63,64] and continued to report considerable clinical success.[65,66]

These initial reports were promising but lacked contemporaneous controls, prompting a call for a more rigorous evaluation. Careful planning for the multicenter RCT that would become the MOMS (Management of Myelomeningocele Study) trial began in 2000. Early leaders agreed that the study should be limited to three centers with no other North American centers offering repair, protocols and techniques should be standardized, and all initial patient assessments should be conducted by an independent center.[5] The landmark MOMS trial was launched in 2002, ending early in 2010 due to a clear superiority of prenatal repair. Although MMC was rare, an adequate number of patients were enrolled with coordination between centers and a prolonged study period.[67] The success of the MOMS trial highlighted the importance of collaboration throughout the field to design and execute a rigorous RCT. MOMS was the first trial to enforce standardization of patient screening, operative techniques, and perioperative management, and in doing so, set a new gold standard for high-quality scientific evidence.

Inspired by the collaborative approach of the MOMS trial, a "Fetal Therapy Working Group" was formed to enable more multi-institutional trials in North America. They would eventually become the North American Fetal Therapy Network (NAFTNet),[68] answering the NIH's call for a cooperative group of investigators and clinicians to oversee the growing field.[69] NAFTNet formed as a research network and partnership among FTCs, similar to the Eurofetus network, to facilitate institutional collaboration and scientifically rigorous RCTs. Today NAFTNet includes 39 centers, with each required to meet standards for clinical and research capabilities—including care by multidisciplinary teams. NAFTNet emphasizes transparency, requiring members to submit annual reports of case numbers and all outcomes of fetal interventions. Lastly, NAFTNet aims to provide research oversight, establishing peer-review and approval processes for study protocols.[70]

The effects of the successful MOMS trials were felt globally. The FETO consortium sought to further substantiate their positive findings from the FETO trial, launching international trials modeled on the MOMS trial. The TOTAL trials (2008–2020) also employed consistent patient selection, strict criteria for FTCs, and standardized surgical techniques and postnatal management.[71]

ADOLESCENT GROWTH SPURTS (AND GROWING PAINS): MAINTAINING INTEGRITY DURING RAPID EXPANSION

The marked success of the MOMS, Eurofetus TTTS, and FETO trials cumulatively spurred a surge of interest in maternal–fetal surgery, leading to a rapid establishment of FTCs—all highly variable in surgeries performed, services offered, terminology, and research capabilities.[72] This inconsistency was an indication of the field growing too quickly, without infrastructure or oversight.

As a result, several societies responded with consensus statements. The same tenets of fetal surgery first proposed in 1982 (transparency, interdisciplinary care, scientific validation before experimental procedures, informed consent) continued to endure, echoed in these guidelines. The National Institute of Child Health and Human Development convened a task force, publishing operational guidelines for FTCs performing prenatal MMC repair.[73] The same year, the American College of Obstetricians and Gynecologists (ACOG) and the American Academy of Pediatrics (AAP) published a joint statement on the broader context of maternal–fetal intervention and FTCs.[74] NAFTNet produced a position paper on innovation in maternal–fetal therapy.[43] In 2017 IFMSS and NAFTNet published a joint opinion on the obligations and minimum standards of FTCs.[75] Contemporary ethical considerations were also proposed in the ACOG-AAP statement and NAFTNet position paper, with emphasis on maternal autonomy, informed consent with limited coercion, and distinguishing between standard therapies and experimental procedures.

A YOUNG ADULT MATURING: IN UTERO THERAPIES AND THE FUTURE OF FETAL THERAPY

Fetal immunity research evolved in parallel with stem cell/gene therapy and gene-editing technologies to usher in the newest article of fetal intervention: *in utero* therapies.[76] *In utero* therapies (IUT) such as stem cell transplantation, gene therapy, and enzyme replacement therapy offer a new realm of possibility beyond structural defects, targeting genetic disorders. Initial human fetal *in utero* stem cell transplantation (IUSCT) experiences were largely disappointing.[77] In 2000 the NIH published a position paper concluding that the available technology and preclinical data were insufficient to justify *in utero* gene therapy (IUGT) clinical trials.[78] Considerable advances were made in the following decades, leading to successful IUT in fetal animal models and pediatric populations.[76] Anticipating that IUT were on the cusp of becoming a reality, an international multidisciplinary conference was held in 2014.

The IFeTIS (International Fetal Transplantation and Immunology Society) was created and, similar to IFMSS, they established early guidelines in anticipation of more clinical IUSCT. They agreed that there was sufficient preclinical evidence to warrant a phase 1 IUSCT clinical trial, and established a patient registry and a forum to provide clinical oversight.[79] Two-phase I IUSCT clinical trials for alpha-thalassemia (NCT02986698) and osteogenesis imperfecta (NCT03706482) were launched in rapid succession. In 2018 X-linked hypohidrotic ectodermal dysplasia was successfully treated *in utero*.[80] IFeTIS followed with consensus statements addressing the scientific, ethical, and clinical issues related to IUGT, and on IUT clinical trials.[81] Phase I trials evaluating IUGT for the treatment of lysosomal storage diseases (NCT04532047) and MMC (NCT04652908) quickly followed. IUT has unique challenges but continues to push forward with rigorous preclinical studies and multidisciplinary efforts.[76]

ADULTHOOD: LOOKING AHEAD TO A BRIGHT FUTURE

Fetal intervention continues to expand, with current clinical trials investigating even more disease processes (hypoplastic left heart syndrome (NCT01736956), Vein of Galen Malformation (NCT04434729). The pool of potential patients grows as diagnostic and therapeutic technologies improve. Despite the profound advancement of the field, the same core tenets and challenges endure. In 1982, the field's pioneers defined a framework that has chiefly remained the same, with necessary revisions and additions as the field evolves. Contemporary guidelines perpetuate the principles of scientific rigor, collaboration, transparency, and accordance—which continue to allow for the deeply personal and rewarding privilege that is fetal intervention. While the 60-year history of maternal–fetal surgery has seen remarkable achievement, the great promise of the future is even more noteworthy.

DISCLOSURE

The authors have no commercial or financial conflicts of interest to disclose.

REFERENCES

1. Liley AW. Intrauterine transfusion of Foetus in haemolytic disease. Br Med J 1963; 2(5365):1107–9.
2. Asensio SH, Figueroa-Longo JG, Pelegrina IA. Intrauterine exchange transfusion. Am J Obstet Gynecol 1966;95(8):1129–33.
3. Adamsons K, Freda VJ, James LS, et al. Prenatal treatment of erythroblastosis Fetalis following hysterotomy. Pediatrics 1965;35(5):848–55.
4. Liggins GC. A self-retaining catheter for fetal peritoneal transfusion. Obstet Gynecol 1966;27(3):323–6.
5. Kitagawa H, Pringle KC. Fetal surgery: a critical review. Pediatr Surg Int 2017; 33(4):421–33.
6. Pringle KC. Fetal surgery: it has a past, has it a future? Fetal Ther 1986;1(1): 23–31.
7. Adamsons K Jr. Fetal surgery. New Engl J Med 1966;275(4):204–6.
8. Hobbins JC, Mahoney MJ. In Utero diagnosis of hemoglobinopathies. Technic for obtaining fetal blood. New Engl J Med 1974;290(19):1065–7.

9. Birnholz JC, Frigoletto FD. Antenatal treatment of hydrocephalus. N Engl J Med 1981;304(17):1021–3.
10. Bang J, Bock JE, Trolle D. Ultrasound-guided fetal intravenous transfusion for severe rhesus haemolytic disease. Br Med J (Clinical Res ed) 1982;284(6313): 373–4.
11. Rodeck CH, Nicolaides KH, Warsof SL, et al. The management of severe rhesus isoimmunization by fetoscopic intravascular transfusions. Am J Obstet Gynecol 1984;150(6):769–74.
12. Deprest JA, Flake AW, Gratacos E, et al. The making of fetal surgery. Prenatal Diagn 2010;30(7):653–67.
13. Bruner JP. In Their footsteps. Clin Perinatology 2003;30(3):439–47.
14. Harrison MR, Bressack MA, Churg AM, et al. Correction of congenital diaphragmatic hernia in utero. II. Simulated correction permits fetal lung growth with survival at birth. Surgery 1980;88(2):260–8.
15. Harrison MR, Ross NA, de Lorimier AA. Correction of congenital diaphragmatic hernia in utero. III. Development of a successful surgical technique using abdominoplasty to avoid compromise of umbilical blood flow. J Pediatr Surg 1981;16(6): 934–42.
16. Glick PL, Harrison MR, Adzick NS, et al. Correction of congenital hydronephrosis in utero IV: in utero decompression prevents renal dysplasia. J Pediatr Surg 1984; 19(6):649–57.
17. Glick PL, Harrison MR, Halks-Miller M, et al. Correction of congenital hydrocephalus in utero II: efficacy of in utero shunting. J Pediatr Surg 1984;19(6):870–81.
18. Adzick NS, Harrison MR, Glick PL, et al. Fetal surgery in the primate. III. Maternal outcome after fetal surgery. J Pediatr Surg 1986;21(6):477–80.
19. Michejda M, Hodgen GD. In utero diagnosis and treatment of non-human primate fetal skeletal anomalies. I. Hydrocephalus. Jama 1981;246(10):1093–7.
20. Michejda M, Patronas N, Di Chiro G, et al. Fetal hydrocephalus. II. Amelioration of fetal porencephaly by in utero therapy in nonhuman primates. Jama 1984; 251(19):2548–52 [doi].
21. Michejda M. Intrauterine treatment of spina bifida: primate model. Z Kinderchirurgie : Organ der Deutschen, der Schweizerischen der Osterreichischen Gesellschaft Kinderchirurgie = Surg infancy Child 1984;39(4):259–61.
22. Harrison MR. The University of California at san Francisco fetal treatment center: a personal perspective. Fetal Diagn Ther 2004;19(6):513–24.
23. Golbus MS, Harrison MR, Filly RA, et al. In utero treatment of urinary tract obstruction. Am J Obstet Gynecol 1982;142(4):383–8.
24. Harrison MR, Golbus MS, Filly RA, et al. Fetal surgery for congenital hydronephrosis. New Engl J Med 1982;306(10):591–3.
25. Harrison MR, Anderson J, Rosen MA, et al. Fetal surgery in the primate I. Anesthetic, surgical, and tocolytic management to maximize fetal-neonatal survival. J Pediatr Surg 1982;17(2):115–22.
26. Clewell WH, Johnson ML, Meier PR, et al. A surgical approach to the treatment of fetal hydrocephalus. New Engl J Med 1982;306(22):1320–5.
27. Harrison MR, Filly RA, Golbus MS, et al. Fetal treatment 1982. New Engl J Med 1982;307(26):1651–2.
28. Brink JG. The first human heart transplant and further advances in cardiac transplantation at Groote Schuur Hospital and the University of Cape Town with reference to: the operation. A human cardiac transplant: an interim report of a successful operation performed at Groote Schuur Hospital, Cape Town: historical review article. Cardiovasc J Africa 2009;20(1):30–8.

29. Manning FA, Harrison MR, Rodeck C. Catheter shunts for fetal hydronephrosis and hydrocephalus. Report of the international fetal surgery registry. New Engl J Med 1986;315(5):336–40.
30. Nakayama DK, Harrison MR, Chinn DH, et al. Prenatal diagnosis and natural history of the fetus with a congenital diaphragmatic hernia: initial clinical experience. J Pediatr Surg 1985;20(2):118–24.
31. Adzick NS, Harrison MR, Glick PL, et al. Diaphragmatic hernia in the fetus: prenatal diagnosis and outcome in 94 cases. J Pediatr Surg 1985;20(4):357–61.
32. Adzick NS, Outwater KM, Harrison MR, et al. Correction of congenital diaphragmatic hernia in utero. IV. An early gestational fetal lamb model for pulmonary vascular morphometric analysis. J Pediatr Surg 1985;20(6):673–80.
33. Pringle KC, Turner JW, Schofield JC, et al. Creation and repair of diaphragmatic hernia in the fetal lamb: lung development and morphology. J Pediatr Surg 1984;19(2):131–40.
34. Harrison MR, Adzick NS, Flake AW, et al. Correction of congenital diaphragmatic hernia in utero: VI. Hard-earned lessons. J Pediatr Surg 1993;28(10):1411–8.
35. Harrison MR, Adzick NS, Longaker MT, et al. Successful repair in utero of a fetal diaphragmatic hernia after removal of herniated viscera from the left thorax. New Engl J Med 1990;322(22):1582–4.
36. Harrison MR, Adzick NS, Bullard KM, et al. Correction of congenital diaphragmatic hernia in utero VII: a prospective trial. J Pediatr Surg 1997;32(11):1637–42.
37. DeLia JE, Rogers JG, Dixon JA. Treatment of placental vasculature with a neodymium-yttrium-aluminum-garnet laser via fetoscopy. Am J Obstet Gynecol 1985;151(8):1126–7.
38. De Lia JE, Cruikshank DP, Keye WR Jr. Fetoscopic neodymium:YAG laser occlusion of placental vessels in severe twin-twin transfusion syndrome. Obstet Gynecol 1990;75(6):1046–53.
39. Ville Y, Hecher K, Ogg D, et al. Successful outcome after Nd : YAG laser separation of chorioangiopagus-twins under sonoendoscopic control. Ultrasound Obstet Gynecol 1992;2(6):429–31.
40. De Lia JE, Kuhlmann RS, Harstad TW, et al. Fetoscopic laser ablation of placental vessels in severe previable twin-twin transfusion syndrome. Am J Obstet Gynecol 1995;172(4 Pt 1):1202–11.
41. Endoscopy in Fetal Medicine. Endo Press; 2015.
42. Luks FI, Deprest J, Marcus M, et al. Carbon dioxide pneumoamnios causes acidosis in fetal lamb. Fetal Diagn Ther 1994;9(2):105–9.
43. Luks FI, Johnson A, Polzin WJ. North American fetal therapy N. Innovation in maternal-fetal therapy: a position statement from the North American fetal therapy network. Obstet Gynecol 2015;125(3):649–52.
44. Luks FI, Peers KH, Deprest JA, et al. The effect of open and endoscopic fetal surgery on uteroplacental oxygen delivery in the sheep. J Pediatr Surg 1996;31(2):310–4.
45. Skarsgard ED, Bealer JF, Meuli M, et al. Fetal endoscopic ('Fetendo') surgery: the relationship between insufflating pressure and the fetoplacental circulation. J Pediatr Surg 1995;30(8):1165–8.
46. DiFiore JW, Fauza DO, Slavin R, et al. Experimental fetal tracheal ligation reverses the structural and physiological effects of pulmonary hypoplasia in congenital diaphragmatic hernia. J Pediatr Surg 1994;29(2):248–57.
47. Hedrick MH, Estes JM, Sullivan KM, et al. Plug the lung until it grows (PLUG): a new method to treat congenital diaphragmatic hernia in utero. J Pediatr Surg 1994;29(5):612–7.

48. VanderWall KJ, Bruch SW, Meuli M, et al. Fetal endoscopic ('Fetendo') tracheal clip. J Pediatr Surg 1996;31(8):1101–4.
49. Bealer JF, Skarsgard ED, Hedrick MH, et al. The 'PLUG' odyssey: adventures in experimental fetal tracheal occlusion. J Pediatr Surg 1995;30(2):361–5.
50. Luks FI, Gilchrist BF, Jackson BT, et al. Endoscopic tracheal obstruction with an expanding device in a fetal lamb model: preliminary considerations. Fetal Diagn Ther 1996;11(1):67–71.
51. Deprest JAM, Evrard VA, Van Ballaer PP, et al. Tracheoscopic endoluminal plugging using an inflatable device in the fetal lamb model. Eur J Obstet Gynecol Reprod Biol 1998;81(2):165–9.
52. Mychaliska GB, Bealer JF, Graf JL, et al. Operating on placental support: the ex utero intrapartum treatment procedure. J Pediatr Surg 1997;32(2):227–30.
53. Hirose S, Harrison MR. The ex utero intrapartum treatment (EXIT) procedure. Semin Neonatal 2003;8(3):207–14.
54. VanderWall KJ, Skarsgard ED, Filly RA, et al. Fetendo-clip: a fetal endoscopic tracheal clip procedure in a human fetus. J Pediatr Surg 1997;32(7):970–2.
55. Harrison MR, Mychaliska GB, Albanese CT, et al. Correction of congenital diaphragmatic hernia in utero IX: fetuses with poor prognosis (Liver herniation and low lung-to-head ratio) can be saved by fetoscopic temporary tracheal occlusion. J Pediatr Surg 1998;33(7):1017–23.
56. Harrison MR, Keller RL, Hawgood SB, et al. A randomized trial of fetal endoscopic tracheal occlusion for severe fetal congenital diaphragmatic hernia. New Engl J Med 2003;349(20):1916–24.
57. Deprest J, Gratacos E, Nicolaides KH, et al. Fetoscopic tracheal occlusion (FETO) for severe congenital diaphragmatic hernia: evolution of a technique and preliminary results. Ultrasound Obstet Gynecol : official J Int Soc Ultrasound Obstet Gynecol 2004;24(2):121–6.
58. Deprest J, Jani J, Gratacos E, et al. Fetal intervention for congenital diaphragmatic hernia: the European experience. Semin perinatology 2005;29(2):94–103.
59. Jani JC, Nicolaides KH, Gratacos E, et al. Severe diaphragmatic hernia treated by fetal endoscopic tracheal occlusion. Ultrasound Obstet Gynecol : official J Int Soc Ultrasound Obstet Gynecol 2009;34(3):304–10.
60. Adzick NS. Fetal surgery for spina bifida: past, present, future. Semin Pediatr Surg 2013;22(1):10–7.
61. Copeland ML, Bruner JP, Richards WO, et al. A model for in utero endoscopic treatment of myelomeningocele. Neurosurgery 1993;33(3):542–4.
62. Bruner JP, Tulipan NE, Richards WO. Endoscopic coverage of fetal open myelomeningocele in utero. Am J Obstet Gynecol 1997;176(1 Pt 1):256–7.
63. Adzick NS, Sutton LN, Crombleholme TM, et al. Successful fetal surgery for spina bifida. Lancet (London, England) 1998;352(9141):1675–6.
64. Tulipan N, Hernanz-Schulman M, Bruner JP. Reduced hindbrain herniation after intrauterine myelomeningocele repair: a report of four cases. Pediatr Neurosurg Nov 1998;29(5):274–8.
65. Sutton LN, Adzick NS, Bilaniuk LT, et al. Improvement in hindbrain herniation demonstrated by serial fetal magnetic resonance imaging following fetal surgery for myelomeningocele. Jama 1999;282(19):1826–31.
66. Bruner JP, Tulipan N, Paschall RL, et al. Fetal surgery for myelomeningocele and the incidence of shunt-dependent hydrocephalus. Jama 1999;282(19):1819–25.
67. Adzick NS, Thom EA, Spong CY, et al. A randomized trial of prenatal versus postnatal repair of myelomeningocele. New Engl J Med 2011;364(11):993–1004.

68. Johnson MP. The North American Fetal Therapy Network (NAFTNet): a new approach to collaborative research in fetal diagnosis and therapy. *Semin Fetal Neonatal Med* Feb 2010;15(1):52–7.

69. Chescheir NC, Socol M. The National Institutes of Health Workshop on fetal treatment: needs assessment and future directions. Obstet Gynecol 2005;106(4): 828–33.

70. North American Fetal Therapy Network NAFTNet. North American fetal therapy network. 2020. Available at: https://www.naftnet.org/. Accessed September 24, 2020.

71. Dekoninck P, Gratacos E, Van Mieghem T, et al. Results of fetal endoscopic tracheal occlusion for congenital diaphragmatic hernia and the set up of the randomized controlled TOTAL trial. Early Hum Dev 2011;87(9):619–24.

72. Kett JC, Woodrum DE, Diekema DS. A survey of fetal care centers in the United States. J neonatal-perinatal Med 2014;7(2):131–5.

73. Cohen AR, Couto J, Cummings JJ, et al. Position statement on fetal myelomeningocele repair. Am J Obstet Gynecol 2014;210(2):107–11.

74. American College of O, Gynecologists. Committee on E, American Academy of Pediatrics.Committee on B. Committee opinion no. 501: maternal-fetal intervention and fetal care centers. Obstet Gynecol 2011;118(2 Pt 1):405–10.

75. Moon-Grady AJ, Baschat A, Cass D, et al. Fetal treatment 2017: the evolution of fetal therapy centers - a joint opinion from the international fetal medicine and surgical society (IFMSS) and the North American fetal therapy network (NAFTNet). Fetal Diagn Ther 2017;42(4):241–8.

76. MacKenzie TC. Future AAVenues for in utero gene therapy. Cell stem cell 2018; 23(3):320–1.

77. Touraine JL, Raudrant D, Royo C, et al. In-utero transplantation of stem cells in Bare Lymphocyte syndrome. Lancet 1989;333(8651).

78. Committee USNIoHRDA. Prenatal gene tranfer: scientific, medical, and ethical issues: a report of the Recombinant DNA Advisory Committee. Hum Gene Ther 2000;11(8):1211–29.

79. MacKenzie TC, David AL, Flake AW, et al. Consensus statement from the first international conference for in utero stem cell transplantation and gene therapy. Front Pharmacol 2015;6:15.

80. Schneider H, Faschingbauer F, Schuepbach-Mallepell S, et al. Prenatal correction of X-linked hypohidrotic ectodermal dysplasia. N Engl J Med 2018; 378(17):1604–10.

81. Almeida-Porada G, Waddington SN, Chan JKY, et al. In Utero gene therapy consensus statement from the IFeTIS. Mol Ther 2019;27(4):705–7.

Molecular and Cellular In Utero Therapy

Cara L. Berkowitz, MD, Valerie L. Luks, MD, Marcelina Puc, BA,
William H. Peranteau, MD*

KEYWORDS

- *In utero* therapy • *In utero* gene editing • Maternal–fetal medicine
- In utero enzyme replacement therapy • In utero stem cell transplantation

KEY POINTS

- *In utero* therapies have the potential to treat genetic disorders before the onset of irreversible disease pathology.
- *In utero* therapies offer potential advantages over postnatal therapies due to the unique properties of fetal development, including small fetal size, a tolerant immune system, and an abundance of accessible progenitor cells, allowing for the treatment of highly morbid disorders with limited postnatal treatment options.
- Safety and ethical considerations are important to examine prior to evaluation in clinical trials.

INTRODUCTION

Significant advances in maternal–fetal medicine and gene sequencing technology have allowed genetic disorders to be identified earlier in pregnancy and with greater accuracy. Given these advances, a new frontier of *in utero* molecular and cellular therapeutics is on the horizon, including gene editing, enzyme replacement therapy and stem cell transplantation therapies with the potential to treat single-gene mutations (monogenic disorders) with limited postnatal treatment strategies. *In utero* therapies offer potential advantages to postnatal therapies due to the unique properties of fetal development, including small fetal size, a tolerant immune system, an abundance of accessible progenitor cells, and the ability to intervene prior to the onset of irreversible disease pathology, which potentially allows for the treatment of highly morbid disorders with limited postnatal treatment strategies.[1]

In the following sections, we will review recent advances in prenatal diagnosis that have allowed for the early diagnosis of monogenic disorders. We will then discuss the

Division of Pediatric General, Thoracic and Fetal Surgery, Children's Hospital of Philadelphia, 3401 Civic Center Boulevard, Philadelphia, PA 19104, USA
* Corresponding author. Division of Pediatric General, Thoracic, and Fetal Surgery, Leonard and Madlyn Abramson Pediatric Research Center, 3615 Civic Center Boulevard, Philadelphia, PA 19104, USA
E-mail address: peranteauw@chop.edu

Clin Perinatol 49 (2022) 811–820
https://doi.org/10.1016/j.clp.2022.06.005

benefits of *in utero* therapies compared to the postnatal counterpart and review advances, predominantly in preclinical animal models, in different molecular and cellular *in utero* therapies, including gene editing, enzyme replacement therapy, and stem cell transplantation. Finally, we will address safety and ethical considerations related to *in utero* therapies, which must be fully evaluated for each therapy prior to clinical translation.

ADVANCES IN PRENATAL DIAGNOSIS

Monogenic disorders result in significant morbidity and mortality worldwide and can be diagnosed earlier and with greater accuracy due to advances in maternal–fetal medicine and gene sequencing technology. Two of the most common diagnostic tests that have been used to identify genetic disorders are amniocentesis and chorionic villus sampling (CVS). Amniocentesis was first developed in the 1950s and consists of performing ultrasound-guided amniotic fluid aspiration.[2] Amniocentesis can be conducted safely starting around 15 weeks gestational age.[3,4] CVS, a procedure in which chorionic villi from the placenta are biopsied by either a transcervical or transabdominal approach, can be performed even earlier, starting around 10 weeks gestational age.[3,5] In both procedures, the amniotic fluid or sampled chorionic villi can then be used to evaluate for genetic abnormalities in the fetus. However, both CVS and amniocentesis are invasive procedures and thus are associated with a small risk to the mother and fetus.[5]

Noninvasive prenatal testing/screening (NIPT/NIPS) was first described in 1997. Short segments of extra-cellular DNA derived from trophoblastic cells, known as cell-free DNA (cfDNA), were found circulating in maternal serum.[5,6] cfDNA can be analyzed for genetic disorders in the fetus and is clinically available as early as 9 weeks gestational age.[3,7,8] While originally only able to detect de novo mutations or paternally inherited mutations distinct from circulating maternal cfDNA, advances in next-generation sequencing, specifically the use of relative mutation dosing and relative haplotype dosing, have allowed for greater fidelity in diagnosing maternally derived mutations.[5] While cfDNA is currently only used to detect chromosomal anomalies and limited genetic mutations, it offers the potential for noninvasively diagnosing a vast array of genetic disorders in the future.

ADVANTAGES OF *IN UTERO* THERAPY

The ability to diagnose fetal monogenic disorders early in pregnancy combined with the fact that some genetic diseases cause significant morbidity or mortality before or shortly after birth highlights the potential to treat these disorders *in utero*. There are several advantages to *in utero* therapy. The smaller fetal size allows for the optimization of the dose of the therapeutic per weight of the recipient and alleviates constraints on the manufacturing and production of therapies.[1,9] Additionally, in contrast to the postnatal recipient, there is increased access to stem and progenitor cells of multiple organs in the fetus.[10–12] For example, hematopoietic stem cells (HSCs) are readily accessible in the fetal liver compared to the postnatal counterpart after undergoing migration to the bone marrow.[12] This is especially important to consider when utilizing gene editing or gene replacement therapy for which the goal is to propagate the therapeutic correction to subsequent daughter cells.[1,12]

In addition, physical and immune barriers in the fetus are not as robust as they are after birth. As an example, the blood–brain barrier (BBB) prevents many enzymes and drugs from entering the central nervous system (CNS) after birth. Neuronopathic Gaucher disease is a lysosomal storage disorder caused by insufficient glucocerebrosidase (GCA) enzyme activity, leading to *in utero* onset of neurodegeneration and early childhood mortality.[13] While the BBB has limited the efficacy of postnatal enzyme replacement therapy, *in utero* GCA gene delivery was able to restore neuronal GCA expression, reduce neurodegeneration, and increase survival in mice.[13] The immune system of the fetus is also tolerogenic, thus posing less of a barrier to immunogenic therapies than the postnatal environment. This is best exemplified by the many studies demonstrating successful allogenic HSC transplants without immunosuppressive or myeloablative conditioning associated with the induction of donor-specific tolerance in fetal mouse and large animal models.[14–17] Gene therapy and gene-editing approaches often rely on a viral vector (adeno-associated virus, AAV) to deliver a potentially immunogenic transgene (an unmade protein due to a genetic mutation or a bacterially derived Cas9 for gene-editing approaches). Many adults already possess antibodies to AAV due to natural exposure, with the development of this immunity documented before six months of life.[18] Similarly, 78% of adults have humoral or cell-mediated immunity to Staphylococcus aureus Cas9 (SaCas9) and 58% to Streptococcus Pyogenes Cas9 (SpCas9), which may render gene-editing therapies less effective.[19] *In utero* gene therapy or gene editing before the second half of the second trimester, when maternal immunoglobulins begin to cross into fetal circulation, would mitigate a preexisting immune barrier.[20] Additionally, the development of an immune response to the viral vector or transgene product after therapy may also limit postnatal gene therapy effectiveness including the ability to readminister the therapy.[18,21,22] Instead, the fetal immune system tends to induce immune tolerance to the transgene product, allowing for repeat doses after birth.[23–25]

Finally, the biggest potential advantage of *in utero* cell and molecular therapies is the ability to intervene before the onset of irreversible disease pathology. For example, in patients with spinal muscular atrophy (SMA), motor neurons are affected during the prenatal period and animal studies have demonstrated increased motor neurons, reduced muscle atrophy, and increased survival after fetal intracranial injection of an AAV packaged with the human survival motor neuron gene.[26] Postnatal studies have demonstrated a clear benefit of earlier treatments for patients with SMA and, thus, the biologic rationale for a prenatal treatment of SMA, assuming it is demonstrated to be safe for both mother and fetus, is clear.

Overall, *in utero* molecular and cellular therapies have vast potential for treating many disease pathologies that currently have limited postnatal treatments. In the following sections, we will discuss various strategies for *in utero* therapies, including gene editing, enzyme replacement therapy, and stem cell transplantation.

IN UTERO GENE EDITING

Advances in gene-editing technology have presented the unique opportunity to target and potentially cure diseases at the genomic level. Programmable nucleases, including the gene-editing technology Clustered Regularly Interspaced Short Palindromic Repeats-Cas9 (CRISPR-Cas9), have significant potential for therapeutic gene editing.[27] In the CRISPR-Cas9 system, a Cas9 endonuclease will create a site-specific double-stranded DNA break (DSB) based on the presence of an appropriate protospacer adjacent motif (PAM) at the DNA target site and guide RNA (gRNA) provided with the Cas9. After the creation of a DSB, one of the 2 editing approaches can occur. Normal DNA repair mechanisms will repair the DSB site, often in an imprecise way with the insertion and deletion of bases (indels). This approach, nonhomologous end joining (NHEJ), is the most efficient editing approach and can result in the silencing of a gene or removal of a segment of DNA (if 2 gRNAs are used). Alternatively, if a DNA repair template is provided with the Cas9 and gRNA, homology-directed repair (HDR) can result in the targeted replacement of a segment of DNA with that in the repair template.[28] HDR is less efficient than NHEJ and requires proliferating cells.

Alternative, potentially safer, and more efficient approaches to gene editing have been developed. CRISPR-mediated base editors consist of an enzymatically impaired Cas9 that is unable to make DSBs fused to a cytosine[29] or adenine[30] deaminase. Together with a gRNA, base editors can make site-specific purine to purine or pyrimidine to pyrimidine changes in the DNA. They do not require proliferating cells and thus, together with the lack of a need for DSBs, are potentially safer and more efficient than traditional CRISPR-Cas9 NHEJ and HDR. Prime editing is a newer technology that allows for even more adaptability in gene editing. Prime editing utilizes an enzymatically impaired Cas9 endonuclease (unable to make DSBs) that is fused to a reverse transcriptase and a prime editing guide RNA (pegRNA) to target selected sites within the genome and reverse transcribe the desired edit contained within the pegRNA.[31] Prime editing has more versatility than traditional CRISPR-Cas9 or base editing as it can perform insertions, deletions and all 12 types of point mutations at targeted locations. Mouse studies have demonstrated the feasibility of *in utero* CRISPR-mediated editing including the ability of *in utero* NHEJ to rescue the neonatal lethal model of a genetic surfactant deficiency,[32] and in utero base editing to rescue the phenotype of the metabolic liver disease hereditary tyrosinemia type 1[33] as well as the multi-organ lysosomal storage disease mucopolysaccharidosis type 1 (Hurler syndrome).[34]

As gene-editing strategies have progressed, so have the mechanisms for delivery. Viral and nonviral vectors can be used to deliver gene-editing technologies in vivo. Viral vectors are able to achieve high-efficiency gene delivery and expression, yet limitations exist with the most commonly used viruses. Adenovirus vectors have the largest DNA-carrying capacity, have very high transduction efficiency in both dividing and quiescent cells, and have a rapid onset of action.[35] However, adenovirus vectors have high immunogenicity and can stimulate severe systemic inflammatory responses. Adeno-associated viruses (AAV) conversely have low immunogenicity and agreeable safety profiles but are limited by the size of the transgene that can be inserted.[35] Lentiviral vectors have an intermediate carrying capacity and, as integrating vectors, they have the potential for long-term transgene expression. However, the concern for insertional mutagenesis as an off-target effect has limited its use to mostly ex vivo gene therapy trials. Furthermore, for gene-editing approaches, persistent expression of the Cas9 transgene, as would occur following lentiviral delivery, is not desirable as it increases the risk of unwanted mutagenesis.

Due to limitations with viral vectors, interest in nonviral delivery mechanisms has exploded in recent years. Unlike viruses, nonviral vectors have lower antigenicity, cytotoxicity, and potential for mutagenesis; however, these vectors have also faced challenges surrounding transduction efficiency and safety.[36] Some of the most common vehicle materials include polymers, lipids, and peptides. The chemical structures and physical properties of these materials can be altered to change the functionality of the particles and thereby modified for unique uses. DNA, RNA, and proteins have all been packaged into nanoparticle delivery systems for gene-editing purposes, which may allow for more versatility.[36–38] In an example of a nonviral approach to *in utero* gene editing, polymeric nanoparticles containing peptide nucleic acids were successfully injected intravenously with the correction of the disease-causing mutation and long-term phenotypic improvement in a beta-thalassemia mouse model.[39]

In addition to modifying the vector, the route of delivery of gene-editing constructs can also target different cells and organs. For example, intravenous injection through the vitelline vein, which drains directly into the fetal portal system, allows for high delivery and uptake in the liver.[33] In addition to targeting fetal hepatocytes, the *in utero* vitelline vein injection targeting the liver can also deliver the therapeutic to HSCs which are found in the fetal liver during development.[12] *In utero* intraamniotic or direct intratracheal injections can be used to target pulmonary epithelium.[32,40] *In utero* direct intracranial or intraventricular injections have been successfully used for brain delivery in animal models with neurocognitive disorders.[41]

Overall, while not yet approved for human application, there have been numerous positive developments in *in* utero gene editing in animal models. Continued studies are needed to help advance the field and potentially provide breakthroughs that may lead to advances in clinical translation.

IN UTERO ENZYME REPLACEMENT THERAPY

Enzyme replacement therapy (ERT) involves administering a deficient or absent enzyme that an individual is not able to produce on their own. ERT was first described in 1965 and is currently available for several genetic disorders, including mucopolysaccharidosis (MPS) type I, MPSII, Gaucher disease, Fabry disease, and Pompe disease.[42,43]

As ERT only replaces a missing enzyme, it is not a one-time treatment and most diseases will require ongoing doses. One of the potential problems with ERT is that patients can develop antibodies against the replacement enzyme leading to the rejection of the treatment. One potential advantage of *in utero* ERT is to minimize the development of antibodies against the therapy as the fetal immune system is more naïve. Clinical trials are actively investigating the efficacy of *in utero* ERT including a phase 1 clinical trial evaluating *in utero* ERT in various lysosomal storage disorders (LSDs).[44] In this trial, fetuses with MPS types 1, 2, 4a, 6, 7, infantile-onset Pompe disease, neuronopathic Gaucher disease type 2 and 3, or Wolman disease between the ages of 18 to 35 weeks gestation will be given ERT every 2–4 weeks in weight-based dosing via the umbilical vein. Following birth, patients will continue postnatal ERT per current standard of care guidelines and will be followed through 5 years of age. In addition, a phase 2 clinical trial is investigating *in utero* ERT for X-linked hypohydrotic ectodermal dysplasia (XLHED).[45] XLHED is a rare disorder resulting from a mutation in the ectodysplasin A gene that results in a sweating disorder manifesting with hypo or anhidrosis, oligo or anodontia, and hypotrichosis. This phase 2 clinical trial involves intraamniotic delivery of the ER004 protein which has high-affinity binding to the ectodysplasin A receptor. This trial is based on early encouraging results following the *in utero* treatment of 3 XLHED fetuses.[46] The results of these clinical trials will provide additional information about the relative value of this form of *in utero* therapy for future applications.

IN UTERO STEM CELL TRANSPLANTATION

In utero stem cell transplantation has the potential to treat many lethal or highly morbid hematologic, immune or genetic disorders. *In utero* HSC transplantation (IUHCT) is an approach that allows for the transplantation of healthy donor HSCs to the fetus without the need for myeloablative or immunosuppressive therapy due to the tolerant fetal immune system.[47] Despite the promise of IUHCT, it has only been consistently demonstrated to correct the clinical phenotype for one disorder, severe combined immunodeficiency (SCID). Patients with SCID suffer from lymphoid hypoplasia, T cell depletion, and hypogammaglobulinemia that result in high susceptibility to infection and failure to thrive.[48] In one of the first clinical examples of IUHCT, Flake and colleagues[14] performed 3 intraperitoneal injections of paternally derived bone marrow cells into a fetus with SCID resulting in the enrichment of hematopoietic cell progenitors and long-term survival to at least 11 months of age. More recently, a clinical trial of IUHCT for alpha thalassemia major is underway.[49] Alpha thalassemia major is an attractive target disease for *in utero* therapies as fetuses often develop severe anemia leading to intrauterine fetal demise if a fetal blood transfusion is not performed. In the current clinical trial, an IUHCT is performed with maternal donor cells at the time of a fetal blood transfusion. In the 2 reported patients, fetal hydrops resolved with the fetal blood transfusions, and long-term results of the engraftment of the maternal donor cells are pending. Both patients continue to receive monthly transfusions and are doing well with normal development and neurologic testing at one year of age with no unanticipated safety events for the mother or child.

In addition to hematologic or immune disorders, IUHCT can also be used for genetic disorders in which transplanted stem cells can produce a missing or deficient enzyme, which occurs in lysosomal storage disorders. HCT has become one of the mainstays of treatment of children with MPSI.[50] The success of HCT in disorders such as MPSI is in part based on the principle of cross-correction, in which cells with restored enzymatic ability secrete lysosomal enzymes into the extra-cellular space, which can be taken up and utilized by other cells.[51] However, the ability of the HCT to mitigate the disease phenotype is most effective if performed before the development of neurocognitive decline.[52] Although encouraging, postnatal HCT is limited by the morbidity associated with the transplant and requisite peri-transplant conditioning as well as the lack of available matched donors. These limitations could potentially be mitigated through *in utero* applications.

Although HSCs have generated a high level of clinical interest, other types of stem cells can also be transplanted, such as mesenchymal stem cells (MSCs). Osteogenesis imperfecta (OI), also known as brittle bone disease, is a multi-system congenital disorder with severe effects on the skeletal system. OI results from the absence or deficiency in type 1 collagen, which results in soft, brittle bones that break easily and can result in fetal demise in the most severe forms.[53] The clinical trial Boost Brittle Bones Before Birth (BOOSTB4) aims to evaluate the safety and efficacy of MSC transplantation in 2 types of OI, comparing *in utero* to postnatal therapy.[54]

MSCs are also being used for in utero repair of myelomeningocele (MMC), a disorder for which the inferior aspect of the spinal cord is exposed and can lead to impaired movement, bowel, and bladder function.[55] One of the current treatments involves performing surgery on the fetus to close the defect. A new clinical trial is investigating the addition of an MSC patch to the repair,[55] which has been shown in animal studies to protect the spinal cord and improve movement and developmental outcomes.[56] The outcomes of these clinical trials for MSCs will provide further information on the effectiveness of in utero stem cell transplantation as a promising in utero therapeutic.

SAFETY AND ETHICAL CONSIDERATIONS

While the application of *in utero* therapy continues to expand, several safety and ethical considerations need to be addressed. Two patients are involved in all prenatal therapies—the fetus and the mother—with the safety of the mother being the utmost priority. A panel was held at the International Fetal Transplantation and Immunology Society (IFeTIS) annual meeting to review risks and ethical considerations associated with *in utero* therapies.[57] These risks include the potential for procedural risks to the mother and fetus, potential for germline alteration, and potential for off-target effects with mutagenesis at other genomic sites when considering gene editing. For most molecular and cellular therapeutics, it is anticipated that the procedural risks will be low and similar to that associated with amniocentesis or umbilical vein transfusion. In a large retrospective review of umbilical vein transfusions for fetal anemia, the risk of complications was noted to be approximately 1.2% without any increased risk to subsequent pregnancies.[58] While early studies do not indicate that *in utero* gene editing performed in mid to late gestation fetuses affects the germline or maternal tissues, more studies are needed to further evaluate this as well as the potential for other unwanted mutagenesis following *in utero* gene editing or replacement gene therapy.[33,39] For this reason, it is critical to perform further studies in small and large animal models prior to translation to humans.

SUMMARY

Genetic disorders are being diagnosed earlier in pregnancy and with greater accuracy due to significant advances in maternal–fetal medicine and gene sequencing technology. This has allowed for the development of new technologies to potentially treat and cure monogenic disorders *in utero* before the onset of irreversible disease pathology. These therapies take advantage of the unique properties of fetal development, including small fetal size, a tolerant immune system, an abundance of accessible progenitor cells, and the ability to intervene before disease pathology develops. The advent of CRISPR-Cas9 gene editing presents an unprecedented opportunity for therapeutic gene correction. While there have not been any *in utero* trials to date, initial animal studies have demonstrated the significant potential for this therapy for future clinical application. *In utero* ERT is also well underway in clinical trials and may be significantly beneficial for LSDs and XLHED. Finally, IUHCT has been successful in the treatment of SCID, while MSCs are innovatively being utilized for OI and myelomeningocele. To realize the potential of prenatal therapies and provide hope to those with genetic diseases currently with limited treatment options, the safety and efficacy of *in utero* molecular and cellular therapies must continue to be rigorously studied in small and large animal models to facilitate translation to the clinic.

Best practices

What is the current practice for In Utero Molecular and Cellular Therapies?

In utero molecular and cellular therapies have significantly progressed over the past decade. There are active clinical trials investigating *in utero* stem cell transplantation and enzyme replacement therapy for highly morbid monogenic disorders. While there are currently no clinical trials for *in utero* gene editing or gene therapy, advances in preclinical studies are offering hope for the clinical application of these approaches in the future.

What changes in current practice are likely to improve outcomes?

Outcomes of current investigational studies and clinical trials will provide further information on the effectiveness of *in utero* therapies for future clinical translation.

Major recommendations

Continued robust preclinical large animal studies, including those in nonhuman primates, are required to assess the safety of prenatal molecular and cellular therapies, especially gene therapy and gene editing.

DISCLOSURE

This work was supported by grants 5R01HL151352, 5R01DK123049, and DP2HL152427 from the United States National Institute of Health (NIH).

REFERENCES

1. Peranteau W, Flake A. The future of in utero gene therapy. Mol Diagn Ther 2020; 24(2):135–42.
2. Serr D, Sachs L, Danon M. The diagnosis of sex before birth using cells from the amniotic fluid (a preliminary report). Bull Res Counc Isr 1955;5B(2):137–8.
3. Jelin A, Sagaser K, Wilkins-Haug L. Prenatal genetic testing options. Pediatr Clin North Am 2019;66(2):281–93.
4. Alfirevic Z, Navaratnam K, Mujezinovic F. Amniocentesis and chorionic villus sampling for prenatal diagnosis. Cochrane Database Syst Rev 2017;9(9):CD003252.
5. Mellis R, Chandler N, Chitty L. Next-generation sequencing and the impact on prenatal diagnosis. Expert Rev Mol Diagn 2018;18(8):689–99.
6. Lo Y, Corbetta N, Chamberlain P, et al. Presence of fetal DNA in maternal plasma and serum. Lancet (London, England) 1997;350(9076):485–7.
7. Carlson L, Vora N. Prenatal diagnosis: screening and diagnostic tools. Obstet Gynecol Clin North Am 2017;44(2):245–56.
8. Scotchman E, Shaw J, Paternoster B, et al. Non-invasive prenatal diagnosis and screening for monogenic disorders. Eur J Obstet Gynecol Reprod Biol 2020;253: 320–7.
9. Witt R, MacKenzie T, Peranteau W. Fetal stem cell and gene therapy. Semin Fetal Neonatal Med 2017;22(6):410–4.
10. Endo M, Henriques-Coelho T, Zoltick PW, et al. The developmental stage determines the distribution and duration of gene expression after early intra-amniotic gene transfer using lentiviral vectors. Gene Ther 2009;17(1):61–71.
11. Karda R, Buckley S, Mattar C, et al. Perinatal systemic gene delivery using adeno-associated viral vectors. Front Mol Neurosci 2014;0:89.
12. Waddington S, Kramer M, Hernandez-Alcoceba R, et al. In utero gene therapy: current challenges and perspectives. Mol Ther 2005;11(5):661–76.
13. Massaro G, Mattar C, Wong A, et al. Fetal gene therapy for neurodegenerative disease of infants. Nat Med 2018;24(9):1317–23.
14. Flake A, Roncarolo M, Puck J, et al. Treatment of X-linked severe combined immunodeficiency by in utero transplantation of paternal bone marrow. N Engl J Med 1996;335(24):1806–10.
15. Kim H, Shaaban A, Milner R, et al. In utero bone marrow transplantation induces donor-specific tolerance by a combination of clonal deletion and clonal anergy. J Pediatr Surg 1999;34(5):726–9.
16. Peranteau W, Hayashi S, Hsieh M, et al. High-level allogeneic chimerism achieved by prenatal tolerance induction and postnatal nonmyeloablative bone marrow transplantation. Blood 2002;100(6):2225–34.
17. Flake AW, Harrison MR, Adzick NS, Zanjani ED. Transplantation of fetal hematopoietic stem cells in utero: the creation of hematopoietic chimeras. Science 1986 Aug 15;233(4765):776–8. https://doi.org/10.1126/science.2874611. PMID: 2874611.
18. Calcedo R, Morizono H, Wang L, et al. Adeno-associated virus antibody profiles in newborns, children, and adolescents. Clin Vaccin Immunol 2011;18(9):1586–8.
19. Charlesworth C, Deshpande P, Dever D, et al. Identification of preexisting adaptive immunity to Cas9 proteins in humans. Nat Med 2019;25(2):249–54.
20. Simister N. Placental transport of immunoglobulin G. Vaccine 2003;21(24): 3365–9.
21. Basner-Tschakarjan E, Bijjiga E, Martino A. Pre-clinical assessment of immune responses to adeno-associated virus (AAV) vectors. Front Immunol 2014;5:28.

22. Moss R, Milla C, Colombo J, et al. Repeated aerosolized AAV-CFTR for treatment of cystic fibrosis: a randomized placebo-controlled phase 2B trial. Hum Gene Ther 2007;18(8):726–32.
23. Tran N, Porada C, Almeida-Porada G, et al. Induction of stable prenatal tolerance to beta-galactosidase by in utero gene transfer into preimmune sheep fetuses. Blood 2001;97(11):3417–23.
24. Davey M, Riley J, Andrews A, et al. Induction of immune tolerance to foreign protein via adeno-associated viral vector gene transfer in mid-gestation fetal sheep. PLoS One 2017;12(1):e0171132.
25. Sabatino D, Mackenzie T, Peranteau W, et al. Persistent expression of hF.IX after tolerance induction by in utero or neonatal administration of AAV-1-F.IX in hemophilia B mice. Mol Ther 2007;15(9):1677–85.
26. Rashnonejad A, Amini Chermahini G, Gündüz C, et al. Fetal gene therapy using a single injection of recombinant AAV9 rescued SMA phenotype in mice. Mol Ther 2019;27(12):2123–33.
27. Bak R, Gomez-Ospina N, Porteus M. Gene editing on center stage. Trends Genet 2018;34(8):600–11.
28. Doudna J, Charpentier E. Genome editing. The new frontier of genome engineering with CRISPR-Cas9. Science 2014;346(6213):1258096.
29. Kim D, Lim K, Kim S, et al. Genome-wide target specificities of CRISPR RNA-guided programmable deaminases. Nat Biotechnol 2017;35(5):475–80.
30. Gaudelli N, Komor A, Rees H, et al. Programmable base editing of A•T to G•C in genomic DNA without DNA cleavage. Nature 2017;551(7681).
31. Anzalone A, Randolph P, Davis J, et al. Search-and-replace genome editing without double-strand breaks or donor DNA. Nature 2019;576(7785):149–57.
32. Alapati D, Zacharias WJ, Hartman HA, Rossidis AC, Stratigis JD, Ahn NJ, Coons B, Zhou S, Li H, Singh K, Katzen J, Tomer Y, Chadwick AC, Musunuru K, Beers MF, Morrisey EE, Peranteau WH. In utero gene editing for monogenic lung disease. Sci Transl Med 2019 Apr 17;11(488):eaav8375. https://doi.org/10.1126/scitranslmed.aav8375. PMID: 30996081; PMCID: PMC6822403.
33. Rossidis AC, Stratigis JD, Chadwick AC, et al. In Utero CRISPR-mediated therapeutic editing of metabolic genes. Nat Med 2018;24(10):1513–8.
34. Bose SK, White BM, Kashyap MV, et al. In utero adenine base editing corrects multi-organ pathology in a lethal lysosomal storage disease. Nat Commun 2021;12(1):1–16.
35. Bulcha J, Wang Y, Ma H, et al. Viral vector platforms within the gene therapy landscape. Signal Transduction Targeted Ther 2021;6(1):1–24.
36. Morille M, Passirani C, Vonarbourg A, et al. Progress in developing cationic vectors for non-viral systemic gene therapy against cancer. Biomaterials 2008; 29(24–25):3477–96.
37. Zu H, Gao D. Non-viral vectors in gene therapy: recent development, challenges, and prospects. AAPS J 2021;23(4):78.
38. Schuh RS, Poletto E, Fachel FNS, et al. Physicochemical properties of cationic nanoemulsions and liposomes obtained by microfluidization complexed with a single plasmid or along with an oligonucleotide: implications for CRISPR/Cas technology. J Colloid Interface Sci 2018;530:243–55.
39. Ricciardi A, Bahal R, Farrelly J, et al. In Utero nanoparticle delivery for site-specific genome editing. Nat Commun 2018;9(1):1–11.
40. Peddi N, Ramesh H, Gude S, et al. Intrauterine fetal gene therapy: is that the future and is that future now? Cureus 2022;14(2):e22521.

41. Hu S, Yang T, Wang Y. Widespread labeling and genomic editing of the fetal central nervous system by in utero CRISPR AAV9-PHP.eB administration. Development 2021;148(2):dev195586.
42. Neufeld E. Enzyme replacement therapy – a brief history. In: Atul Mehta, Michael Beck, Gere Sunder-Plassmann, editors. Fabry disease: perspectives from 5 years of FOS. Oxford: Oxford PharmaGenesis; 2006.
43. Ries M. Enzyme replacement therapy and beyond-in memoriam Roscoe O. Brady, M.D. (1923-2016). J Inherit Metab Dis 2017;40(3):343–56.
44. ClinicalTrials.gov. In utero enzyme replacement therapy for lysosomal storage diseases - identifier: NCT04532047 national library of medicine (US). 2020. Available at: https://clinicaltrials.gov/ct2/show/NCT04532047. Accessed June 3, 2022.
45. ClinicalTrials.gov. Intraamniotic administrations of ER004 to male subjects with X-linked hypohidrotic ectodermal dysplasia- identifier: NCT04980638. National Library of Medicine (US); 2021. Available at: https://clinicaltrials.gov/ct2/show/NCT04980638. Accessed June 3, 2022.
46. Schneider H, Faschingbauer F, Schuepbach-Mallepell S, et al. Prenatal correction of X-Linked hypohidrotic ectodermal dysplasia 2018;378:1604–10. https://doi.org/10.1056/NEJMoa1714322.
47. Peranteau W. In utero hematopoietic cell transplantation: induction of donor specific immune tolerance and postnatal transplants. Front Pharmacol 2014;5:251.
48. Fischer A. Severe combined immunodeficiencies. Immunodefic Rev 1992;3(2):83–100.
49. Mackenzie T, Frascoli M, Sper R, et al. In utero stem cell transplantation in patients with alpha thalassemia major: interim results of a phase 1 clinical trial | request PDF. Blood 2022;136:1.
50. Hobbs J, Hugh-Jones K, Barrett A, et al. Reversal of clinical features of Hurler's disease and biochemical improvement after treatment by bone-marrow transplantation. Lancet 1981;2(8249):709–12.
51. Fratantoni J, Hall C, Neufeld E. Hurler and Hunter syndromes: mutual correction of the defect in cultured fibroblasts. Science 1968;162(3853):570–2.
52. Tanaka A, Okuyama T, Suzuki Y, et al. Long-term efficacy of hematopoietic stem cell transplantation on brain involvement in patients with mucopolysaccharidosis type II: a nationwide survey in Japan. Mol Genet Metab 2012;107(3):513–20.
53. Rowe D. Osteogenesis imperfecta. 3rd edition. Amsterdam: Elsevier; 2008.
54. ClinicalTrials.gov. Boost brittle bones before birth - identifier: NCT03706482 national library of medicine (US). 2018. Available at: https://clinicaltrials.gov/ct2/show/NCT03706482. Accessed June 3, 2022.
55. ClinicalTrials.gov. Cellular therapy for in utero repair of myelomeningocele - the CuRe trial - identifier: NCT04652908 national library of medicine (US). 2020. Available at: https://clinicaltrials.gov/ct2/show/NCT04652908. Accessed June 3, 2022.
56. Wang A, Brown E, Lankford L, et al. Placental mesenchymal stromal cells rescue ambulation in ovine myelomeningocele. Stem Cells Translational Med 2015;4(6):659–69.
57. Almeida-Porada G, Waddington S, Chan J, et al. In utero gene therapy consensus statement from the IFeTIS. Mol Ther 2019;27(4):705–7.
58. Zwiers C, Lindenburg I, Klumper F, et al. Complications of intrauterine intravascular blood transfusion: lessons learned after 1678 procedures. Ultrasound Obstet Gynecol 2017;50(2):180–6.

Fetal and Neonatal Anesthesia

Marla B. Ferschl, MD[a],*, Ranu R. Jain, MD[b]

KEYWORDS

• Fetal anesthesia • Neonatal anesthesia • Fetal physiology • Neonatal physiology
• EXIT procedure

KEY POINTS

- Anesthesia for fetal surgery requires a coordinated team-based approach to ensure the optimal care of the pregnant patient and the fetus.
- A thorough understanding of maternal and fetal physiology as well as pharmacology are essential considerations during fetal and Ex-Utero Intrapartum Treatment procedures.
- Neonates undergo a profound transition following birth; these changes may not proceed normally in the setting of physiologic stress.

INTRODUCTION

Fetal and neonatal anesthesia are complicated subspecialties of anesthesia and require specialized experience and training. Neonatal anesthesia is most often performed by fellowship-trained pediatric anesthesiologists; fetal anesthesia by pediatric or obstetric fellowship-trained anesthesiologists. A thorough understanding of maternal, fetal, and neonatal anatomy and physiology as well as anesthetic pharmacology is essential for the provider caring for these patients. Several important anesthetic concepts are important to both fetal and neonatal anesthetic cases. These include an understanding of the fetal circulation, the role of temperature management, and the concept of anesthetic neurotoxicity and its effect on the developing brain.

The Fetal Circulation

In utero, three fetal shunts optimize the delivery of oxygenated blood to the tissues and minimize unnecessary blood flow through the non-ventilated lungs. These include the foramen ovale, the ductus arteriosus, and the ductus venosus (**Fig. 1**). In utero, the pulmonary vascular resistance (PVR) is relatively high, whereas the systemic vascular

a Department of Anesthesia and Perioperative Care, University of California San Francisco, 550 16th St. San Francisco, CA 94143, USA; b Department of Anesthesiology, University of Texas HSC at Houston, 6431 Fannin St. Houston, TX 77030, USA
* Corresponding author.
E-mail address: Marla.Ferschl@ucsf.edu

Clin Perinatol 49 (2022) 821–834
https://doi.org/10.1016/j.clp.2022.07.001
0095-5108/22/© 2022 Elsevier Inc. All rights reserved.

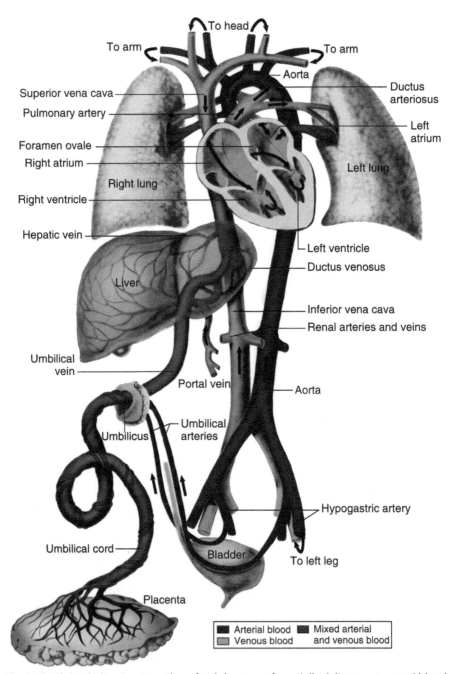

To head

To arm

To arm

Aorta

Superior vena cava

Ductus arteriosus

Pulmonary artery

Left atrium

Foramen ovale

Right atrium

Left lung

Right lung

Right ventricle

Left ventricle

Hepatic vein

Ductus venosus

Liver

Inferior vena cava

Renal arteries and veins

Umbilical vein

Portal vein

Aorta

Umbilicus

Umbilical arteries

Hypogastric artery

Umbilical cord

Bladder

To left leg

Placenta

Arterial blood	Mixed arterial
Venous blood	and venous blood

Fig. 1. Fetal circulation: In utero, three fetal shunts preferentially deliver oxygenated blood to the fetal brain and body: the ductus venosus, the foramen ovalae, and the ductus arteriosus. (*From* Jooste EH, Machovec KA, Greeley WJ. Anesthesia for pediatric cardiac surgery. In: Gropper MA, Cohen NH, Eriksson LI, Fleisher LA, Leskie K, Wiener-Kronish JP, editors. Miller's Anesthesia Volume II. Philadelphia: Elsevier 2020. p 2461; with permission. (Figure 78.1 in original).)

resistance (SVR) is relatively low. At birth, this relationship switches with the clamping of the placenta and the neonate's first breath, which delivers blood to the lungs and results in an increased left atrial volume and pressure. However, this transition can be dynamic; especially during periods of acidosis, hypoxia, or hypothermia, the neonatal PVR can increase, leading to right to left shunting, worsened hypoxemia, and acidosis. In general, the pulmonary vascular pressures can remain high or reactive for at least 2 months following delivery. Cardiac output, blood pressure, and heart rate mature more gradually over the first few years of life.[1]

Both the fetus and the neonate have a cardiac output that depends on heart rate, as the myocardium is stiff and non-compliant and cannot easily augment its stroke volume. A normal fetus has a combined ventricular output that ranges from 425 to 550 mL/kg/min[2] and normal neonatal cardiac output is approximately 300 cc/kg/min. As this baseline cardiac output is already quite high, newborns are minimally able to respond to increased cardiac demand or compensate for changes in preload or afterload.[3]

Blood volume increases over the course of gestation. It is estimated to be 110 to 160 mL/kg at mid-gestation; 1/3 of this blood is in the fetus and 2/3 is contained in the placenta.[4] Hemoglobin levels rise in a linear fashion from 11 g/dL in a 17-wk fetus to 18 g/dL in a term infant at birth.

Temperature Regulation

Intrauterine temperatures are generally 20° F warmer than the ambient environment. Exposure of the fetus or the neonate to cooler temperatures results in an increased caloric expenditure, oxygen consumption, and cellular metabolism. Heat loss can occur from radiation, convection, evaporation, and conduction. Heat loss is further exacerbated by lack of subcutaneous fat, a large body surface to body weight ratio, and the inability to shiver. To compensate, non-shivering thermogenesis can occur after approximately 25 weeks of gestation. This process of triglyceride and fatty acid metabolism is stimulated by thyroid stimulating hormone and circulating catecholamines.[5]

In the setting of hypothermia, oxygen consumption, and pulmonary and peripheral vascular resistance are increased, whereas the cardiac output is decreased, leading to metabolic acidosis. Neonates with neurologic injury or sepsis are more prone to hypothermia. Prolonged periods of hypothermia can lead to inadequate oxygen delivery and cardiovascular collapse.[6] During open fetal procedures, even limited fetal hypothermia can lead to fetal bradycardia and demise.[7,8]

Therefore, maintaining a neutral thermal environment for the fetus and neonate undergoing anesthesia is essential to maintain normal physiologic homeostasis. The ambient operating room temperature should be elevated for both fetal and neonatal procedures. In fetal procedures, warmed crystalloid solutions should be used for irrigation to preserve temperature, and maternal forced warm-air devices should be used to maintain maternal temperature.[9] For neonates, the use of forced-air warming devices, hats, and plastic sheets are useful to help maintain body temperature.[10] In both types of procedures, careful monitoring of temperature should occur to avoid overhearing the fetus/neonate, as this can be detrimental as well.[11]

Neurotoxicity

On December 14, 2016, the US Food and Drug Administration (FDA) issued a "Drug Safety Communication" warning that multiple exposures or prolonged exposure (more than 3 h) to general anesthesia and sedation drugs to children less than 3 years of age or pregnant women in their third trimester "may affect the development of children's brains."[12] This warning was published in response to multiple studies in non-human animal models that showed learning and memory deficits as well as histologic evidence of neuroapoptosis following to prolonged or repeated exposure to anesthetic agents, including volatile anesthetic agents, midazolam, propofol, and ketamine.[13,14] However, the effect of anesthetic agents on the human brain are less conclusive. Two prospective trials have evaluated the effect of a single short anesthetic on cognitive outcomes in neonates undergoing surgery and have not found any significant neurodevelopmental consequences.[15,16] There are limited data about neurotoxicity in the human fetal population. One study has examined the exposure of general anesthesia to the fetus during a cesarean section and found no neurodevelopmental consequences at age 5.[17] An international clinical registry for fetal surgery patients has been created to assess long-term neurodevelopmental outcomes following exposure to general anesthesia (ClinicalTrials.gov identifier NCT02591745). Unfortunately, many patients who undergo fetal procedures are born prematurely and may also need anesthesia after birth, making the data analysis complicated. Providers should consider the impact of anesthetic medications during maternal-fetal and neonatal cases and minimize anesthetic exposure when possible.

ANESTHESIA FOR FETAL PROCEDURES
The Pregnant Patient

Pregnancy is accompanied by a host of physiologic changes due to hormonal and anatomic alternations. Important cardiopulmonary changes seen in pregnancy are summarized in **Box 1**. Pregnancy results in progressive increases in maternal oxygen consumption and minute ventilation, as well as a decreased pulmonary residual volume and functional residual capacity.[18] These changes can make adequate oxygenation and perfusion of the mother and the fetoplacental unit a challenge during maternal general anesthesia. During periods of apnea or hypoventilation, the pregnant patient is prone to rapid desaturation and hypercapnia.[19] The pregnant airway

---

Box 1
Physiologic changes of pregnancy

Pulmonary
　Decreased functional residual capacity
　Increased minute ventilation
　Increased oxygen consumption
　Decreased Pa_{CO_2}
　Upper airway edema and capillary engorgement

Cardiovascular
　Increased cardiac output
　Decreased systemic vascular resistance
　At risk for aortocaval compression

Gastrointestinal
　Decreased lower esophageal sphincter tone

Renal
　Increased glomerular filtration rate

Hematologic
　Increased plasma volume
　Physiologic anemia
　Hypercoagulable state

presents additionally anatomic challenges due to mucosal edema and tissue friability. Deliberate and meticulous airway management strategies are essential to avoid hypercarbia and hypoxemia. The induction of and emergence from anesthesia with inhalational anesthetics occurs faster in pregnant patients than in nonpregnant patients because the combination of increased alveolar ventilation and decreased functional residual capacity speedsdenitrogenation and the rate at which inspired and alveolar concentrations of inhalational anesthetics reach equilibrium.[20] Pregnant patients are at risk for pulmonary edema due to a decrease in colloid oncotic pressure that occurs during pregnancy coupled with the use of tocolytic agents (eg, magnesium or β-adrenoceptor agonists), and as a result excessive intravenous fluid administration should be avoided.

From a cardiovascular standpoint, maternal cardiac output increases by 35% to 40% by the end of the first trimester and continues to increase steadily throughout the second trimester until it reaches a level 50% greater than the cardiac output of nonpregnant women.[21] Heart rate increases 15% to 25% and stroke volume increases 25% to 30% compared with pre-pregnancy values by the end of the second trimester, after which they both remain stable until term.[22] Aortocaval compression by the gravid uterus can decrease cardiac output; lesser decreases occur in the sitting or semi-recumbent positions. Left lateral uterine displacement should be performed to optimize fetal-placental circulation during fetal procedures.[23] Under anesthesia, maternal blood pressure should be maintained within 10% of baseline, using intravenous ephedrine or phenylephrine; often a phenylephrine infusion is necessary to maintain normotension in the setting of high volatile anesthetic agent use.

Anesthetic drug pharmacokinetics and pharmacodynamics are affected by the physiologic changes of pregnancy. Volume of distribution is altered by an increase in total body water and adipose tissue, as well as a decrease in plasma protein concentration. Renal drug elimination is enhanced by an increased renal blood flow and glomerular filtration rate (GFR). Hepatic metabolism of some drugs may have a greater clearance associated with the increased basal metabolic rate, whereas others may be inhibited by competition with steroid hormones during pregnancy. Most maternally administered medications, including volatile anesthetics and opioids cross the placenta. Transplacental drug diffusion is influenced by lipid solubility, the pH of both maternal and fetal blood, the degree of ionization, protein binding, perfusion, placental area and thickness, and drug concentration.[24]

Other important physiologic changes for the anesthesiologist to consider include: (1) decreased lower esophageal sphincter tone, making the pregnant patient more prone to aspiration and (2) a physiologic anemia of pregnancy, with average hemoglobin levels around 11.6 g/dL.

Fetal Pain Perception

An understanding of the development of fetal pain perception is essential when performing fetal procedures. The first fetal spinal reflexes may be present as early as 8 weeks of gestation, and neuronal proliferation rapidly occurs between 8 and 18 weeks' gestation.[25] Synaptogenesis occurs first peripherally and then centrally, at approximately 20 weeks' gestation.[26] Nociceptive sensory receptors proliferate in parallel with the development of the central nervous system, and are present throughout all of the skin and mucosal surfaces by 20 weeks' gestation.[27] Initially, these nociceptive receptors are involved in local reflex movements at the spinal cord level without higher cortical integration. With time, these reflex responses become more complex and involve the brainstem, through which other responses, such as increases in heart rate and blood pressure, are mediated. However, these reflexes to noxious stimuli do not involve the cortex and, thus, do not result in conscious pain perception.[28,29]

When considering fetal intervention, one must consider whether being subjected to surgical stress during early development might permanently alter physiology. This concept is known as *programming,* and is defined as "the process whereby a stimulus or insult at a critical, sensitive period of development has permanent effects on structure, physiology, and metabolism."[30,31] Animal studies have shown increased basal and stress-induced cortisol concentrations in antenatally stressed animals that persist into adulthood. Behavioral changes, such as poor coping behaviors, have also been observed.[31] Consequently, though it is unlikely that the fetus can perceive pain at the gestational age of most *in utero* procedures, it is recommended by both the American Society of Anesthesiologists and the Society of Maternal Fetal Medicine that opioid analgesia be administered to the fetus during invasive fetal procedures to attenuate the fetal stress response and its deleterious consequences.[32,33] Typically, intramuscular opioid (eg, fentanyl 10–20 mcg/kg) is administered along with a muscle relaxant (eg, rocuronium 2–3 mg/kg), with or without an anticholinergic (atropine 20 mcg/kg) to reduce the possibility of bradycardia associated with opioid administration. Alternatively, maternal administration of remifentanil has been shown to transfer opioids to the fetus.[34] The umbilical cord and placenta do not have pain receptors, so procedures only involving these tissues (eg, laser ablation for TTTS) do not require the administration of opioid analgesics.

Minimally Invasive Procedures

Most minimally invasive fetal procedures (placental laser ablation for Twin–Twin Transfusion Syndrome (TTTS), selective reduction by radiofrequency ablation (RFA) or bipolar cord coagulation (BPC), Intrauterine blood transfusion (IUBT), Shunts— Thoracic and Bladder, and Fetoscopic Endotracheal Occlusion (FETO)) are percutaneous needle-guided or fetoscope guided.[35] These procedures are generally performed under monitored anesthesia care, with local anesthetic administered by the surgeon at the port insertion sites. Most cases are supine, with a left or right lateral displacement of the uterus based on the location of the umbilical cord placental insertions and/or fetal position.[36] The anesthetic technique frequently involves minimal maternal sedation, with a combination of midazolam, fentanyl, remifentanil, and/or propofol. It is important to avoid deep sedation, which may cause deep breathing, excessive abdominal movement, and unwanted motion on the surgical field, as well as risk maternal aspiration. Neuraxial techniques can also be used, though, this may result in longer procedure times, increased fluid administration, and more maternal hypotension.[37] The patient should be given intravenous famotidine and oral sodium citrate before the procedure. The fetus may require intramuscular pain medication and paralysis for procedures on the fetus like fetal shunts and FETO.

Open Mid-Gestation Procedures

The most commonly performed open fetal procedure is fetal myelomeningocele (MMC) repair. Fetal MMC repair can be done hysteroscopically generally following a laparotomy, or via open fetal surgery. Both techniques require profound uterine relaxation to prevent uterine contractions and preterm labor and delivery. Open fetal procedures involve greater fetal and maternal risk, as well as a higher likelihood of hemodynamic compromise. The team must be prepared for maternal and fetal blood loss, the need for fetal and/or maternal resuscitation, and the potential for emergent delivery.[9]

A thorough preoperative evaluation, including a detailed history and physical of the mother, as well as a complete fetal workup is essential before open fetal procedures to exclude contraindications to the surgical intervention. Extensive maternal counseling on the risks, benefits, and alternatives of the planned intervention is paramount. A discussion regarding the plan for fetal resuscitation and delivery (in the event of unsuccessful resuscitation) should occur with the patient, family, and perioperative team.

Before entering the operating room, the patient should be given citric acid/sodium citrate and famotidine, indomethacin for tocolysis, and a preoperative anxiolytic if necessary. A preoperative low thoracic epidural or regional blocks (bilateral transversus a abdominus plane bvlocks) can be done for postoperative pain control. Fetal drugs are prepared based on estimated fetal weight by ultrasound and dispensed to the scrub technician in a sterile fashion before the patient is brought to the operating room. These include a including a fetal cocktail consisting of a muscle relaxant (rocuronium 2.5 mg/kg or vecuronium 0.25 mg/kg), fentanyl 10 to 20 mcg/kg, +/− atropine 20 mcg/kg, and fetal resuscitation medications including epinephrine 10 mcg/kg and atropine 20 mcg/kg. Maternal and fetal blood products are prepared for emergency administration.[38]

General endotracheal anesthesia is usually the anesthetic of choice for these procedures. Left uterine displacement, sequential compression devices, and a forced air warming blanket should be used, and fetal well-being assessed before induction. A rapid sequence induction and intubation should be performed following adequate preoxygenation. Care must be taken to maintain maternal physiology close to the preanesthetic baseline; end-tidal carbon dioxide levels should be 28 to 32. Because uteroplacental perfusion is not autoregulated and depends on maternal systemic blood pressure, the maternal systemic blood pressure is tightly maintained (within 10% of baseline) with titration of a phenylephrine intravenous infusion for optimal uteroplacental perfusion. Additional large bore intravenous access ± an arterial line should be placed. At most centers, a 6-g intravenous bolus of magnesium sulfate is administered over 30 minutes after induction, followed by a continuous infusion of 2 g/h to provide tocolysis.[39] High-dose volatile anesthetic agents are used to provide uterine relaxation for the surgical procedure. Supplemental intravenous infusions of propofol and remifentanil can also be considered.[40,41] Uterine tone is clinically assessed by direct visualization and palpation of the uterus by the surgeon. If uterine relaxation is not adequate, the amount of sevoflurane may be increased, and/or doses of IV or sublingual nitroglycerin can be administered if necessary to augment uterine relaxation. Intraoperative fetal heart rate is monitored continuously by an ultrasonographer; often fetal cardiac output and umbilical arterial blood flow are also monitored.[42,43] During the hysterotomy, careful attention should be paid to maternal blood loss, as it can be rapid and difficult to detect. Once the hysterotomy is complete, warmed saline irrigation is continuously instilled into the uterine cavity to prevent fetal hypothermia and preserve umbilical cord blood flow. Following completion of the surgical procedure, anesthetic agents are weaned, and the epidural is activated for postoperative pain control. The patient is extubated when fully away once adequate neuromuscular recovery and hemodynamic stability are verified.

Ex-Utero Intrapartum Treatment Procedure

The Ex-Utero Intrapartum Treatment (EXIT) procedure is a unique delivery performed on a near-term fetus, usually with anticipated airway obstruction. The goal of the procedure is to secure the fetal airway and establish adequate ventilation before the delivery of the fetus via cesarean section.[44] The EXIT procedure is most commonly used in cases where there is a concern for establishing an airway immediately after birth.

Before the procedure, a multidisciplinary team meeting is essential to establish a plan and ensure all necessary providers and equipment are available. From an anesthetic standpoint, fetal medications should be prepared, including weight-based doses of fetal epinephrine, atropine, muscle relaxant, and narcotic. A sterile fetal pulse oximeter should be available for fetal monitoring during the procedure. Fetal airway equipment must be prepared, including a sterile ventilation circuit with a pressure manometer, multiple sizes of endotracheal tubes and laryngoscopes, as well as rigid and flexible bronchoscopes. Sterile IV starting kits should be placed on the field for fetal intravenous access if necessary. O-negative blood, that is leukocyte-depleted, CMV-negative, and maternally crossmatched should be prepared for the fetus (40 mL/kg). Maternal blood should also be readily available in case of uterine hemorrhage.

General endotracheal anesthesia is usually employed for these cases, though neuraxial techniques have been described.[45] A high lumbar epidural can be placed preoperatively to provide postoperative pain control, or alternatively, bilateral transversus abdominis plane blocks can be done. Following induction and tracheal intubation, large bore maternal intravenous access should be established, and an arterial line considered. Because maintenance of maternal hemodynamics is essential for uteroplacental and fetal perfusion, maternal blood pressure should be kept within 10% of baseline using phenylephrine infusions or other vasopressors. Like open fetal surgery, uterine relaxation is ensured with high dose volatile anesthetic agents (>2 MAC) with the addition of nitroglycerin (100–250 mcg bolus dose or 1–10 mcg/kg/min infusion) as necessary. Some practitioners also use a maternal remifentanil infusion (0.1–0.3 mcg/kg/min) to supplement the anesthetic and provide fetal analgesia, as remifentanil rapidly crosses the placenta.[46,47]

The EXIT procedure typically involves the delivery of the fetal head and neck and one arm through a hysterotomy while maintaining the uteroplacental circulation through the umbilical cord. A sterile fetal pulse oximeter can be placed following the hysterotomy to allow for continuous fetal monitoring. Care must be taken to maintain fetal temperature, usually with a warm ambient room temperature and the use of warmed irrigation fluids. The umbilical cord must also be evaluated to avoid compression and/or kinking. After the fetal airway is secured and oxygenation and ventilation are confirmed, the umbilical cord is clamped and cut. An oxytocin infusion is started following delivery of the fetus to increase uterine tone, and uterotonics such as methergine or hemabate may be required to further reduce uterine atony. Volatile anesthetic agent levels are immediately decreased and nitroglycerin is promptly discontinued following delivery to diminish the risk of maternal hemorrhage and the uterine incision is quickly closed.[44] Following the completion of the procedure, the patient is extubated when hemodynamically stable and fully awake.

NEONATAL ANESTHESIA

Neonatal anesthesia is challenging because of these patients' complicated and evolving physiology as well as their distinct anatomy. In addition to the challenges posed by their transitional circulation, inadequate temperature regulation, and risk of neurotoxicity, as discussed above, the neonate poses additional challenges for the anesthesiologist once separated from the uteroplacental circulation. These include anatomically different airways, altered glucose and electrolyte regulation, differential metabolism of commonly administered anesthetic medications, and the occurrence of apnea and bradycardia following general anesthesia.

The Neonatal Airway

The pediatric airway, particularly in newborns, is different. Understanding these differences is important when managing the pediatric airway. The larynx is situated more cephalad at the third and fourth cervical vertebrae (C3–C4) level in the infant and migrates to the adult C5 level by 6 years of age. Because the infant's larynx is more rostral (higher), the tongue is located closer to the palate and more easily opposes the palate.

The neonatal epiglottis is long, stiff, and often described as Ω or U-shaped. It projects posteriorly above the glottis at a 45° angle. Because the epiglottis is more obliquely angled, visualization of the vocal cords may be difficult during direct laryngoscopy. It may be necessary to lift the tip of the epiglottis with a laryngoscope blade to visualize the vocal cords. Straight laryngoscope blades are often preferred for this reason. The glottic opening and the subvocal cord level are the narrowest portions of the infant's airway, and the airway is more cylindrical in shape. It is important not to have a tight-fitting endotracheal tube as it may compress the mucosa at this level and may lead to subglottic stenosis.

Direct laryngoscopy involves alignment of the oral, pharyngeal, and laryngeal axes to visualize the glottis (**Fig. 2**). Because the larynx is situated in a more cephalad position and the occiput is large, the sniffing position in infants does not assist in visualization of the larynx. The infant should be positioned with the head in a neutral position with the neck neither flexed nor extended. A small shoulder or neck roll may be beneficial. Optimum external laryngeal manipulation should also be used with a poor laryngoscopic view to improve visualization.[48]

Glucose, Fluid, and Blood Replacement

Intraoperative neonatal fluid replacement should be guided by three needs: meeting maintenance fluid requirements, replacing preoperative deficits, and fulfilling ongoing surgical loss. The hourly maintenance requirement for children follows the "4-2-1" rule, whereby a neonate should get 4 mL/kg of fluid per hour, though this formula may overestimate the fluid requirement for a critically ill infant.[49] In neonates, the amount of insensible water loss is inversely proportional to gestational age, due to skin permeability, metabolic demand, and the ratio of body surface area to weight. Neonates are unable to concentrate or dilute their urine, so isotonic fluids with sodium concentrations similar to plasma are recommended. Care should be taken to not over administer intravenous fluid to neonates with volume limiting devices. No prospective,

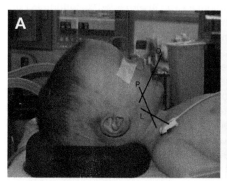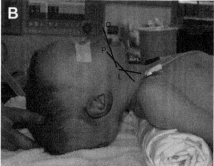

Fig. 2. Head position for intubation. Optimal positioning for laryngoscopy requires the alignment of the oral (O), pharyngeal (P) and laryngeal (L) axes. A flexed or sniffing position (A) prevents this alignment, whereas a small shoulder roll (B) improves this alignment. (Karsli C. Managing the challenging pediatric airway: Continuing Professional Development. Can J Anesth/J Can Anesth 62, 1000–1016 (2015). https://doi.org/10.1007/s12630-015-0423-y.)

randomized studies support the role for colloids vs crystalloids for volume expansion or fluid replacement in neonates. However, albumin is frequently used to maintain colloid osmotic pressure in the setting of hypovolemia.[50]

Neonatal hypoglycemia is generally defined as a blood glucose level <47 mg/dL.[51] Neonatal hypoglycemia is associated with neurologic injury and neurodevelopmental disorders.[52,53] Because the neonatal liver lacks glycogen stores, a dextrose continuing fluid should be used for maintenance replacement intraoperatively to avoid hypoglycemia. An infusion of 10% dextrose at 4 mL/kg/h provides 6.6 mg/kg/min of dextrose, sufficient to maintain euglycemia.

Preterm infants have a blood volume of 90 to 100 mL/kg, whereas term infants have a blood volume of 80 to 90 mL/kg. A current threshold for red blood cell (RBC) transfusion in neonates does not exist. The need for transfusion should balance the clinical need with the risks of transfusion including intravascular volume overload (TACO) and transfusion-induced lung injury (TRALI).[54] When given, RBCs should be screened for infectious agents (including CMV) and irradiated for leukocyte depletion. RBCs can also be washed before transfusion to minimize potassium load.

Medication Metabolism

The premature and term neonates have significant differences in drug absorption, distribution, metabolism, and elimination as compared with older children and adults.

Drug Absorption and Distribution

Drug absorption in neonates is largely affected by the maturation process of organ systems. Oral absorption is slower in neonates than older children. A higher gastric pH alters medication ionization, and delayed gastric emptying time, decreased intestinal motility and a reduction in bile acid synthesis all affect the oral absorption of drugs. Rectal absorption of drugs is generally also increased in the neonate as compared with children and adults. However, variability in the depth of insertion of drug in the rectum can affect the absorption. Drugs administered deep in the rectum undergo first-pass metabolism in the liver through the superior rectal veins whereas shallow administration will be absorbed by systemic circulation directly through the inferior and middle rectal veins. Neonates have less muscle mass, perfusion, and decreased contractility, which alters intramuscular drug absorption. Variations in cardiac output can also alter the absorption of drugs given intramuscularly. The transdermal absorption of drugs is increased in premature neonates as the skin is very thin and has more water content. The neonatal central nervous system has less myelination is the neonates, which results in increased permeability in the blood–brain barrier; this can be exacerbated by hypoxia, sepsis, and ischemia.

Compared with children and adults, the total body water is 80% in newborns, which decreases to 60% by 1 year. Hydrophilic drugs have decreased plasma concentration because of increased volume of distribution. The body fat in premature neonates is about 1% to 2% in preterm as compared with term neonates who have 10% to 15%. By the age of 1 year the body fat increases to and 20% to 25%. Lipophilic drugs will have increased plasma concentration because of decreased volume of distribution. Protein binding in neonates is low due to lower levels in circulation. Albumin levels are directly proportional to the gestational age. α-1-acid glycoprotein levels are significantly low in preterm neonate. This will result in higher concentration of unbound drug in plasma. The drugs can also compete and displace bilirubin from binding which will result in increased levels of unconjugated bilirubin and risk of kernicterus in neonates.[55]

Drug Metabolism and Elimination

The rate of hepatic drug metabolism is typically low at birth despite reduced protein binding and can sometimes lead to unpredictiblre unpredictableb metabolic clearance of drugs. Mechanisms of renal excretion affected by these factors are GFR, active tubular secretion, and tubular reabsorption. The renal clearance of drugs increases with gestational age, postnatal age, and weight gain. The GFR is significantly lower in the neonates and even less in the premature neonates due to delayed immature nephrogenesis.[56] The term neonate shows a rapid rise in the GFR in the first 2 weeks of life and reaches the adult levels at 1 year of age. Maturation of active tubular secretion increases steadily and reaches the adult values by 6 to 12 months of life. Maturation of tubular reabsorption shows a steep rise between 1 and 3 y of age and continues slowly to reach the mature levels by adolescence.

Apnea and Bradycardia of Prematurity

The development of postoperative apnea and bradycardia is a major concern with surgery in neonates. An apneic spell is defined as a cessation of breathing for 20 seconds or longer or if shorter, apnea which is accompanied by bradycardia (<100 beats per minute), cyanosis, or pallor. The cause of episodes in preterm patients can be central or obstructive or both. The risk of apnea and bradycardia are multifactorial. Common causes include prematurity (less than 37 weeks post-conception), a prior history of apnea and bradycardia, chronic lung disease, multiple congenital anomalies, and anemia (hematocrit < 30%). A decreased ventilatory response to hypoxia and hypercarbia due to immature nervous system development may be potentiated by anesthetic agents.

Different institutions have different age post-conceptual age guidelines for admission after general anesthesia in neonates. The incidence of significant apnea and bradycardia is highest in the first 4 to 6 h after surgery but has been reported up to 12 h after surgery. The most accepted guideline is to monitor premature infants who are less than 50 to 60 weeks post-conceptual age for at least 12 h after surgery. Physicians should be encouraged to delay elective outpatient surgery on premature infants who are less than 50 weeks post-conceptual age.

SUMMARY

Anesthesia for fetal and neonatal surgery requires subspecialized knowledge and expertise. Attention to important anatomic, physiologic, and metabolic differences seen in pregnancy and at birth are essential for the optimal care of these patients. Thorough preoperative evaluations, tailored intraoperative strategies, and careful postoperative management are critical when devising the anesthetic approach for each of these cases.

CLINICS CARE POINTS

- A thorough understanding of the anatomy and physiology of the pregnant patient, fetus, and neonate is essentail for the anesthesiologist
- Minimally invasive fetal proceudres can often be performed with monitored anesthesia care, while open fetal procedures and neonatal procedures usually require general anesthesia.
- When anesthtizing a neonatal patient, careful attention to temperature, fluid resusitation, airway management, and drug metabolism are essential considerations.

DISCLOSURE

The authors have nothing to disclose.

REFERENCES

1. AM R. The fetal circulation. In: Congenital diseases of the heart. West Sussex, UK: Wiley-Blackwell; 2009. p. 1–24.
2. Rychik J. Fetal cardiovascular physiology. Pediatr Cardiol 2004;25(3):201–9.
3. Thornburg KL, Louey S. Uteroplacental circulation and fetal vascular function and development. Curr Vasc Pharmacol 2013;11(5):748–57.
4. Morris JA, Hustead RF, Robinson RG, et al. Measurement of fetoplacental blood volume in the human previable fetus. Am J Obstet Gynecol 1974;118(7):927–34.
5. Stern L, Lees MH, Leduc J. Environmental temperature, oxygen consumption, and catecholamine excretion in newborn infants. Pediatrics 1965;36(3):367–73.
6. Adamson SK Jr, Towell ME. Thermal homeostasis in the fetus and newborn. Anesthesiology 1965;26:531–48.
7. Aboud E, Neales K. The effect of maternal hypothermia on the fetal heart rate. Int J Gynecol Obstet 1999;66(2):163–4.
8. Mann DG, Nassr aa, Whitehead we, et al. Fetal bradycardia associated with maternal hypothermia after fetoscopic repair of neural tube defect. Ultrasound Obstet Gynecol 2018;51(3):411–2.
9. Ferschl MB, Rollins MD, Chatterjee D. Error traps in anesthesia for fetal interventions. Paediatr Anaesth 2021;31(3):275–81.
10. Buisson P, Bach V, Elabbassi EB, et al. Assessment of the efficiency of warming devices during neonatal surgery. Eur J Appl Physiol 2004;92(6):694–7.
11. Stanger R, Colyvas K, Cassey JC, et al. Predicting the efficacy of convection warming in anaesthetized children. Br J Anaesth 2009;103(2):275–82.
12. FDA Drug Safety Communication: FDA review results in new warnings about using general anesthetics and sedation drugs in young children and pregnant women. 2016. Available at: https://wayback.archive-it.org/7993/20170111071047/http://www.fda.gov/Drugs/DrugSafety/ucm532356.htm. Accesses January 11, 2021.
13. Brambrink AM, Evers AS, Avidan MS, et al. Isoflurane-induced neuroapoptosis in the neonatal rhesus macaque brain. Anesthesiology 2010;112(4):834–41.
14. Jevtovic-Todorovic V, Hartman RE, Izumi Y, et al. Early exposure to common anesthetic agents causes widespread neurodegeneration in the developing rat brain and persistent learning deficits. J Neurosci 2003;15(3):295–6.
15. Davidson AJ, Disma N, de Graaff JC, et al. Neurodevelopmental outcome at 2 years of age after general anaesthesia and awake-regional anaesthesia in infancy (GAS): an international multicentre, randomised controlled trial. Lancet 2016;387(10015):239–50.
16. Sun LS, Li G, Miller TLK, et al. Association between a single general anesthesia exposure before age 36 Months and neurocognitive outcomes in later childhood. JAMA 2016;315(21):2312–20.
17. Sprung J, Flick RP, Wilder RT, et al. Anesthesia for cesarean delivery and learning disabilities in a population-based birth cohort. Anesthesiology 2009;111(2):302–10.
18. Rosen MA. Management of anesthesia for the pregnant surgical patient. Anesthesiology 1999;91(4):1159–63.
19. Archer GW Jr, Marx GF. Arterial oxygen tension during apnoea in parturient women. Br J Anaesth 1974;46(5):358–60.

20. Norris MC, Kirkland MR, Torjman MC, et al. Denitrogenation in pregnancy. Can J Anaesth 1989;36(5):523-5.
21. Thornburg KL, Jacobson SL, Giraud GD, et al. Hemodynamic changes in pregnancy. Semin Perinatol 2000;24(1):11-4.
22. Hunter S, Robson SC. Adaptation of the maternal heart in pregnancy. Br Heart J 1992;68(6):540-3.
23. Milsom I, Forssman L. Factors influencing aortocaval compression in late pregnancy. Am J Obstet Gynecol 1984;148(6):764-71.
24. Sibley CP, Birdsey TJ, Brownbill P, et al. Mechanisms of maternofetal exchange across the human placenta. Biochem Soc Trans 1998;26(2):86-91.
25. Okado N, Kakimi S, Kojima T. Synaptogenesis in the cervical cord of the human embryo: sequence of synapse formation in a spinal reflex pathway. J Comp Neurol 1979;184(3):491-518.
26. Rabinowicz T, de Courten-Myers GM, Petetot JM, et al. Human cortex development: estimates of neuronal numbers indicate major loss late during gestation. J Neuropathol Exp Neurol 1996;55(3):320-8.
27. SS. Commission of inquiry into fetal sentience. London: CARE; 1996.
28. Verriotis M, Chang P, Fitzgerald M, et al. The development of the nociceptive brain. Neuroscience 2016;338:207-19.
29. Lee SJ, Ralson HJP, Drey EA, et al. Fetal pain: a systematic multidisciplinary review of the evidence. JAMA 2005;294(8):947-54.
30. FC. The astonishing hypothesis: the scientific search for the soul. New York: Simon and Schuster; 1994.
31. Barker DJ, Arendt KW, Moldenhauer JS. In utero programming of cardiovascular disease. Theriogenology 2000;53(2):555-74.
32. Chatterjee D, Arendt KW, Moldenhauer JS, et al. Anesthesia for maternal-fetal interventions: a consensus statement from the American society of anesthesiologists committees on obstetric and pediatric anesthesiology and the north American fetal therapy network. Anesth Analg 2021;132(4):1164-73.
33. Norton ME, Cassidy A, Ralston SJ, et al. Society for Maternal-Fetal Medicine Consult Series #59: the use of analgesia and anesthesia for maternal-fetal procedures. Am J Obstet Gynecol 2021;225(6):B2-8.
34. Van de Velde M, Van Schoubroeck D, Lewi LE, et al. Remifentanil for fetal immobilization and maternal sedation during fetoscopic surgery: a randomized, double-blind comparison with diazepam. Anesth Analg 2005;101(1):251-8.
35. Hoagland MA, Chatterjee D. Anesthesia for fetal surgery. Paediatr Anaesth 2017;27(8):873.
36. Graves CE, Harrison MR, Padilla BE. Minimally invasive fetal surgery. Clin Perinatol 2017;44(4):729-51.
37. Ferschl MB, Feiner J, Vu L, et al. A comparison of spinal anesthesia versus monitored anesthesia care with local anesthesia in minimally invasive fetal surgery. Anesth Analg 2018;130(2):409-15.
38. Ferschl M, Ball R, Lee H, et al. Anesthesia for in utero repair of myelomeningocele. Anesthesiology 2013;118(5):1211-23.
39. Donepudi R, Huynh M, Moise KJ Jr, et al. Early administration of magnesium sulfate during open fetal myelomeningocele repair reduces the dose of inhalational anesthesia. Fetal Diagn Ther 2019;45(3):192-6.
40. Boat A, Mahmoud M, Michelfelder EC, et al. Supplementing desflurane with intravenous anesthesia reduces fetal cardiac dysfunction during open fetal surgery: anesthesia AND FETAL CARDIAC FUNCTION. Pediatr Anesth 2010;20(8):748-56.

41. Marsh BJ, Sinskey J, Whitlock EL, et al. Use of remifentanil for open in utero fetal myelomeningocele repair maintains uterine relaxation with reduced volatile anesthetic concentration. Fetal Diagn Ther 2020;47(11):810–6.

42. Sinskey JL, Rollins MD, Whitlock E, et al. Incidence and management of umbilical artery flow abnormalities during open fetal surgery. Fetal Diagn Ther 2017;43(4): 274–83.

43. Gonser M, Vonzun L, Kandler L, et al. Fetal circulatory redistribution during open spina bifida repair: can loss or reversal of end-diastolic umbilical artery flow be avoided? Ultrasound Obstet Gynecol 2022;59(1):130–1.

44. Moldenhauer JS. Ex utero intrapartum therapy. Semin Pediatr Surg 2013; 22(1):44–9.

45. Rosen MA, Andreae MH, Cameron AG, et al. Nitroglycerin for fetal surgery: fetoscopy and ex utero intrapartum treatment procedure with malignant hyperthermia precautions. Anesth Analg 2003;96(3):698–700.

46. Kan RE, Hughes SC, Rosen MA, et al. Intravenous remifentanil: placental transfer, maternal and neonatal effects. Anesthesiology 1998;88(6):1467–74.

47. Fink RJ, Allen TK, Habib AS. Remifentanil for fetal immobilization and analgesia during the ex utero intrapartum treatment procedure under combined spinal-epidural anaesthesia †. Br J Anaesth 2011;106(6):851–5.

48. Jain RARM. The difficult pediatric airway. In: Hagberg C, editor. Benumof and Hagberg's airway management. Philadelphia: Elsevier; 2017. p. 723–60.

49. Bailey AG, McNaull PP, Jooste E, et al. Perioperative crystalloid and colloid fluid management in children: where are we and how did we get here? Anesth Analg 2010;110(2):375–90.

50. Osborn DA, Evans N. Early volume expansion for prevention of morbidity and mortality in very preterm infants. Cochrane Database Syst Rev 2004;2004(2): Cd002055.

51. Lucas A, Morley R, Cole TJ. Adverse neurodevelopmental outcome of moderate neonatal hypoglycaemia. Bmj 1988;297(6659):1304–8.

52. Wickström R, Sköld B, Petersson G, et al. Moderate neonatal hypoglycemia and adverse neurological development at 2-6 years of age. Eur J Epidemiol 2018; 33(10):1011–20.

53. Burns CM, Rutherford MA, Boardman JP, et al. Patterns of cerebral injury and neurodevelopmental outcomes after symptomatic neonatal hypoglycemia. Pediatrics 2008;122(1):65–74.

54. Iskander IF, Salama KM, Gamaleldin RM, et al. Neonatal RBC transfusions: do benefits outweigh risks? Transfus Apher Sci 2018;57(3):431–6.

55. Anderson BJ, Lerman J, Cote C. Pharmacokinetcs and pharmacology of drugs used in children. In: A practice of anesthesia for infants and children. Elsevier; 2019. p. 100–76.

56. Ku LC, Smith PB. Dosing in neonates: special considerations in physiology and trial design. Pediatr Res 2015;77(1–1):2–9.

Fetal Repair of Neural Tube Defects

Su Yeon Lee, MD[a],*, Ramesha Papanna, MD, MPH[b], Diana Farmer, MD[c],
KuoJen Tsao, MD[d]

KEYWORDS

- Spina bifida • Myelomeningocele • Open neural tube defect • MOMS trial

KEY POINTS

- Fetal surgery is an option for prenatally diagnosed myelomeningocele if eligibility criteria are met.
- The repair involves closure of the skin over the defect, focusing on creating a watertight seal thereby preventing egress of cerebrospinal fluid.
- Prenatal repair of myelomeningocele may reverse hindbrain herniation, reduces the requirement for cerebrospinal fluid shunt placement, and improves distal neurologic function to a degree.
- Clinical trials are currently underway using stem cells and other technologies during prenatal repair to augment the current standard of care by further ameliorating distal motor function.

INTRODUCTION

Spina bifida (SB) is the most common congenital defect of the nervous system. Myelomeningocele (MMC) is the most severe form of SB, whereby congenital neural tube closure failure results in leakage of spinal fluid and progressive spinal cord damage via chemical (amniotic fluid) and mechanical (uterine wall) trauma. This trauma results in hindbrain herniation, loss of lower limb motor function, and bowel and bladder dysfunction. Currently, MMC is the only nervous system defect that can be repaired *in utero* and is the only nonlethal disease for which fetal surgery is offered. MMC was historically treated with postnatal closure of the defect until the Management of

[a] Department of Surgery, Division of Pediatric, Thoracic and Fetal Surgery, University of California Davis Medical Center, 2335 Stockton Boulevard, Room 5107, Sacramento, CA 95817, USA; [b] Department of Obstetrics, Gynecology and Reproductive Sciences, UT Health Science Center at Houston, 6410 Fannin Street, Suite 210, Houston, TX 77030, USA; [c] Department of Surgery, University of California Davis Medical Center, 2335 Stockton Boulevard, Sacramento, CA 95817, USA; [d] Department of Pediatric Surgery, UT Health Science Center at Houston, 6410 Fannin Street, Suite 950, Houston, TX 77030, USA
* Corresponding author.
E-mail address: suyle@ucdavis.edu

Clin Perinatol 49 (2022) 835–848
https://doi.org/10.1016/j.clp.2022.06.004
0095-5108/22/© 2022 Elsevier Inc. All rights reserved.

Abbreviations	
AChe	Acetylcholinesterase
AFAFP	Amniotic fluid alpha-fetoprotein
BMI	Body mass index
CA	Chorioamniotic
CIC	Clean intermittent catheterization
CSF	Cerebrospinal fluid
ECM	Extracellular matrix
HUC	Human umbilical cord
MMC	Myelomeningocele
MOMS	Management of Myelomeningocele Study
MRI	Magnetic resonance imaging
MSAFP	Maternal serum alpha-fetoprotein
NICU	Neonatal Intensive Care Unit
PMSCs	Placental mesenchymal stem cells
SB	Spina bifida
VP	Ventriculoperitoneal

Myelomeningocele Study (MOMS) established fetal repair as an option for improving outcomes for the fetus/child.[1]

Epidemiology

The incidence of SB is variable. In the United States, the rates of SB improved from 1 in 1500 to 2000 to 1 in 2500 to 3000 live births, after the implementation of the US folic acid fortification program in 1998.[2] The birth prevalence of SB has been similar between Hispanic, non-Hispanic white women, and non-Hispanic black women.[3] Additionally, there is a decrease in SB prevalence from lower-middle to high-income countries.[4] Most recent studies have demonstrated an incidence of approximately 4.7 per 10,000 live births worldwide, with the highest prevalence in Ukraine at 10.9 per 10,000 live births.[5,6] Of note, these prevalence are from live births, and must take into account that up to 82% of SB pregnancies are terminated in North America.[7]

Nature of the Problem

MMC results from the incomplete closure of the neural tube, the embryologic structure that forms the brain and spinal cord by the fourth week of gestation. Incomplete tubularization of the caudal neuropore forms a placode on the back of the fetus, whereby the incomplete vertebral neural arches and agenesis of overlying skin leave the spinal cord exposed. The two-hit hypothesis of injury for MMC describes anatomic abnormalities in the development of the spinal cord (1st hit), which results in secondary damage from chemical and mechanical trauma from exposure to the *in utero* environment (2nd hit). This trauma results in increased apoptosis of motor neurons in the spinal cord.[8,9]

The development of MMC is likely multifactorial. While the genetic component is thought to contribute to approximately 60% to 70% of the risk of neural tube defects, the specific genes have yet to be elucidated.[10] Chromosomal anomalies including trisomy 13, trisomy 18 and triploidy are associated with MMC 10% of the time.[11] Family history of MMC is one of the strongest risk factors, with familial aggregation studies demonstrating 3% to 8% and 1% to 2% increase in risk with first degree and second degree relatives respectively.[10,12] MMC is also linked to genetic conditions, including Waardenburg syndrome, VATER syndrome, PHAVER syndrome, and x-linked neural tube defects.[13] Additionally, maternal obesity (BMI >29 kg/m2) has been demonstrated to have 2.2 to 3.5 fold increase risk for MMC in the fetus.[14–17] Factors including reduced folic acid intake, paternal exposure to agent orange, maternal antiepileptic use, maternal diabetes, and maternal hyperthermia also increase risk to varying degrees.[13,17] However, less than 50% of cases are attributable to known risk factors.[18]

Diagnosis

MMC is traditionally diagnosed with a combination of ultrasound and biochemical screening. Routine second-trimester fetal anatomy scan has a detection rate of over 90% for MMC.[19] Ultrasound will best show the level of the lesion with splayed vertebral arches. Secondary to cerebrospinal fluid (CSF) leakage, patients will develop Arnold–Chiari II malformation with crowded posterior fossa seen as "lemon sign" (scalloping of frontal bones) and "banana sign" (obliteration of cisterna magna with postero-caudal displacement of cerebellar vermis).[20] (**Fig. 1**) Varying degrees of ventriculomegaly can be seen. Additionally, a second-trimester ultrasound can reveal additional anomalies. With improvements in first-trimester ultrasound technology, an increasing number of MMC cases are being detected or suspected before these second-trimester prenatal tests.[21] However, the diagnosis should be confirmed with second-trimester ultrasound. Fetal magnetic resonance imaging (MRI) is not recommended for routine evaluation or as a primary screening modality.[22]

Second-trimester prenatal blood tests drawn between 15 to 20 weeks gestation include maternal serum alpha-fetoprotein (MSAFP) to screen for open neural tube defects. Elevated MSAFP in conjunction with second-trimester ultrasound is able to detect 96% of MMC cases, compared with 75% of cases detected with abnormal MSAFP only.[23] As such, diagnosis should be confirmed by targeted ultrasound or amniocentesis. Amniotic fluid alpha-fetoprotein (AFAFP) and acetylcholinesterase (AChe) can also be measured with amniocentesis. In combination, elevated AFAFP and AChe can detect MMC 100% of the times with less than 0.05% false positive rate.[24] Amniocentesis results can also reveal crucial information, such as chromosomal and genetic abnormalities that will preclude patients from fetal surgery.

Anatomy

As previously described, MMC is a result of incomplete neurulation of the posterior neuropore. As such, the central canal of the closed spinal cord splays opens at the superior midline margin of the MMC lesion through which CSF leaks (**Fig. 2**). From the midline embryonic ventral sulcus, ventral motor nerve roots exit through basal plates. Laterally, alar plate carries sensory nerves. The outer edge of the lesion is attached to the meninges and skin.

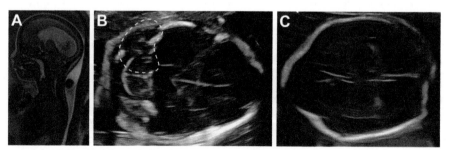

Fig. 1. Prenatal imaging findings of Arnold–Chiari II malformation secondary to myelomeningocele. (*A*) Sagittal section of fetal MRI demonstrating crowded posterior fossa with hindbrain herniation. Fetal ultrasound showing (*B*) Banana sign and (*C*) Lemon sign.

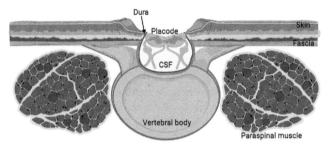

Fig. 2. Cross-section schematic of myelomeningocele defect.

Preoperative/Preprocedure Planning for Open Fetal Surgical Repair

Patients should be evaluated at a fetal therapy center as defined by the MMC Maternal–Fetal Management Task Force, which includes an experienced fetal care team, multidisciplinary SB program, obstetric team capable of caring for maternal–fetal surgery complications, Level IIIC Neonatal Intensive Care Unit (NICU), institutional review board and ethics committee, maternal–fetal advocate, and capacity for long-term follow-up.[25] Individualized counseling should be given with options including termination, expectant management with postnatal repair, and fetal repair when appropriate. Included in the counseling should be maternal considerations including the possibility of uterine dehiscence and the need for cesarean section for all pregnancies after open fetal surgery. In one study, 16% of patients were not able to receive fetal intervention due to delays in presentation.[26] This highlights the importance of timely evaluations.

Fetal MRI is obtained for preoperative assessment to definitively establish abnormalities of the posterior fossa, any other congenital anomalies, and for comparison after fetal surgery.[20] Additionally, it can help guide patient counseling as spinal findings on MRI with higher and larger lesions are associated with wheelchair dependence and dysphagia, and absent covering membrane are associated with scoliosis and bladder dysfunction.[27] The candidacy at most centers for fetal surgery is determined using the same inclusion and exclusion criteria as MOMS protocol, as recommended by the MMC Maternal–Fetal Management Task Force.[25] (**Table 1**). Repair occurs between 19^0 to 25^6 weeks of gestation.

Prep and Patient Positioning

Patient undergoes general and epidural anesthesia. Patient is placed supine with lateral tilt to prevent obstruction of the maternal IVC with the gravid uterus (**Fig. 3**). A Foley catheter is placed. Preinduction ultrasound confirms the position and viability of fetus, and site of placental attachment. Throughout the procedure, the fetus is monitored by maternal–fetal medicine or pediatric cardiologist with fetal echocardiogram. Perioperative indomethacin and magnesium sulfate infusion are given for tocolysis.

Procedural Approach for Open Fetal Surgery

The current standard of care open fetal repair for MMC is described later in discussion:

1) The uterus is exposed in a typical fashion.
2) The position of the fetus and placenta is determined with ultrasound. If the fetus is in the breech position, cephalic version is performed to move the MMC defect toward the uterine fundus.

Table 1
Inclusion and exclusion criteria for in utero repair of MMC for MOMS trial

Inclusion	Exclusion
• MMC at levels T1 to S1 with hindbrain herniation confirmed by US and fetal MRI • Maternal age ≥18 y • Gestational age between 19^0 to 25^6 weeks • Normal karyotype	• Nonresident of the United States • Nonsingleton pregnancy • Unrelated fetal anomaly • Fetal kyphosis >30° • Maternal conditions for preterm delivery (pregestational insulin-dependent diabetes, uncontrolled hypertension, HIV, hepatitis B, or hepatitis C status) • Increased risk for preterm delivery (short cervix, current or history of incompetent cervix, prior spontaneous premature singleton delivery) • Placenta previa or placental abruption • BMI >35 • Maternal–fetal Rh isoimmunization, Kell sensitization, or history of neonatal alloimmune thrombocytopenia • Uterine anomaly • Maternal contraindication to surgery or general anesthesia • Lack of social support • Maternal psychosocial limitations • Limitations to follow-up

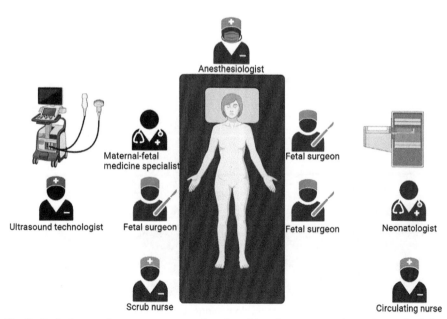

Fig. 3. Typical operating room personnel and position for open myelomeningocele defect repair.

3) A small hysterotomy of 6 to 8 cm is made with an absorbable uterine stapling device.
4) The fetus is positioned with the MMC defect exposed through the hysterotomy (**Fig. 4**A). Fetal anesthesia comprised of fentanyl and a nondepolarizing neuromuscular blocker is administered.
5) The fetal skin is sharply incised to the level of fascia around the neural placode, and the neural elements are allowed to descend into the spinal canal.
6) The dura is separated by a mix of sharp and hydro-dissection using an angiocath with lactated ringer under the dura-covered fascia. The dura is dissected free and is closed as a separate layer or a dural patch is used if needed. The spinal cord is re-tubularized in some centers.
7) The skin is mobilized and closed primarily using a running monofilament suture (**Fig. 4**B). If there is insufficient amount of tissue or too much tension, relaxing flank incisions can be made with or without the addition of acellular dermal allograft.
8) The hysterotomy is closed with a combination of full thickness interrupted and running monofilament suture. Before final closure, antibiotics are instilled in the amniotic cavity.
9) The maternal laparotomy incision is closed in layers in a typical fashion.

Fetoscopy

There is a large variation in the operative approach and technique for fetoscopic repair, which is gaining popularity, as compared with the standardized open repair. Three to 4 trocars are placed percutaneously or after uterine exposure. The uterus is partially insufflated with carbon dioxide. Dissection of the placode occurs in a similar fashion with the possible use of a dural graft. A myofascial flap or dermal allograft is closed with running or interrupted stitch.

Recovery and Rehabilitation

Postsurgical management largely follows the MOMS protocol. The patient remains in the hospital for 3 to 5 days postoperatively and is discharged on tocolytics and

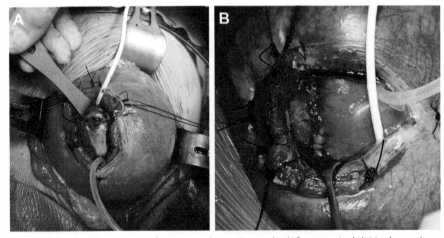

Fig. 4. Intraoperative images of open myelomeningocele defect repair. (*A*) Myelomeningocele defect can be seen through hysterotomy. Temperature probe and irrigation tubing w inserted into the uterus. (*B*) Fetus with completed repair.

modified activity. They receive weekly scheduled follow-up with ultrasound monitoring. Patient must remain close to a center that can manage postoperative complications including preterm labor, and NICU that can support preterm and term infants with MMC. Patients are planned for cesarian section at 37 weeks.

In the original MOMS trial, mothers receiving prenatal surgery had significantly more chorioamniotic (CA) membrane separation, placental abruption, spontaneous membrane rupture, and maternal transfusion at delivery, with CA membrane separation being the most common.[28] There were also significantly more premature deliveries, with only 18.7% patients delivering after 37 weeks.[28,29] Additionally, oligohydramnios was seen significantly more often with *in utero* repair and was a risk factor for preterm delivery.[28,29]

Mothers should also be made aware that every subsequent childbirth should be the cesarian section. Additionally, while fertility does not seem to be affected by open fetal surgery, there is a higher risk of uterine dehiscence or rupture in subsequent pregnancies if patients are allowed to labor.[30] In addition, it is recommended for women to delay conception for a minimum of 18 to 24 months from the date of delivery of the fetus that received fetal repair to minimize complications related to hysterotomy.[25,31]

Management of Babies with Spina Bifida

For patients who are not eligible for fetal repair, management currently includes surgery within the first 48 hours of birth to minimize infection risk. Unfortunately, spinal cord damage accrued *in utero* cannot be reversed in these cases. In any case, patients with MMC require a multidisciplinary team comprised of several pediatric subspecialties including pediatric surgery, neurosurgery, gastroenterology, orthopedics, urology, physical therapist, social workers, and case coordinators. Family involvement is integral to managing both physical and social aspects of this disease.

Hydrocephalus may result in the need for ventriculoperitoneal (VP) shunting in these patients even after fetal MMC repair although the need is reduced in patients with fetal surgery (40% needing shunts versus 80% without fetal surgery). More cephalad lesions had significantly higher rates of shunting.[32] Endoscopic third ventriculostomy-choroid plexus cauterization has been shown as an alternative to VP shunt and has decreased maintenance compared with VP shunt.[33] With the advent of prenatal repair and reversal of hindbrain herniation, patients with cerebellar and upper cervical nerve dysfunction are becoming less frequent. These patients may present with abnormalities in oculomotor function, swallowing, vocal cord motion dysfunction, with airway obstruction from vocal cord paralysis or central hypoventilation needing oxygen supplementation, and upper extremity sensorimotor loss.[34] These children may undergo additional surgery for foramen magnum decompression or dural augmentation, but symptom improvement was largely through adequate ventricular drainage.[34,35]

Given the disruption of the low sacral nerves in MMC, many of these patients also suffer from bowel dysfunction and neurogenic bladder. Urologic issues are particularly important as urologic complications are among the leading causes of long-term mortality.[36] Both expectant and proactive management aims to prevent upper urinary tract changes through clean intermittent catheterization (CIC) and anticholinergics.[37] Bladder augmentation and reconstruction are indicated with renal deterioration despite maximal medical therapy and to facilitate continence to enhance the quality of life.[37]

Bowel dysfunction has a significant impact on the quality of life for patients with MMC and their families.[38] Neurogenic bowel dysfunction can present as constipation or fecal incontinence from alterations in colorectal motility, abnormal anal sphincter function, and decreased sensation.[39] Step-wise, age appropriate bowel management is recommended; conservative therapy with fiber bulking agents, oral laxatives and suppositories and enemas, to antegrade continence enemas with surgically created conduits.[39,40]

The degree of mobility depends largely on the level of the lesion. The more distal the defect, the more lower extremity motor function that is preserved. In all cases, patients undergo extensive rehabilitation with physical therapy. Almost all patients with MMC will experience issues with foot deformity, including 30% to 50% with clubfoot deformity, which additionally impacts ambulation.[41] Scoliosis is also another common orthopedic condition seen in about 50% of all patients with MMC and up to 90% of patients with MMC with thoracic functional level.[42] Continued evaluation and rehabilitation by a skilled physical therapist, and early interventions with casting and bracing possibly preventing surgical interventions for correction.

Outcomes

With advances in medical therapies and fortification of folic acid in food, infant mortality and MMC case fatality has declined over time.[43] The overall first-week mortality was 6.9%, with majority occurring on the first day of life.[6] One-year survival has improved to more than 88%.[44] Notably, there was an increased risk of mortality for black and Hispanic children, compared with white children. Of note, birth weight remains the strongest predictor of infant mortality even after adjusting for a race with lower birth weights associated with poor survival.[44]

Fetal repair of MMC decreases the need for VP shunt, compared with postnatal repair. The MOMS trial was stopped early because of the significant decrease in the primary outcome of fetal or neonatal death and the need for VP shunt by 12 months in the prenatal surgery group (68%), compared with the postnatal surgery group (98%).[1] In long-term follow-up of outcomes at school-age, the prenatal repair group had significantly fewer shunts placed (49% vs 85%) and significantly fewer shunt revisions (47% vs 70%) than those in postnatal group.[45] Prenatal repair of MMC also improved the frequency and severity of hindbrain herniation. At 12 months, there were significantly more infants with complete reversal of Arnold Chiari II malformation in the prenatal group compared with the postnatal group (36% vs 4%).[1] Additionally, only 25% of patients in the prenatal group had moderate or severe hindbrain (vs 67%).

The MOMS trial also looked at a composite assessment of early cognitive and language development, and motor ability. At 30 months, both Bayley Scales of Infant Development II mental developmental index and Function Independence Measure for Children cognitive scores were similar between the 2 groups.[46] In school-aged children, there was also no meaningful difference in cognitive function. While prenatally repaired children did score significantly higher on the KBIT-2 and reading composite of Woodcock–Johnson test, both groups were in the average range and did not show a difference in other measures.[45] However, fetal repair improved motor function and increased rates of independent ambulation. At 30 months of age, 38% of the prenatally repaired patients had improved motor function compared with the anatomic level of the defect (vs 19% in the postnatal repair group).[46] 44% of prenatally repaired children were walking independently at 30 months (vs 23.9% in the postnatal repair group).[46] At school-age, 29% in the prenatal group were able to walk independently, significantly greater than 11% in the postnatal group.[45] While these results were promising, 55% of prenatally repaired children were still unable to walk independently at 30 months and more become dependent on mobility aids as they grew older. Knee movement at screening ultrasound, lesion below L3, and absent sac over lesion on MRI were associated with independent walking at 30 months, with absent sac also associated with motor function greater than 2 levels better than anatomic lesion.[46] Children ages 5 to 10 in the MOMS trial in the prenatal repair group continued to demonstrate better motor function compared with their anatomic lesion level, as well as being 70% more likely to ambulate independently.[47] Fewer prenatally repaired patients needed assistive devices to ambulate (45% vs 69%) or needed bracing compared with postnatally repaired patients (15% vs 32%).

With regards to urologic outcomes, at 30 months of age there was no statistical difference in the rate of children who were voiding by CIC between prenatally repaired and postnatally repaired patients (38% vs 51%).[48] By school-age, significantly less patients in the prenatal surgery group were voiding by CIC compared with postnatal surgery group (62% vs 87%).[49] 24% of patients who underwent fetal MMC repair were able to void volitionally, compared with only 4% of patients who underwent postnatal repair.[49] Additionally, significantly more children who received postnatal surgery were also on anticholinergic medication compared with children who received prenatal surgery (67% vs 44%).[49] Although there was significant improvement in CIC rates and volitional voiding by school-age children who underwent prenatal repair, the CIC rate remains high with most of the patients incontinent of urine.

While comprehensive bowel function outcomes were not reported for MOMS trial, 59% of prenatally repaired patients were reported to have one or more bowel accidents per week at 30 months of age, similar to postnatally repaired patients (56%).[1] Studies before the MOMS trial reported variable functional outcomes after prenatal repair. One study reports 31% of patients having normal bowel function at a median age of 10 years, with more than half of the patients on a bowel regimen.[50]

Current Controversies

With MOMS trial, open fetal repair of MMC with watertight dural and skin closure became the gold standard. During the MOMS trial, fetoscopic MMC repair was paused in the US, to standardize the open technique. However, there has been continued development of minimally invasive methods in other parts of the world to reduce rates of obstetric complications of open fetal surgery. There was no significant difference between open and fetoscopic approaches in combined fetal and postnatal mortality, VP shunt placement rate, hindbrain herniation reversal, CA membrane separation, and placental abruption in a recent meta-analysis.[51–53] However, there was a higher rate of MMC site dehiscence requiring treatment, premature membrane rupture, and preterm birth after fetoscopic repair compared with open repair.[52–54] Open repair had higher rates of uterine dehiscence.[52–54] Fetoscopic repair does allow for mothers to deliver vaginally, with the index and subsequent pregnancies. Preliminary data show that there is no significant difference in VP shunt rates at 12 months between the 2 groups.[55] However, there has not been a randomized control trial to directly compare the outcomes between open and fetoscopic surgery. Additionally, given the relatively recent development of fetoscopic surgery, long-term follow-up is needed for outcomes of MMC children repaired fetoscopically.

Future Developments

Stem cell therapy has generated significant interest in the last 2 decades during prenatal repair for MMC. As previously mentioned, while the prenatal repair of MMC prevents hindbrain herniation and improvements in motor scores compared with postnatal repair, more than half the patients are unable to ambulate independently. Wang *and colleagues* demonstrated that the *in utero* application of regenerative placental mesenchymal stem cells (PMSCs) seeded on a clinical-grade extracellular matrix (ECM) to the exposed fetal spinal cord reverses the lower extremity paralysis associated with MMC in the ovine model.[56–58] This improvement in motor function correlated with increased large neuron density, suggesting neuroprotective effects of PMSC-ECM.[58,59] Currently, there is a Phase 1/2a clinical trial (CuRe Trial: Cellular Therapy for In Utero Repair of Myelomeningocele, NCT04652908) of the PMSC-ECM product for use in fetal MMC repair.

Papanna and colleagues are investigating a human umbilical cord (HUC) patch as a skin patch material for MMC repair.[60] The study in the ovine model showed higher sensorimotor function in groups repaired with HUC compared with primary skin closure or patch repair, potentially from reduced inflammation.[60] The use of HUC in fetoscopic MMC repair is currently being investigated as a phase 1 clinical trial (Fetoscopic NEOX Cord 1K Spina Bifida Repair, NCT04243889). Furthermore, a concentrated intra-amniotic injection of MSCs is being studied as an option for prenatal skin coverage of MMC.[61] It is currently in the preclinical phase, with promising results showing improvement in hindbrain herniation in rodent and rabbit models after injection.[61,62]

Lastly, robot-assisted endoscopic fetal repair is being investigated. Full-thickness skin lesions have been created and repaired using a robotic system in an ovine model.[63–65] Robotic approach could be advantageous given the limited intrauterine space and the articulation required for suturing. Further study is needed in insufflation techniques, robotic instrument size, and duration of the surgery with docking of the robotic arms.

SUMMARY

MMC is the first nonlethal condition to be considered for fetal surgery and is now the most common open fetal surgery performed. The MOMS trial showed fetal repair of MMC to reverse Arnold–Chiari II malformation, reduce VP shunting, and improve distal motor function. These effects persevered in long-term follow-up studies. The fetoscopic approach is becoming more popular but still needs to be further studied. Efforts are being made to further address distal neurologic function, with a current clinical trial adding stem cells to the prenatal repair.

CLINICS CARE POINTS

- Prompt evaluation and fetal surgery should be performed in designated centers with resources and expertise.
- Advantages of fetoscopic repair on future pregnancies and uterine dehiscence must be balanced with increased risk for premature rupture of membrane, premature birth, need for postnatal revision of repair, and unknown long-term outcomes for the children
- Management of neurogenic bladder to prevent upper tract changes is important to prevent long-term morbidity and mortality of these patients

ACKNOWLEDGEMENT

Author DLF has projects funded by Shriners Hospital for Children research grants (72008-NCA-21, 85135-NCA-21, 85108-NCA-19), California Institute for Regenerative Medicine's (CIRM) Clinical Trial Stage Projects CLIN2 grant (CLIN2-12129), and NIH/NINDS grant (1R01NS115860-01A1, 1R01NS100761-01A1). Author RP has projects funded by NIH/NICHD grant (R21HD092754, 5R01HD105173). The content is solely the responsibility of the authors and does not necessarily represent the official views of the respective funding agencies.

REFERENCES

1. Adzick NS, Thom EA, Spong CY, et al. A randomized trial of prenatal versus post-natal repair of myelomeningocele. N Engl J Med 2011;364(11):993–1004.
2. Centers for Disease Control and Prevention (CDC). Spina bifida and anencephaly before and after folic acid mandate–United States, 1995-1996 and 1999-2000. MMWR Morb Mortal Wkly Rep 2004;53(17):362–5.
3. Centers for Disease Control and Prevention (CDC). Racial/ethnic differences in the birth prevalence of spina bifida - United States, 1995-2005. MMWR Morb Mortal Wkly Rep 2009;57(53):1409–13.
4. Zaganjor I, Sekkarie A, Tsang BL, et al. Describing the prevalence of neural tube defects Worldwide: a systematic literature review. PLOS ONE 2016;11(4): e0151586.
5. Parker SE, Mai CT, Canfield MA, et al. Updated National Birth Prevalence estimates for selected birth defects in the United States, 2004-2006. Birth Defects Res A Clin Mol Teratol 2010;88(12):1008–16.
6. Bakker MK, Kancherla V, Canfield MA, et al. Analysis of mortality among Neonates and children with spina bifida: an International Registry-Based study, 2001-2012. Paediatr Perinat Epidemiol 2019;33(6):436–48.
7. Johnson CY, Honein MA, Dana Flanders W, et al. Pregnancy termination following prenatal diagnosis of anencephaly or spina bifida: a systematic review of the literature. Birth Defects Res A Clin Mol Teratol 2012;94(11):857–63.
8. Sival DA, van Weerden TW, Vles JSH, et al. Neonatal loss of motor function in human spina bifida aperta. Pediatrics 2004;114(2):427–34.
9. Stiefel D, Meuli M. Scanning electron microscopy of fetal murine myelomeningocele reveals growth and development of the spinal cord in early gestation and neural tissue destruction around birth. J Pediatr Surg 2007;42(9):1561–5.
10. Lupo PJ, Agopian AJ, Castillo H, et al. Genetic epidemiology of neural tube defects. J Pediatr Rehabil Med 2017;10(3–4):189–94.
11. Kennedy D, Chitayat D, Winsor EJ, et al. Prenatally diagnosed neural tube defects: ultrasound, chromosome, and autopsy or postnatal findings in 212 cases. Am J Med Genet 1998;77(4):317–21.
12. Partington MD, McLone DG. Hereditary factors in the Etiology of neural tube defects. PNE 1995;23(6):311–6.
13. Shaer CM, Chescheir N, Schulkin J. Myelomeningocele: a review of the epidemiology, genetics, risk factors for conception, prenatal diagnosis, and Prognosis for affected Individuals. Obstetrical Gynecol Surv 2007;62(7):471–9.
14. Shaw GM, Todoroff K, Finnell RH, et al. Spina bifida phenotypes in infants or fetuses of obese mothers. Teratology 2000;61(5):376–81, 200005)61:5<376:: AID-TERA9>3.0.CO;2.
15. Watkins ML, Rasmussen SA, Honein MA, et al. Maternal obesity and risk for birth defects. Pediatrics 2003;111(5 Pt 2):1152–8.
16. Stothard KJ, Tennant PWG, Bell R, et al. Maternal overweight and obesity and the risk of congenital anomalies: a systematic review and meta-analysis. JAMA 2009; 301(6):636–50.
17. Donnan J, Walsh S, Sikora L, et al. A systematic review of the risks factors associated with the onset and natural progression of spina bifida. Neurotoxicology 2017;61:20–31.
18. Agopian AJ, Tinker SC, Lupo PJ, et al. Proportion of neural tube defects attributable to known risk factors. Birth Defects Res A Clin Mol Teratol 2013;97(1):42–6.

19. Sivarajah K, Relph S, Sabaratnam R, et al. Spina bifida in pregnancy: a review of the evidence for preconception, antenatal, intrapartum and postpartum care. Obstet Med 2019;12(1):14–21. https://doi.org/10.1177/1753495X18769221.

20. Sepulveda W, Wong AE, Sepulveda F, et al. Prenatal diagnosis of spina bifida: from intracranial translucency to intrauterine surgery. Childs Nerv Syst 2017; 33(7):1083–99.

21. Chen FCK, Gerhardt J, Entezami M, et al. Detection of spina bifida by first trimester screening - results of the Prospective Multicenter Berlin IT-study. Ultraschall Med 2017;38(2):151–7.

22. Practice Bulletin No. 187. Neural tube defects. Obstet Gynecol 2017;130(6): e279–90.

23. Norem CT, Schoen EJ, Walton DL, et al. Routine ultrasonography compared with maternal serum alpha-fetoprotein for neural tube defect screening. Obstet Gynecol 2005;106(4):747–52.

24. Loft AG, Høgdall E, Larsen SO, et al. A comparison of amniotic fluid alpha-fetoprotein and acetylcholinesterase in the prenatal diagnosis of open neural tube defects and anterior abdominal wall defects. Prenat Diagn 1993;13(2): 93–109.

25. Cohen AR, Couto J, Cummings JJ, et al. Position statement on fetal myelomeningocele repair. Am J Obstet Gynecol 2014;210(2):107–11.

26. Mazzone L, Moehrlen U, Casanova B, et al. Open spina bifida: Why not fetal surgery? FDT 2019;45(6):430–4.

27. Chao TT, Dashe JS, Adams RC, et al. Fetal spine findings on MRI and associated outcomes in children with open neural tube defects. Am J Roentgenology 2011; 197(5):W956–61.

28. Johnson MP, Bennett KA, Rand L, et al. MOMS: obstetrical outcomes and risk factors for obstetrical complications following prenatal surgery. Am J Obstet Gynecol 2016;215(6):778.e1–9.

29. Licci M, Guzman R, Soleman J. Maternal and obstetric complications in fetal surgery for prenatal myelomeningocele repair: a systematic review. Neurosurg Focus 2019;47(4):E11.

30. Wilson RD, Lemerand K, Johnson MP, et al. Reproductive outcomes in subsequent pregnancies after a pregnancy complicated by open maternal-fetal surgery (1996–2007). Am J Obstet Gynecol 2010;203(3):209.e1–6.

31. Moldenhauer JS, Flake AW. Open fetal surgery for neural tube defects. Best Pract Res Clin Obstet Gynaecol 2019;58:121–32.

32. Rintoul NE, Sutton LN, Hubbard AM, et al. A New Look at myelomeningoceles: functional level, vertebral level, shunting, and the Implications for fetal intervention. Pediatrics 2002;109(3):409–13.

33. Norkett W, McLone DG, Bowman R. Current management Strategies of Hydrocephalus in the child with open spina bifida. Top Spinal Cord Inj Rehabil 2016; 22(4):241–6.

34. Messing-Jünger M, Röhrig A. Primary and secondary management of the Chiari II malformation in children with myelomeningocele. Childs Nerv Syst 2013;29(9): 1553–62.

35. Talamonti G, Marcati E, Mastino L, et al. Surgical management of Chiari malformation type II. Childs Nerv Syst 2020;36(8):1621–34.

36. Oakeshott P, Hunt GM, Poulton A, et al. Expectation of life and unexpected death in open spina bifida: a 40-year complete, non-selective, longitudinal cohort study. Dev Med Child Neurol 2010;52(8):749–53.

37. Snow-Lisy DC, Yerkes EB, Cheng EY. Update on urological management of spina bifida from prenatal diagnosis to Adulthood. J Urol 2015;194(2):288–96.
38. Rocque BG, Bishop ER, Scogin MA, et al. Assessing health-related quality of life in children with spina bifida. J Neurosurg Pediatr 2015;15(2):144–9.
39. Beierwaltes P, Church P, Gordon T, et al. Bowel function and care: Guidelines for the care of people with spina bifida. J Pediatr Rehabil Med 2020;13(4):491–8.
40. Velde SV, Biervliet SV, Bruyne RD, et al. A systematic review on bowel management and the success rate of the various treatment modalities in spina bifida patients. Spinal Cord 2013;51(12):873–81.
41. Swaroop VT, Dias L. Orthopaedic management of spina bifida—part II: foot and ankle deformities. J Child Orthop 2011;5(6):403–14.
42. Bradko V, Castillo H, Fremion E, et al. What is the Role of scoliosis surgery in Adolescents and Adults with myelomeningocele? A systematic review. Clin Orthopaedics Relat Research® 2022. https://doi.org/10.1097/CORR.0000000000002087.
43. Ho P, Quigley MA, Tatwavedi D, et al. Neonatal and infant mortality associated with spina bifida: a systematic review and meta-analysis. PLoS One 2021; 16(5):e0250098.
44. Shin M, Kucik JE, Siffel C, et al. Improved survival among children with spina bifida in the United States. J Pediatr 2012;161(6):1132–7.
45. Houtrow AJ, Thom EA, Fletcher JM, et al. Prenatal repair of myelomeningocele and school-age functional outcomes. Pediatrics 2020;145(2):e20191544.
46. Farmer DL, Thom EA, Brock JW, et al. The Management of Myelomeningocele Study: full cohort 30-month pediatric outcomes. Am J Obstet Gynecol 2018; 218(2):256.e1–13.
47. Houtrow AJ, MacPherson C, Jackson-Coty J, et al. Prenatal repair and physical functioning among children with myelomeningocele: a secondary analysis of a randomized clinical trial. JAMA Pediatr 2021;175(4):e205674.
48. Brock JW, Carr MC, Adzick NS, et al. Bladder function after fetal surgery for myelomeningocele. Pediatrics 2015;136(4):e906–13.
49. Brock JW, Thomas JC, Baskin LS, et al. Effect of prenatal repair of myelomeningocele on urological outcomes at school age. J Urol 2019;202(4):812–8.
50. Danzer E, Thomas NH, Thomas A, et al. Long-term neurofunctional outcome, executive functioning, and behavioral adaptive skills following fetal myelomeningocele surgery. Am J Obstet Gynecol 2016;214(2):269.e1–8.
51. Araujo Júnior E, Tonni G, Martins WP. Outcomes of infants followed-up at least 12 months after fetal open and endoscopic surgery for meningomyelocele: a systematic review and meta-analysis. J Evid Based Med 2016;9(3):125–35.
52. Joyeux L, Engels AC, Russo FM, et al. Fetoscopic versus open repair for spina bifida aperta: a systematic review of outcomes. FDT 2016;39(3):161–71.
53. Kabagambe SK, Jensen GW, Chen YJ, et al. Fetal surgery for myelomeningocele: a systematic review and meta-analysis of outcomes in fetoscopic versus open repair. Fetal Diagn Ther 2018;43(3):161–74.
54. Araujo Júnior E, Eggink AJ, van den Dobbelsteen J, et al. Procedure-related complications of open vs endoscopic fetal surgery for treatment of spina bifida in an era of intrauterine myelomeningocele repair: systematic review and meta-analysis. Ultrasound Obstet Gynecol 2016;48(2):151–60.
55. Cortes MS, Chmait RH, Lapa DA, et al. Experience of 300 cases of prenatal fetoscopic open spina bifida repair: report of the International Fetoscopic Neural Tube Defect Repair Consortium. Am J Obstet Gynecol 2021;225(6):678.e1–11.

56. Wang A, Brown EG, Lankford L, et al. Placental mesenchymal stromal cells Rescue ambulation in ovine myelomeningocele. Stem Cells Transl Med 2015; 4(6):659–69.
57. Kabagambe S, Keller B, Becker J, et al. Placental mesenchymal stromal cells seeded on clinical grade extracellular matrix improve ambulation in ovine myelomeningocele. J Pediatr Surg 2017. S0022-3468(17)30654-1.
58. Vanover M, Pivetti C, Lankford L, et al. High density placental mesenchymal stromal cells provide neuronal preservation and improve motor function following in utero treatment of ovine myelomeningocele. J Pediatr Surg 2019;54(1):75–9.
59. Theodorou CM, Stokes SC, Jackson JE, et al. Efficacy of clinical-grade human placental mesenchymal stromal cells in fetal ovine myelomeningocele repair. J Pediatr Surg 2021. S0022-3468(21)00435-8.
60. Mann LK, Won JH, Patel R, et al. Allografts for skin closure during in utero spina bifida repair in a sheep model. J Clin Med 2021;10(21):4928.
61. Dionigi B, Brazzo JA, Ahmed A, et al. Trans-amniotic stem cell therapy (TRASCET) minimizes Chiari-II malformation in experimental spina bifida. J Pediatr Surg 2015;50(6):1037–41.
62. Shieh HF, Tracy SA, Hong CR, et al. Transamniotic stem cell therapy (TRASCET) in a rabbit model of spina bifida. J Pediatr Surg 2019;54(2):293–6.
63. Aaronson OS, Tulipan NB, Cywes R, et al. Robot-assisted endoscopic intrauterine myelomeningocele repair: a Feasibility study. PNE 2002;36(2):85–9.
64. Kohl T, Hartlage MG, Kiehitz D, et al. Percutaneous fetoscopic patch coverage of experimental lumbosacral full-thickness skin lesions in sheep. Surg Endosc 2003; 17(8):1218–23.
65. Knight CG, Lorincz A, Johnson A, et al. Robot-enhanced fetoscopic surgery. J Pediatr Surg 2004;39(10):1463–5.

Fetal Therapy for Renal Anhydramnios

Jena L. Miller, MD[a],*, Ahmet A. Baschat, MD[a], Meredith A. Atkinson, MD, MHS[b]

KEYWORDS

- Amnioinfusion • Anhydramnios • Bilateral renal agenesis • Fetal intervention
- Fetal megacystis • Fetal renal failure • Lower urinary tract obstruction
- Oligohydramnios

KEY POINTS

- Severe fetal congenital anomalies of the kidneys and urinary tract that result in early onset anhydramnios are considered lethal due to pulmonary hypoplasia without intervention during pregnancy.
- Detailed prenatal imaging with ultrasound or magnetic resonance imaging, diagnostic amnioinfusion, and genetic testing IS necessary to evaluate for associated anomalies, prognosis and determine candidacy for fetal treatment.
- Fetal intervention aims to restore amniotic fluid volume either mechanically via vesicoamniotic shunting or cystoscopy in cases of urinary obstruction, or with serial amnioinfusions when fetal urine production is absent or insufficient, thereby supporting pulmonary development.
- Neonates with sufficient pulmonary function after birth require ongoing treatment of the underlying renal disease. Newborns with end-stage renal disease need chronic dialysis as a bridge to renal transplant for longer-term survival.
- The success rate of serial amnioinfusions to promote pulmonary survival and allow the initiation of chronic dialysis in patients with early pregnancy renal anhydramnios is one measure currently being evaluated in the multi-center Renal Anhydramnios Fetal Therapy (RAFT) trial.

Conflicts of Interest: The Authors receive funding from the National Institutes of Health NICHD R01HD100540 for the Renal Anhydramnios Fetal Therapy Trial. The authors have no commercial interests to report.

[a] Department of Gynecology and Obstetrics, The Johns Hopkins Center for Fetal Therapy, 600 North Wolfe Street, Nelson 228, Baltimore, MD 21287, USA; [b] Division of Pediatric Nephrology, Johns Hopkins University School of Medicine, 200 North Wolfe Street, Room 3064, Baltimore, MD 21287, USA
* Corresponding author.
E-mail address: jmill260@jhmi.edu
Twitter: @drjenamiller (J.L.M.)

INTRODUCTION

Congenital anomalies of the kidneys and urinary tract complicate about 1 in 2,500 pregnancies and comprise approximately 20% of all prenatally identified anomalies.[1,2] Renal abnormalities may be unilateral or bilateral and range from mild to severe based on their impact on renal function in fetal life. Severe congenital renal malformations can render the fetus anuric and fall into 3 major categories: bilateral renal agenesis, fetal renal failure, or lower urinary tract obstruction (**Table 1**).[3–5] Although fetal urine production begins between 8 and 10 weeks of gestation, its magnitude is negligible and the amniotic fluid that fills the amniotic cavity in the first trimester is predominantly from transudate across the placenta and fetal tissues. By 16 weeks, this transitions to fetal urine as the primary contributor to amniotic fluid.[6] Regardless of the underlying etiology of fetal anuria, the final common pathway results in a progressive decrease in amniotic fluid and ultimately oligohydramnios or anhydramnios. Morbidity and mortality associated with fetal renal disease are related to the degree of reduction in amniotic fluid volume.

NATURE OF THE PROBLEM

Amniotic fluid is required for normal fetal lung development. When anhydramnios develops, fluid produced in the tracheobronchial tree escapes during normal opening and closing of the fetal glottis. This depressurization of the fetal airway prevents the lungs from growing normally and can result in lethal pulmonary hypoplasia when anhydramnios develops prior to 22 weeks of pregnancy.[7] Therefore, the presence of severe fetal renal disease almost invariably results in a multisystem disorder affecting both respiratory and renal function after birth. The combined impact on these 2 organ systems leads to lethality due to severe fetal renal conditions. Restoring amniotic fluid around the fetus is the principle goal of fetal therapy for early pregnancy renal anhydramnios (EPRA). This aims to maintain the back pressure on the fetal tracheobronchial tree and allow normal lung development and convert an inherently multisystem disorder at birth to a clinical scenario where the primary treatment is focused on addressing the renal etiology. The goal of this approach is to improve survival, but many unanswered questions remain about the effectiveness of fetal interventions for this indication.[8] The underlying cause of anhydramnios must be addressed secondarily.

Imaging of the Fetal Urinary System

Ultrasound is the primary imaging modality for the fetal urinary system as it is cost-effective and widely available as part of the standard of care for prenatal anomaly

Table 1
Causes and diagnosis of early pregnancy renal anhydramnios

Category	Imaging Findings	Differential Diagnosis
Renal agenesis	No identifiable fetal kidneys, bladder, or renal arteries with color Doppler	Unilateral or bilateral Pelvic kidney
Fetal renal failure	Kidneys may be small or large, cystic, or echogenic	Polycystic kidney disease Multicystic dysplastic kidneys Renal dysplasia
Lower urinary tract obstruction	Urinary tract dilation Dilated bladder	Posterior urethral valve Urethral atresia Cloacal abnormality

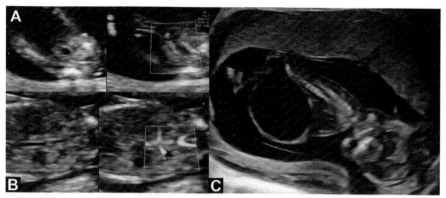

Fig. 1. First-trimester ultrasound assessment of the fetal urinary system. Transverse view of the fetal bladder and umbilical arteries at the level of the pelvis (*A*). Coronal view of the kidneys and renal arteries with color Doppler (*B*). Dilated bladder with "keyhole sign" (*C*).

screening. The fetal kidneys are visible as early as 9 weeks in gestation but are identified in up to 92% of pregnancies with either transvaginal or transabdominal ultrasound by 13 weeks.[9–11] The hyperechoic renal cortex and hypoechoic renal pelvis can be identified lateral to the spine in both the transverse and coronal planes.[12,13] By 12 weeks, bladder filling should be identified in the pelvis and increased bladder dimensions can point toward the presence of bladder outlet obstruction[14] (**Fig. 1**). If no bladder filling is observed by 15 weeks, this is considered abnormal, and the absence of functional renal tissue must be considered. Conversely, bladder distention and absence of amniotic fluid volume are suggestive of lower urinary tract obstruction. Accordingly, preliminary ultrasound diagnosis of severe renal tract abnormalities can be achieved in the early second trimester. International guidelines recommend the assessment of the kidneys and bladder as an essential component of the mid-trimester anatomy scan.[15] The fetal ureters are typically not visible unless they are dilated.

Fetal magnetic resonance imaging (MRI) can be an important adjunct to prenatal ultrasound in selected cases,[16–18] particularly when there are technical limitations to ultrasound, such as oligohydramnios/anhydramnios or maternal obesity.[19] MRI sequences are not limited by fetal position and allow the evaluation of the fetal anatomy in multiple planes, enhance differentiation between tissues and may identify additional morphological abnormalities.[20,21] This can be particularly helpful to distinguish characteristics of renal tissue from the surrounding abdominal organs. These benefits may help to refine the diagnosis and impact management planning.[20] Although the data regarding the assessment of total lung volumes are limited in the setting of fetal genitourinary anomalies, this measure may also provide another data point in evaluating the risk for pulmonary hypoplasia.[22] Newer techniques involving 3D reconstruction of the fetal genitourinary system and functional imaging of the fetal kidneys are under development and may provide additional clinical utility in the future.[19]

Differential Diagnosis of Renal Anhydramnios

Renal agenesis
Congenital bilateral renal agenesis (CoBRA) occurs in 0.1–0.3 per 1000 births and must be suspected when the fetal kidneys are not visible in the renal fossa. Color Doppler ultrasonography is a useful adjunct to assess the presence of the renal arteries branching from each side of the aorta in the posterior coronal view (see

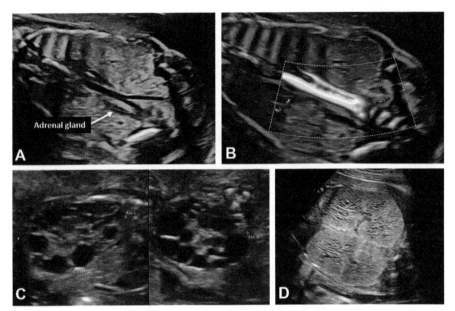

Fig. 2. Ultrasound appearance of common etiologies of early pregnancy renal anhydramnios. Coronal view of the renal fossa without evidence of kidneys or renal arteries as well as lying down the appearance of the adrenal gland on grey-scale (*A*) and color Doppler (*B*). Multicystic dysplastic kidney with multiple noncommunicating cysts of varying sizes and echogenic parenchyma (*C*). Massively enlarged echogenic kidneys with microcysts consistent with autosomal recessive polycystic kidney disease (*D*).

Fig. 1).[11,23] If no kidneys or bladder filling are identified in combination with anhydramnios after 16 weeks, bilateral renal agenesis is probable. Lack of amniotic fluid or maternal obesity may negatively impact the visualization of the urinary tract and the remainder of the fetal anatomy. Additionally, the renal fossa may be obscured by fetal bowel. The fetal adrenal glands can be enlarged or have a more longitudinal appearance and may be confused with the kidneys. As such, a detailed evaluation of the renal fossae is critical to confirming the diagnosis [24] (**Fig. 2**). The sensitivity of second-trimester ultrasound to detect bilateral renal agenesis was 83.7% in a cohort where the diagnosis was confirmed postnatally.[2]

In cases of unilateral renal agenesis, the contralateral kidney may be hypertrophied, but normal bladder filling and amniotic fluid are expected. These cases are not at increased risk for perinatal mortality. In parents with unilateral renal agenesis, the risk for CoBRA in offspring is increased to 4%. Thus, when CoBRA is diagnosed in pregnancy, parental kidneys should be examined reflexively.

CoBRA is considered universally fatal without prenatal intervention due to prolonged anhydramnios and resulting pulmonary hypoplasia. For this reason, intensive prenatal or neonatal management is not offered.[25] Newborns exposed to anhydramnios through the second and third trimesters also may display fetal deformations attributable to prolonged intrauterine compression including flattened facies, low-set ears, and clubbed feet described as the Potter sequence.[6]

Fetal renal failure

Intrinsic kidney disease and prenatal renal failure can have several etiologies including cystic kidney disease, nephronophthisis, ciliopathies, and renal dysplasia. Polycystic kidney disease can have an autosomal recessive or dominant inheritance pattern. Autosomal recessive polycystic kidney disease (ARPKD) typically presents prenatally, and autosomal dominant polycystic kidney disease (ADPKD) typically has a milder impact on renal function and more commonly emerges clinically in adulthood, although in some cases cysts may be noted prenatally.

ARPKD is a disease characterized by the transformation of the collecting tubules of the kidneys into elongated cysts. The degree of renal failure is related to the proportion of nephrons that are affected. The cysts may be microscopic, so the kidneys appear echogenic on ultrasound and progressively enlarge over time (see **Fig. 2**). The increased size of the kidney can cause upward displacement of the diaphragm contributing to pulmonary hypoplasia. In some cases, there is also associated biliary dysgenesis and hepatic fibrosis.[26,27] Thus, ARPKD is considered a multi-organ disease and not considered a candidate condition for fetal therapy. In contrast, ADPKD develops more slowly and typically presents in adulthood and is not a common cause of prenatal renal failure.

Multicystic dysplastic kidney disease (MCDK) may be unilateral or bilateral and is characterized by multiple noncommunicating anechoic macrocysts within the dysplastic renal parenchyma (see **Fig. 2**). The kidneys may enlarge initially and then shrink when no urine is produced. When unilateral, amniotic fluid is preserved due to the normal functioning contralateral kidney and the prognosis is good. Bilateral MCDK with anhydramnios is anticipated to be fatal.[4]

Lower urinary tract obstruction

Lower urinary tract obstruction (LUTO) most commonly occurs due a mechanical blockage at the level of the urethra due to posterior urethral valves, urethral stenosis or atresia.[28] Posterior urethral valves are the most common etiology in males, but, in women, urethral atresia or urinary tract obstruction related to more complex anomalies of the genitourinary system including cloacal abnormalities are more likely.[29,30] When the obstruction is complete, the bladder can become severely distended, and a classic keyhole sign can be observed (see **Fig. 1**). Additional findings such as bladder wall thickening, hydroureter or hydronephrosis, and oligohydramnios support diagnosis of LUTO.[31,32] A systematic review and meta-analysis of the predictive accuracy of ultrasound findings to identify LUTO revealed that the keyhole sign was only a modest predictor of LUTO so its presence or absence cannot be reliably used to make the diagnosis.[33] Increased pressure in the kidneys due to the obstruction or urinary reflux may also lead to the development of cortical cysts in the kidneys or renal dysplasia and ultimately fetal renal failure.[5,34]

When LUTO is associated with oligohydramnios or anhydramnios, the perinatal mortality rate can be up to 90% without treatment. For cases that have a sufficient respiratory reserve to allow survival into infancy, renal replacement therapy is required in up to 50% of cases.[35–38]

Diagnostic Testing

Whenever oligohydramnios is identified during pregnancy, a thorough history should be obtained to assess the likelihood of prelabor rupture of membranes (PROM) as a cause. The next step is a detailed ultrasound assessment of the fetal anatomy including fetal echocardiogram to evaluate the urinary tract as well as other associated anomalies. Diagnostic amnioinfusion can be helpful to confirm intact membranes and allow better evaluation of the fetal anatomy in greater detail.[39]

Genetic counseling and diagnostic testing by either karyotype or chromosomal microarray are imperative as genetic abnormalities including aneuploidy, copy number variants, or single gene disorders can be present in 20–30% of cases.[40–42] In the setting of oligohydramnios or anhydramnios, genetic testing by either chorionic villus sampling or fetal blood sampling are often the only options, and the choice is often determined by technical considerations for the procedure. Several genetic syndromes are associated with CoBRA, fetal renal failure, or LUTO. Patients must be counseled that additional extrarenal anomalies may be identified after birth. Targeted gene panels or whole exome sequencing may provide greater insight into the cause of EPRA. Further research is required to determine if genetic findings may be beneficial to stratify patients that may be most suitable for fetal treatment.[42]

For cases of urinary tract obstruction with a distended bladder, fetal vesicocentesis using ultrasound guidance can be considered to evaluate the genetics and urinary electrolytes (sodium, chloride, osmolality, beta-2 microglobulin) as a surrogate for fetal renal function.[43,44] Up to 3 sequential assessments of urinary electrolytes as well as the assessment of bladder refilling after vesicocentesis are commonly used to evaluate renal function.[5] A systematic review of 23 studies including 572 women revealed that none of the studied urinary electrolytes can accurately predict poor renal function.[45] As such, use of urinary electrolyte values to determine candidacy for fetal intervention remains controversial. However, the absence of bladder refilling after vesicocentesis, points toward oligohydramnios or anuria associated with unfavorable prognosis.[5]

Therapeutic Options

In cases of LUTO with suspected preserved renal function, potential fetal interventions include vesicoamniotic shunting and fetal cystoscopy[35] to overcome the blockage and allow natural replenishment of amniotic fluid volume by fetal urination. Both procedures are conducted under ultrasound guidance with local or regional anesthesia. The most common type of shunt utilized in the United States is a double pigtail silicone catheter (Harrison/Rodeck). Amnioinfusion is first performed to create space within the amniotic cavity to allow shunt deployment. Next, the shunt introducer is inserted into the amniotic cavity percutaneously using ultrasound guidance. The proximal portion of the shunt is deployed inside the fetal bladder and the distal end is released into the amniotic cavity. As the shunts are not fixed in the abdominal wall, they are prone to dislodgement due to migration tendencies or grasped by the fetus. An alternative shunt device to decrease the chance for dislodgement during the pregnancy is of a smaller caliber made of nitinol wire mesh in a silicone membrane with a parasol shape on either end (SOMATEX).[46] The aim of shunting is to bypass the urinary obstruction and allow the urine to drain from the bladder into the amniotic cavity, thereby decompressing the urinary tract and maintaining amniotic fluid volume.

Fetal cystoscopy is performed by inserting a small trochar through the maternal abdominal wall into the uterine cavity and then into the fetal bladder under ultrasound guidance. Once inside the fetal bladder, a small fetoscope can be introduced to perform cystoscopy. The fetoscope is directed to the posterior urethra. If a posterior urethral valve is visualized, the location of the valve can be verified with a guidewire and laser fulguration can be performed. The goal of this intervention is to create a patent urethra and decompress the bladder.[47,48] If urethral atresia is identified, then the need for a working shunt is required to allow bladder decompression.

Clinical Outcomes

A systematic review of 369 fetuses that were evaluated for bladder drainage by either vesicoamniotic shunting, open fetal bladder surgery, or cystoscopy observed that perinatal survival was improved for ongoing pregnancies in fetuses undergoing intervention compared to no intervention (OR 2.43, 95% CI 1.18–5.02, I^2 5.3%) particularly in the subgroup of patients with an initial poor prognosis (OR 8.05; 95% CI 1.23, 52.9; I^2 0%).[49] The multi-centered randomized PLUTO (Percutaneous shunting in Lower Urinary Tract Obstruction) trial aimed to assess the effectiveness of shunting on survival and renal function. Unfortunately, the trial was stopped for poor recruitment. Although there seemed to be a survival advantage in fetuses undergoing shunting with 50% surviving until 28 days (RR 3.20, 1.06–9.62; p = 0.03), assessment of the treatment effect remained limited due to the small sample size.[50] A more recent meta-analysis of 117 patients, reported pooled two-year survival after vesicoamniotic shunting was 40%.[51] In a retrospective cohort study of 30 cystoscopies, two-year survival was 54% with 73% of survivors having normal renal function.[29] Both vesicoamniotic shunting or cystoscopy may have a range of complications including but not limited to PROM, miscarriage, shunt failure, dislodgment, or procedure failure.[49,51] Urinary fistulas are complications unique to fetal cystoscopy related to iatrogenic tissue damage that is peripheral to the posterior urethral valve.[52]

Serial Amnioinfusions

For the subset of pregnancies affected by bilateral renal agenesis, fetal renal failure, or LUTO the ability of the fetus to physiologically correct the amniotic fluid volume after in-utero treatment is absent and therefore these patients have not been considered candidates for conventional fetal intervention. Artificial replacement of amniotic fluid volume by serial amnioinfusions to prevent pulmonary hypoplasia has been investigated in these circumstances. Case reports and small series have suggested the potential for improved respiratory function after serial amnioinfusions performed either percutaneously or via an implanted port.[53–55] For newborns who do not have pulmonary hypoplasia after this intervention, renal replacement therapy with chronic dialysis is obligatory for the management of end-stage renal disease as a bridge to kidney transplant. A systematic review of 17 fetuses undergoing serial amnioinfusions for renal causes of anhydramnios demonstrated that the overall survival for the first week of life was 64.7% (11/17) with 56.2% (9/16) initiating peritoneal dialysis and 44.4% (4/9) undergoing renal transplant.[56] A series of 8 pregnancies complicated by bilateral fetal renal agenesis and treated with serial amnioinfusions (range 3–26 infusions per patient) at a single-center reported 6 neonatal deaths shortly after delivery and 2 infants who survived > 30 days, but subsequently died of sepsis while on dialysis.[57] Lack of reported selection criteria for patients undergoing serial amnioinfusions and the potential selection bias in these series are major limitations to understanding the confounding factors and survival outcomes. Reporting of procedure-related risks is limited and all that underwent serial amnioinfusions delivered prematurely with the median gestational age at birth of 32 weeks and 2 days (N = 17; IQR, 30 to 35.9 weeks).[56]

Renal Anhydramnios Fetal Therapy Trial

In light of reports that maintaining normal amniotic fluid levels during pregnancies affected by EPRA can subvert pulmonary hypoplasia followed by successful postnatal dialysis and transplantation,[53,58] this intervention generated much interest in the lay community and controversy within the medical community. In 2016, the National Institute of Diabetes and Digestive and Kidney Diseases and The *Eunice Kennedy Shriver* National Institute of Child Health and Human Development (NICHD) of the National Institutes of Health held a workshop to develop a research agenda for addressing early pregnancy renal anhydramnios based on the available evidence.[8] A national ethics symposium was also held to address the complexity of risk/benefit analysis, informed consent, counseling, conflicts of interest, impacts on providers, institutions and society of amnioinfusions for this indication[59] and informed the design of the renal anhydramnios fetal therapy (RAFT) trial (NCT03101891).[60]

The RAFT trial is a NICHD-funded multicenter trial aimed to determine the safety, feasibility, and efficacy of serial amnioinfusions for early pregnancy anhydramnios caused by bilateral renal agenesis or fetal renal failure, as well as the quality of life of survivors and their families (R01HD100540). Each participating center must have maternal–fetal medicine specialists with expertise in performing amnioinfusions in the setting of anhydramnios as well as neonatal and pediatric expertise in dialysis and kidney transplantation. The study population consists of 70 maternal–fetal dyads with either isolated fetal bilateral renal agenesis (n = 35) or fetal renal failure (n = 35). The sample size was calculated based on available case report data generating the hypothesis that 25% of patients who undergo serial amnioinfusions may initially survive.

A multidisciplinary approach is used for patients undergoing evaluation prior to participation in the RAFT trial. Detailed ultrasound assessment, fetal MRI, diagnostic amnioinfusion, and genetic testing with either karyotype or chromosomal microarray are performed during the screening phase to confirm the diagnosis and exclude associated structural or genetic abnormalities. Consultations with maternal–fetal medicine, genetic counseling, neonatology, pediatric surgery, nephrology, transplant surgery, and social work are conducted to address the obstetric risks of serial amnioinfusions and postnatal challenges and complications of chronic dialysis and renal transplant.[42,60] Multidisciplinary support is critical given the demands that infant dialysis treatment places on caregivers. The limited societal support available to families to address physical, psychological, social, and financial burdens requires study and clinical care team members to be transparent about these factors when discussing study enrollment and the potential challenges of caring for an infant with end-stage kidney disease to support the decision-making process. If all criteria are met, then enrollment is offered (**Table 2**). An expectant management arm to document the natural history of EPRA is an available alternative for patients that meet eligibility, but do not desire to undergo the termination of pregnancy or serial amnioinfusions.

Once enrolled, serial amnioinfusions of isotonic solution with or without antibiotics according to the local institutional protocol approximately 1–3 times weekly based on the case characteristics. Timing of subsequent infusions aims to avoid recurrent anhydramnios. Amnioinfusions are continued until confirmed PROM occurs or if there is an obstetric indication for delivery. Delivery must occur at a RAFT center to facilitate smooth transition to neonatal intensive care. The primary efficacy outcome measure is the proportion of neonates that achieve successful use of a dialysis catheter for equal to or greater than 14 continuous days. For survivors that are discharged on chronic dialysis, long-term follow-up data are captured with the North American Pediatric Renal Trials and Collaborative Studies (NAPRTCS) registry. Study participants remain in the study until fetal/pediatric death or four years after transplant (**Fig. 3**).

Renal Replacement Therapy

Expertise in neonatal renal replacement therapy for children with isolated end-stage renal disease has advanced to the degree that nearly all children are offered chronic dialysis.[60,61] Data from the NAPRTCS registry show that 3-year survival for neonates initiating dialysis is 78.6%, which is comparable to those who start dialysis between 1 and 12 months of age.[62] Additionally, for children who proceed to kidney transplant, 3-year graft survival of 92.1% was reported.[62] One important limitation of this database is that the entry criteria require a child to have transitioned to outpatient dialysis, so it does not capture mortalities that occur during the initial hospitalization and thus may

Table 2 Inclusion and exclusion criteria for the RAFT trial	
Inclusion Criteria	**Exclusion Criteria**
Maternal age ≥ 18 years	Multiple gestation
Anhydramnios < 22 weeks GA for fetal renal failure or confirmed CoBRA	Cervical shortening < 25 mm or history of preterm labor
No other anomalies	Pathogenic finding on karyotype or chromosomal microarray
Termination of pregnancy declined	Chorioamnionitis or placental abruption
Multi-specialty consults completed	Prelabor rupture of membranes or significant chorion-amnion separation
Intervention arm -Willingness to undergo intervention and delivery at a RAFT center	Severe maternal medical condition or depression
Expectant management arm-Willingness to return to a RAFT center for fetal MRI and echocardiogram at 32 weeks	Technical limitations precluding amnioinfusion

overestimate survival for the population of neonates with end-stage renal disease requiring dialysis.

Despite favorable contemporary survival rates, chronic dialysis has a significant risk profile for the infant as well as incurs substantial effort and financial burden for the family. Infants are at increased risks for complications including, but not limited to catheter malfunction, dialysis access-related infections and sepsis, need for multiple surgeries, failure to thrive, impaired neurodevelopment as well as additional complications if born prematurely or with additional comorbidities.[63] Caregivers must have substantial training and dedication to administer home peritoneal dialysis, which is administered nightly over 8–14 hours, and bear a substantial cost burden.[64] Although peritoneal dialysis is the first-line approach to neonatal dialysis given its feasibility as a home therapy, for infants in whom peritoneal dialysis is not an option, hemodialysis is considered. Hemodialysis can be complicated by issues of vascular access in very small neonates, although there has been progress in dialysis technology. For these reasons, there is variability among pediatric nephrologists' willingness to start neonates on chronic dialysis. In an international survey of pediatric nephrologists, only 30% offer renal replacement therapy to all neonates with additional abnormalities as the most common reason for withholding dialysis.[61] For these reasons, the decision to initiate renal replacement therapy in the neonatal period versus a palliative care approach requires shared decision-making as well as informed consent or refusal for treatment, for which the goals of care for the family and treatment team are aligned considering the child's additional needs.[65,66]

Questions and Controversies

One of the important considerations for designing eligibility criteria for fetal therapies rests on the balance of maternal risks of interventions measured against the benefits for the fetus and ultimately the infant. There is a range of potential maternal risks of repeated installation of fluid by ultrasound-guided needle puncture of the amniotic cavity that includes preterm rupture of membranes, intra-amniotic infection progressing to maternal sepsis, and other rare complications that may not yet be recognized due to under-reporting.[60] An alternative approach of placing a subcutaneous port to instill amniotic fluid in fetuses with EPRA has been reported.[55] Although this approach

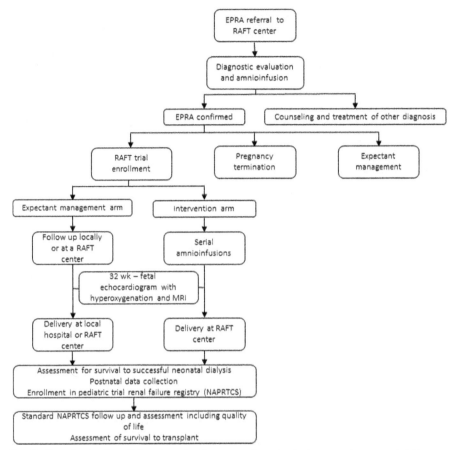

Fig. 3. Flowchart of participant evaluation, enrollment, study procedures, and follow-up period for the RAFT trial.

aims to avoid multiple invasive procedures to the uterus, it incurs additional maternal risk for device placement and is described at a time where the full range of amnioinfusion-related risks has not yet been defined. The critical information that is also lacking is the generalizable benefits and risks for the fetus and infant.

Because fetal renal disease has often been considered lethal, prenatal interventions were not offered. As such, the potential benefits are hard to estimate. The RAFT trial will be able to produce generalizable knowledge about the extent to which life-sustaining pulmonary function can be achieved by artificial correction of the amniotic fluid volume. Although survival may be possible, the range of morbidities that may affect individuals with severe prenatally acquired renal impairment or even the absence of renal tissue altogether cannot yet be estimated. Considering the multiple functions of the kidneys after birth it is likely simplistic to view renal agenesis as a single organ disease for several reasons. First, the genetics of renal disease may be more complex than previously anticipated and the expansion to whole exome or genome testing may reveal mutations that have multi-organ functional impacts, Second, the kidneys play a central role in blood pressure and hematopoietic control. This is likely to require multidisciplinary or currently uncharted management approaches that fall outside the current practice of neonatal and pediatric standards of care. Complications that may arise as a result of cardiovascular and hematologic dysregulation may be remote from delivery or too infrequent to accurately delineate in the context of the current RAFT trial. Yet, result in significant health impacts. Noting the potential range of health outcomes in patients with renal agenesis, it will be critical to identify other potential therapies to support other organ systems.

Despite these significant issues a robust scientific approach to assess the benefits and risks of fetal therapy for severe renal disease is required to acquire generalizable knowledge based on a representative cohort rather than individual or single-center outcomes. The near future holds promise to better understand this new cohort of patients and steer fetal treatments for renal disease in a meaningful direction.

Best practices

- Pregnancies affected by congenital anomalies of the kidney and urinary tract require detailed prenatal ultrasound assessment, genetic counseling and consideration of diagnostic testing for comprehensive evaluation.

- For cases of early pregnancy renal anhydramnios caused by suspected fetal renal failure, serial amnioinfusions to prevent pulmonary hypoplasia are being investigated as a part of the NICHD-funded multicenter Renal Anhydramnios Fetal Therapy (RAFT) trial.

REFERENCES

1. Queißer-Luft A, Stolz G, Wiesel A, et al. Malformations in newborn: results based on 30940 infants and fetuses from the Mainz congenital birth defect monitoring system (1990–1998). Arch Gynecol Obstet 2002;266(3):163–7.
2. Grandjean H, Larroque D, Levi S. The performance of routine ultrasonographic screening of pregnancies in the Eurofetus Study. Am J Obstet Gynecol 1999; 181(2):446–54.
3. Isaksen CV, Eik-Nes SH, Blaas HG, et al. Fetuses and infants with congenital urinary system anomalies: correlation between prenatal ultrasound and postmortem findings. Ultrasound Obstet Gynecol 2000;15(3):177–85.
4. Balasundaram M, Chock VY, Wu HY, et al. Predictors of poor neonatal outcomes in prenatally diagnosed multicystic dysplastic kidney disease. J Perinatol 2018; 38(6):658–64.
5. Ruano R, Safdar A, Au J, et al. Defining and predicting "intrauterine fetal renal failure" in congenital lower urinary tract obstruction. Pediatr Nephrol 2016;31(4):605–12.
6. Rosenblum S, Pal A, Reidy K. Renal development in the fetus and premature infant. Semin Fetal Neonatal Med 2017;22(2):58–66.
7. Hislop A, Hey E, Reid L. The lungs in congenital bilateral renal agenesis and dysplasia. Arch Dis Child 1979;54(1):32–8.
8. Moxey-Mims M, Raju TNK. Anhydramnios in the setting of renal malformations: the national institutes of health workshop summary. Obstet Gynecol 2018; 131(6):1069–79.
9. Rosati P, Guariglia L. Transvaginal sonographic assessment of the fetal urinary tract in early pregnancy. Ultrasound Obstet Gynecol 1996;7(2):95–100.
10. Souka AP, Pilalis A, Kavalakis Y, et al. Assessment of fetal anatomy at the 11-14-week ultrasound examination. Ultrasound Obstet Gynecol 2004;24(7):730–4.
11. Dias T, Sairam S, Kumarasiri S. Ultrasound diagnosis of fetal renal abnormalities. Best Pract Res Clin Obstet Gynaecol 2014;28(3):403–15.

12. Tudorache S, Cara M, Iliescu DG, et al. Fetal kidneys ultrasound appearance in the first trimester - clinical significance and limits of counseling. Curr Health Sci J 2016;42(1):19–30.
13. von Kaisenberg CS, Kuhling-von Kaisenberg H, Fritzer E, et al. Fetal transabdominal anatomy scanning using standard views at 11 to 14 weeks' gestation. Am J Obstet Gynecol 2005;192(2):535–42.
14. Salomon LJ, Alfirevic Z, Bilardo CM, et al. ISUOG practice guidelines: performance of first-trimester fetal ultrasound scan. Ultrasound Obstet Gynecol 2013;41(1):102–13.
15. Salomon LJ, Alfirevic Z, Berghella V, et al. Practice guidelines for performance of the routine mid-trimester fetal ultrasound scan. Ultrasound Obstet Gynecol 2011;37(1):116–26.
16. Cassart M, Massez A, Metens T, et al. Complementary role of MRI after sonography in assessing bilateral urinary tract anomalies in the fetus. AJR Am J Roentgenol 2004;182(3):689–95.
17. Abdelazim IA, Abdelrazak KM, Ramy ARM, et al. Complementary roles of prenatal sonography and magnetic resonance imaging in diagnosis of fetal renal anomalies. Aust N Z J Obstet Gynaecol 2010;50(3):237–41.
18. Barseghyan K, Jackson HA, Chmait R, et al. Complementary roles of sonography and magnetic resonance imaging in the assessment of fetal urinary tract anomalies. J Ultrasound Med 2008;27(11):1563–9.
19. Chalouhi GE, Millischer AÉ, Mahallati H, et al. The use of fetal MRI for renal and urogenital tract anomalies. Prenat Diagn 2020;40(1):100–9.
20. Millischer AE, Grevent D, Rousseau V, et al. Fetal MRI compared with ultrasound for the diagnosis of obstructive genital malformations. Prenat Diagn 2017;37(11):1138–45.
21. Chauvin NA, Epelman M, Victoria T, et al. Complex genitourinary abnormalities on fetal MRI: imaging findings and approach to diagnosis. AJR Am J Roentgenol 2012;199(2):W222–31.
22. Zaretsky M, Ramus R, McIntire D, et al. MRI calculation of lung volumes to predict outcome in fetuses with genitourinary abnormalities. AJR Am J Roentgenol 2005;185(5):1328–34.
23. DeVore GR. The value of color Doppler sonography in the diagnosis of renal agenesis. J Ultrasound Med 1995;14(6):443–9.
24. Bronshtein M, Amit A, Achiron R, et al. The early prenatal sonographic diagnosis of renal agenesis: techniques and possible pitfalls. Prenat Diagn 1994;14(4):291–7.
25. Thomas AN, McCullough LB, Chervenak FA, et al. Evidence-based, ethically justified counseling for fetal bilateral renal agenesis. J Perinat Med 2017;45(5):585–94.
26. Wilson PD. Polycystic kidney disease. N Engl J Med 2004;350(2):151–64.
27. Hartung EA, Guay-Woodford LM. Autosomal recessive polycystic kidney disease: a hepatorenal fibrocystic disorder with pleiotropic effects. Pediatrics 2014;134(3):e833–45.
28. Robyr R, Benachi A, Daikha-Dahmane F, et al. Correlation between ultrasound and anatomical findings in fetuses with lower urinary tract obstruction in the first half of pregnancy. Ultrasound Obstet Gynecol 2005;25(5):478–82.
29. Sananes N, Cruz-Martinez R, Favre R, et al. Two-year outcomes after diagnostic and therapeutic fetal cystoscopy for lower urinary tract obstruction. Prenat Diagn 2016;36(4):297–303.

30. Pinette MG, Blackstone J, Wax JR, et al. Enlarged fetal bladder: differential diagnosis and outcomes. J Clin Ultrasound 2003;31(6):328–34.
31. Bernardes LS, Aksnes G, Saada J, et al. Keyhole sign: how specific is it for the diagnosis of posterior urethral valves? Ultrasound Obstet Gynecol 2009;34(4): 419–23.
32. Ibirogba ER, Haeri S, Ruano R. Fetal lower urinary tract obstruction: what should we tell the prospective parents? Prenat Diagn 2020;40(6):661–8.
33. Keefe DT, Kim JK, Mackay E, et al. Predictive accuracy of prenatal ultrasound findings for lower urinary tract obstruction: a systematic review and Bayesian meta-analysis. Prenat Diagn 2021;41(9):1039–48.
34. Pringle KC, Zuccollo J, Kitagawa H, et al. Renal dysplasia produced by obstructive uropathy in the fetal lamb. Pathology 2003;35(6):518–21.
35. Ruano R. Fetal surgery for severe lower urinary tract obstruction. Prenat Diagn 2011;31(7):667–74.
36. Freedman AL, Johnson MP, Smith CA, et al. Long-term outcome in children after antenatal intervention for obstructive uropathies. Lancet 1999;354(9176):374–7.
37. Parkhouse HF, Barratt TM, Dillon MJ, et al. Long-term outcome of boys with posterior urethral valves. Br J Urol 1988;62(1):59–62.
38. Anumba DO, Scott JE, Plant ND, et al. Diagnosis and outcome of fetal lower urinary tract obstruction in the northern region of England. Prenat Diagn 2005; 25(1):7–13.
39. Vikraman SK, Chandra V, Balakrishnan B, et al. Impact of antepartum diagnostic amnioinfusion on targeted ultrasound imaging of pregnancies presenting with severe oligo- and anhydramnios: an analysis of 61 cases. Eur J Obstet Gynecol Reprod Biol 2017;212:96–100.
40. Liao AW, Sebire NJ, Geerts L, et al. Megacystis at 10-14 weeks of gestation: chromosomal defects and outcome according to bladder length. Ultrasound Obstet Gynecol 2003;21(4):338–41.
41. Malin G, Tonks AM, Morris RK, et al. Congenital lower urinary tract obstruction: a population-based epidemiological study. BJOG 2012;119(12):1455–64.
42. Jelin AC, Sagaser KG, Forster KR, et al. Etiology and management of early pregnancy renal anhydramnios: is there a place for serial amnioinfusions? Prenat Diagn 2020;40(5):528–37.
43. Ruano R, Sananes N, Wilson C, et al. Fetal lower urinary tract obstruction: proposal for standardized multidisciplinary prenatal management based on disease severity. Ultrasound Obstet Gynecol 2016;48(4):476–82.
44. Haeri S, Ruano SH, Farah LMS, et al. Prenatal cytogenetic diagnosis from fetal urine in lower urinary tract obstruction. Congenit Anom 2013;53(2):89–91.
45. Morris RK, Quinlan-Jones E, Kilby MD, et al. Systematic review of accuracy of fetal urine analysis to predict poor postnatal renal function in cases of congenital urinary tract obstruction. Prenat Diagn 2007;27(10):900–11.
46. Strizek B, Spicher T, Gottschalk I, et al. Vesicoamniotic shunting before 17 + 0 Weeks in fetuses with lower urinary tract obstruction (LUTO): comparison of somatex vs. Harrison Shunt Syst J Clin Med Res 2022;11(9). https://doi.org/10. 3390/jcm11092359.
47. Quintero RA, Hume R, Smith C, et al. Percutaneous fetal cystoscopy and endoscopic fulguration of posterior urethral valves. Am J Obstet Gynecol 1995; 172(1 Pt 1):206–9.
48. Ruano R, Duarte S, Bunduki V, et al. Fetal cystoscopy for severe lower urinary tract obstruction–initial experience of a single center. Prenat Diagn 2010; 30(1):30–9.

49. Morris RK, Malin GL, Khan KS, et al. Systematic review of the effectiveness of antenatal intervention for the treatment of congenital lower urinary tract obstruction. BJOG 2010;117(4):382–90.

50. Morris RK, Malin GL, Quinlan-Jones E, et al. Percutaneous vesicoamniotic shunting versus conservative management for fetal lower urinary tract obstruction (PLUTO): a randomised trial. Lancet 2013;382(9903):1496–506.

51. Nassr AA, Shazly SAM, Abdelmagied AM, et al. Effectiveness of vesicoamniotic shunt in fetuses with congenital lower urinary tract obstruction: an updated systematic review and meta-analysis. Ultrasound Obstet Gynecol 2017;49(6):696–703.

52. Sananes N, Favre R, Koh CJ, et al. Urological fistulas after fetal cystoscopic laser ablation of posterior urethral valves: surgical technical aspects. Ultrasound Obstet Gynecol 2015;45(2):183–9.

53. Bienstock JL, Birsner ML, Coleman F, et al. Successful in utero intervention for bilateral renal agenesis. Obstet Gynecol 2014;124(2 Pt 2 Suppl 1):413–5.

54. Sheldon CR, Kim ED, Chandra P, et al. Two infants with bilateral renal agenesis who were bridged by chronic peritoneal dialysis to kidney transplantation. Pediatr Transpl 2019;23(6):e13532.

55. Polzin WJ, Lim FY, Habli M, et al. Use of an amnioport to maintain amniotic fluid volume in fetuses with oligohydramnios secondary to lower urinary tract obstruction or fetal renal anomalies. Fetal Diagn Ther 2017;41(1):51–7.

56. Warring SK, Novoa V, Shazly S, et al. Serial amnioinfusion as regenerative therapy for pulmonary hypoplasia in fetuses with intrauterine renal failure or severe renal anomalies: systematic review and future perspectives. Mayo Clin Proc Innov Qual Outcomes 2020;4(4):391–409.

57. Riddle S, Habli M, Tabbah S, et al. Contemporary outcomes of patients with isolated bilateral renal agenesis with and without fetal intervention. Fetal Diagn Ther 2020;47(9):675–81.

58. Werner EF, Han CS, Burd I, et al. Evaluating the cost-effectiveness of prenatal surgery for myelomeningocele: a decision analysis. Ultrasound Obstet Gynecol 2012;40(2):158–64.

59. Sugarman J, Anderson J, Baschat AA, et al. Ethical considerations concerning amnioinfusions for treating fetal bilateral renal agenesis. Obstet Gynecol 2018; 131(1):130–4.

60. O'Hare EM, Jelin AC, Miller JL, et al. Amnioinfusions to treat early onset anhydramnios caused by renal anomalies: background and rationale for the renal anhydramnios fetal therapy trial. Fetal Diagn Ther 2019;45(6):365–72.

61. Teh JC, Frieling ML, Sienna JL, et al. Attitudes of caregivers to management of end-stage renal disease in infants. Perit Dial Int 2011;31(4):459–65.

62. Carey WA, Martz KL, Warady BA. Outcome of patients initiating chronic peritoneal dialysis during the first year of life. Pediatrics 2015;136(3):e615–22.

63. Neu AM, Sander A, Borzych-Duzalka D, et al. Comorbidities in chronic pediatric peritoneal dialysis patients: a report of the International Pediatric Peritoneal Dialysis Network. Perit Dial Int 2012;32(4):410–8.

64. Lantos JD, Warady BA. The evolving ethics of infant dialysis. Pediatr Nephrol 2013;28(10):1943–7.

65. Ethics and the care of critically ill infants and children. American academy of pediatrics committee on Bioethics. Pediatrics 1996;98(1):149–52.

66. Galla JH. Clinical practice guideline on shared decision-making in the appropriate initiation of and withdrawal from dialysis. The Renal Physicians Association and the American Society of Nephrology. J Am Soc Nephrol 2000;11(7):1340–2.

In Utero Therapy for Congenital Diaphragmatic Hernia

Marisa E. Schwab, MD[a,b], Hanmin Lee, MD[a], KuoJen Tsao, MD[c,*]

KEYWORDS

- In utero therapy • Congenital diaphragmatic hernia • Fetal surgery

KEY POINTS

- Congenital diaphragmatic hernia is associated with high mortality and long-term morbidity, making it an ideal disease for fetal intervention.
- The Tracheal Occlusion To Accelerate Lung growth trial showed that fetal endoscopic tracheal occlusion significantly improved survival for fetuses with severe but not moderate congenital diaphragmatic hernia.
- Fetal endoscopic tracheal occlusion is still associated with high rates of prematurity.
- Technical improvements in fetal endoscopic tracheal occlusion and preclinical studies of medical therapies such as sildenafil, amniotic fluid stem cell-derived extracellular vesicles, and transamniotic stem cell therapy are promising.

INTRODUCTION

Congenital diaphragmatic hernia (CDH) is an embryological defect in the diaphragm that allows abdominal viscera to herniate into the thoracic cavity. CDH is thought to occur in approximately 2.6 to 3.2 per 10,000 live births.[1,2] The exact pathogenesis of CDH remains poorly understood; the current leading hypothesis is that a defect in the retinoid signaling occurs before 10 weeks of gestation, leading to developmental abnormalities of the pleuropulmonary fold.[3] There is increasing evidence that genetic variants can play a role in the pathogenesis of CDH. Approximately one-third of patients are now thought to have an identifiable genetic etiology, such as cytogenetic abnormalities, copy number variants, and single gene variants.[4–6]

[a] Division of Pediatric Surgery, University of California San Francisco, 550 16th Street, San Francisco, San Francisco, CA 94158, USA; [b] Department of Surgery, University of California, San Francisco, 505 Parnassus Avenue, San Francisco, CA 94143, USA; [c] Department of Pediatric Surgery and Obstetrics, Gynecology & Reproductive Sciences, McGovern Medical School at the University of Texas Health Science Center at Houston, 6410 Fannin Street, Suite 950, Houston, TX 77030, USA
* Corresponding author.
E-mail address: KuoJen.tsao@uth.tmc.edu

Clin Perinatol 49 (2022) 863–872
https://doi.org/10.1016/j.clp.2022.07.008
0095-5108/22/© 2022 Elsevier Inc. All rights reserved.

The mortality for fetuses diagnosed with CDH remains high despite advances in perinatal care and the introduction of extracorporeal membrane oxygenation (ECMO) as a bridge to surgical repair. In the United States, survival is approximately 70% at specialized tertiary care centers.[7,8] However, published survival rates often do not account for the hidden mortality of fetuses with CDH who die in utero or at birth.[9,10]

Fetuses with CDH have abnormal lung development and resulting pulmonary hypertension, which lead to persistent fetal circulation (also known as persistent pulmonary hypertension), cardiorespiratory failure, and fetal or neonatal death. The severity of pulmonary hypoplasia and hypertension are the main determinants of survival, and extensive research has been dedicated to improving the growth of the hypoplastic lungs before they are needed for gas exchange at birth. Given the prenatal diagnosis and disease severity associated with significant long-term morbidities, CDH was one of the first congenital anomalies to be targeted for fetal intervention, at the University of California, San Francisco (UCSF) in 1990.[11,12]

PRENATAL DIAGNOSIS OF CONGENITAL DIAPHRAGMATIC HERNIA

Establishing the severity of disease and associated prognosis prenatally is critical because it can inform what, if any, fetal therapies are available. Prenatal diagnosis has been associated with decreased mortality.[13] Historically, given the risks of fetal intervention such as preterm premature rupture of the membranes and preterm birth, only women pregnant with a fetus with a severe or lethal prognosis were offered fetal intervention options.

As prenatal imaging has improved over time, it has enhanced the ability to diagnose fetuses with congenital anomalies and enable the risk stratification of fetuses with CDH. Additionally, care must be taken on all prenatal imaging studies to look for additional anomalies that may be present in fetuses with CDH. Ultrasound examination has been the gold standard imaging technique for the diagnosis of CDH with a prenatal detection rate of more than 60%.[14] Ultrasound examination is useful to evaluate characteristics such as lung size, liver and stomach position, and the lung-to-head ratio (LHR). However, ultrasound examination is limited by user dependency and the lack of standardized ultrasound methods and reporting. Several groups have attempted to standardize ultrasound evaluations and reports for CDH.[15,16]

Fetal MRI is a more recent imaging modality that is not as user dependent and less affected by fetal movement and maternal body habitus.[17] MRI also provides more accurate lung volumes, liver position, and herniation volumes.[14] Moreover, MRI provides a detailed evaluation of the size and location of the diaphragmatic defect.[18] However, MRI remains costly and not widely available, and has not been widely studied in the CDH population. Ultrasound examination thus remains the most commonly used imaging modality to screen for and diagnose CDH.[18]

Ultrasound examination is used to calculate the LHR, defined as the area of the contralateral lung at the level of the 4-chamber view of the heart divided by the head circumference. Because the fetal lung and head grow at different speeds, the LHR increases with advancing gestational age. An LHR of less than 1.0 with liver herniated in the chest at 24 weeks gestation has traditionally been the threshold for a high likelihood of perinatal mortality.[19,20] The observed-to-expected (o/e) LHR was developed to normalize for gestational age, calculated as a percentage of the expected LHR based on a healthy fetus of the same gestational age.[21] In the Tracheal Occlusion To Accelerate Lung growth (TOTAL) trial, moderate CDH was defined as an o/e LHR of 25.0% to 34.9%, irrespective of liver position, or 35.0% to 44.9%

with intrathoracic liver herniation, and severe CDH was defined as an o/e LHR of less than 25%, irrespective of liver position.[22,23]

Other measurements that can be performed using ultrasound or MRI are total fetal lung volume (TFLV), percent-predicted lung volume, and o/e TFLV. These measurements are more accurate with MRI and when corrected for gestational age (o/e TFLV). Recent studies suggest lung volumes may more accurately predict the severity of pulmonary hypoplasia with regards to survival and defect type compared with the o/e LHR.[24]

However, there is wide variability among fetal treatment centers in the prenatal assessment of patients with CDH.[25] A survey of all 36 members of the North American Fetal Therapy Network revealed that the method of measuring LHR varied, with 58% of centers using a trace method, 25% using the longest axis, and 17% using an anterior–posterior method. Moreover, although 78% used fetal MRI, there was significant variability in how fetal lung volumes were measured. The authors concluded that there is a strong need for standardization of the prenatal workup of fetuses with CDH.

Other prenatal imaging factors associated with a worse prognosis include liver herniation, the absence of a hernia sac,[26] and intrathoracic stomach herniation.[27,28] However, when agreement for sonographic stomach positioning in left CDH was retrospectively determined across North American Fetal Therapy Network, there was poor agreement among expert participants. Liver herniation, traditionally described as liver up or liver down, can now be quantified as the ratio of herniated liver volume to the thoracic cavity size, or the percentage of liver that is herniated into the thoracic cavity.[14]

Despite the growing amount of research pertaining to the prenatal diagnosis and prognosis of CDH, a recent survey of maternal–fetal medicine specialists revealed that only 45% consider prenatal prediction of neonatal outcomes reliable, yet 80% will still perform a severity assessment in their clinical practice.[29]

IN UTERO THERAPY FOR CONGENITAL DIAPHRAGMATIC HERNIA
History

The first model of CDH was a fetal lamb in which Dr Michael Harrison's group at UCSF created a diaphragmatic defect at 100 days gestation that was corrected at 120 days gestation. These first attempts at in utero correction of CDH were mostly fatal owing to kinking of the umbilical vein after the abdominal viscera were decreased. After an abdominoplasty incision was used to relieve the intra-abdominal pressure, there was improved viability and compensatory lung growth and development, allowing survival of the lamb neonate.[30] Based on these results, Dr Harrison performed the first open surgery in a human fetus with CDH in 1990, which involved the creation of an abdominal silo to accommodate the reduced viscera and prevent compression of the umbilical vessels.[11] Dr Harrison's group subsequently published a prospective trial comparing 4 fetuses treated with open repair with 7 patients repaired postnatally.[12,31] They found no difference in survival between the fetal surgery group and the postnatally treated comparison group (75% vs 86%). Fetal surgery patients were born more prematurely than the comparison group (32 weeks of gestation vs 38 weeks of gestation). Moreover, the duration of ventilatory support and the need for ECMO were equivalent in the fetal surgery group and the postnatally treated comparison group. These results drove the search for less invasive repair methods, as well as better prenatal stratification of disease severity. The concept of tracheal occlusion to stimulate fetal lung development was discovered in the 1970s in a fetal lamb.[32] Harrison and colleagues[33] applied it to the CDH model after observing that pulmonary hyperplasia developed in fetuses with congenital high airway obstruction syndrome. In the fetal lamb model, tracheal occlusion was achieved by suture ligation, foam-cuffed endotracheal tubes, or expandable foam inserts, and led to decreased herniation of abdominal contents, increased lung volume, and improved postnatal cardiopulmonary function.[34–36]

Based on these successful preclinical studies, in utero tracheal occlusion was first applied in humans in 1996: a metallic tracheal clip was placed across the fetal trachea via maternal laparotomy and open hysterotomy.[37] The clip was removed during an ex utero intrapartum therapy procedure, in which placental support was maintained until a patent airway was established. Unfortunately, this approach led to high rates of mortality, morbidity, and preterm labor related to the hysterotomy, as well as tracheal stenosis. A minimally invasive technique for tracheal clipping was introduced in 1997 to decrease the morbidity associated with an open hysterotomy.[38] Yet, clipping was still frequently associated with airway complications, such as stenosis and vocal cord paralysis.

Fetal Endoscopic Tracheal Occlusion

Despite the disappointing results with fetal tracheal clipping, fetal surgeon–scientists continued to believe that tracheal occlusion could improve outcomes of fetuses with severe CDH. Fetal endoscopic tracheal occlusion (FETO) was developed as a minimally invasive method to obstruct the fetal airway, wherein a detachable silicone balloon was placed with the use of fetal bronchoscopy through a single 4- to 5-mm uterine port. Given encouraging initial results,[39] the UCSF group conducted a randomized controlled trial comparing endoscopic tracheal occlusion to standard postnatal care in fetuses with severe CDH (LHR of <1.5 between 22 and 27 weeks, liver up).[40] The trial was closed early after 24 patients had been enrolled, owing to the finding that tracheal occlusion did not improve survival or morbidity rates and was associated with higher rates of premature rupture of the membranes and preterm delivery. The improved survival in the standard postnatal treatment group was thought to be due to improved perinatal care during the observation period. The FETO technique continued to be refined and Deprest and colleagues[41] published the first multicenter study out of Europe of 20 fetuses that underwent FETO. They reported a 50% survival to discharge and found that improved survival coincided with their increasing experience, specifically related to a decreased incidence of postoperative amniorrhexis, later delivery, and a change in the policy on the timing of removal of the balloon from intrapartum to the prenatal period.[41]

In its current form, FETO involves the percutaneous placement of a 3.3-mm cannula through the maternal abdominal wall and uterus, directed toward the fetal mouth.[42] A deflated, detachable balloon is passed through a working channel in the fetoscope. The balloon is inserted past the vocal cords and positioned above the carina before inflation. Ultrasound examination is used to confirm appropriate positioning. The procedure is performed under local maternal anesthetic and fetal anesthesia including neuromuscular blockade. The balloon is placed at 27 to 29 weeks of gestation for severe cases and 30 to 32 weeks for moderate cases.[42] The mother is followed weekly before balloon removal at approximately 34 weeks gestation, ideally. Balloon retrieval is performed using fetoscopic retrieval, ultrasound-guided percutaneous puncture, or tracheoscopic removal on placental circulation during cesarean section or, at last resort, immediately postnatal.[42] The pregnancy can subsequently be managed expectantly with vaginal delivery.

The TOTAL study is the largest multicenter trial to date to evaluate the outcomes of fetuses with CDH treated with FETO compared with fetuses managed expectantly with standard postnatal repair. One arm included fetuses with moderate CDH[22] and the other arm encompassed fetuses with severe CDH.[23] Inclusion criteria were a single fetus with left-sided CDH without chromosomal or other major structural defects, predicted to have severe or moderate lung hypoplasia. Exclusion criteria were maternal medical or anatomic conditions precluding fetal intervention, an increased risk of preterm birth, and psychosocial factors that may impact parents' ability to adhere to the protocol. The primary outcome measure was survival to discharge from the neonatal intensive care unit. For moderate cases, the coprimary outcome variable was survival to 6 months of age without oxygen supplementation. In the moderate CDH group, 196 women were randomized to FETO at 30 to 32 weeks of gestation or to expectant care. There was no significant difference in the survival to discharge (63% in FETO group vs 50% in expectant group) or need for oxygen supplementation at 6 months. However, FETO increased the risk of preterm premature rupture of membranes (4% vs 12%; relative risk, 3.79) and the incidence of preterm birth (64% vs 22%; relative risk, 2.86).[22] In the severe CDH group, 80 women were randomly assigned to FETO at 27 to 29 weeks of gestation or to expectant care.[23] The mean gestational age at birth was 34.6 weeks in the FETO group versus 38.4 weeks in the expectant group. Fetuses who underwent FETO had a 4.5 times higher risk of preterm premature rupture of membranes and 2.6 times higher risk of preterm birth compared with the expectant management group. Major adverse events included 1 case of placental laceration during fetoscopic balloon removal, and 2 fetal deaths owing to the inability to reestablish the airway.[43] The severe CDH arm of the trial was stopped early owing to efficacy: 40% in the FETO group survived to discharge versus 15% in the expectant group. This benefit was sustained at 6 months of age.

Neither arm of the TOTAL trial was adequately powered to assess morbidities, which is critical given the high rate of premature births and known burden of long-term morbidity in the CDH patient population.[43] A second criticism was the low rate of ECMO use in the severe arm of the trial: 2 of 38 in the FETO and 11 of 38 in the control group underwent ECMO. Moreover, the 15% survival rate in the severe expectant group is significantly lower than that seen in some high-volume North American centers, which may be related to expertise in perinatal management.[43] There is concern about the widespread implementation of FETO given the known risk of perinatal death in cases of difficult balloon removal. It is crucial that FETO only be undertaken in specialist centers that have extensive experience in fetoscopy and a sufficient volume of CDH cases, are trained in balloon placement and removal, and have expertise in the management of pulmonary hypertension.[44]

A reanalysis using pooled data from the 2 arms of the TOTAL trial was performed to evaluate the heterogeneity of the treatment effect by observed over expected LHR and to investigate the effect of gestational age at the time of balloon insertion.[45] The adjusted odds ratio of FETO for survival to discharge was 1.78 (95% confidence interval, 1.05–3.01; $P = .031$). The additional effect of early balloon insertion was highly uncertain (adjusted odds ratio, 1.53; 95% confidence interval, 0.60–3.91; $P = .370$). When combining these 2 effects, the adjusted odds ratio of FETO with early balloon insertion was 2.73 (95% confidence interval, 1.15–6.49). The gestational age at delivery was on average 1.7 weeks earlier (95% confidence interval, 1.1–2.3) after FETO with late insertion and 3.2 weeks earlier (95% confidence interval, 2.3–4.1) after FETO with early insertion, compared with expectant management.[45] Deprest and colleagues concluded that the difference between results in the moderate and severe arms of the trial may be due to the difference in timing of balloon insertion. However, this could not be ascertained given the small sample size of confounding effect of disease severity.

Future Directions

There are several exciting therapies currently being investigated in the preclinical realm. Transplacental sildenafil, a phosphodiesterase-5 inhibitor, has been shown to have vasodilatory and anti-remodeling effects on the placental circulation in several CDH animal models.[46,47] Fetal pulmonary administration of amniotic fluid stem cell-derived extracellular vesicles is another promising approach.[48] Amniotic fluid stem cell-derived extracellular vesicles were shown by Zani's group to promote lung development and maturation in fetal rodent models of pulmonary hypoplasia (primary epithelial cells, organoids, explants, and in vivo).[49] Transamniotic stem cell therapy, the intra-amniotic administration of large amounts of select fetal-derived mesenchymal stem cells, is another experimental strategy for fetal treatment of CDH.[50] In a CDH mouse model, transamniotic stem cell therapy led to a significant downregulation of endothelial nitric oxide synthase and endothelin receptor expression, as well as decreased arteriole thickness. Donor amniotic fluid-derived mesenchymal stem cells were found to be circulating in the bone marrow and umbilical cord.[50]

Randomized clinical trials have been difficult to conduct in the field of fetal medicine, owing to tenuous patient recruitment from a small patient population given the rareness and need for timely prenatal diagnosis, the quality of observational studies, and the potential loss of equipoise.[29] Regulatory guidance on what constitutes an appropriate risk–benefit ratio in fetal therapy trials is lacking.[51] The National Institutes of Health recently proposed a new ethical framework for fetal therapy research. They advocate for expanding benefits to include evidence-based psychosocial effects of fetal therapies, such as improved mobility and independent functioning after fetal myelomeningocele repair. Furthermore, instead of the traditional categorical risks and/or benefit thresholds for assessing fetal therapy research (such as limiting fetal intervention to life-threatening conditions), they propose that the individual risks for the pregnant patient and her fetus should be justified by the specific potential benefits to them.[51]

Educating providers about the nuances of fetal interventions is also essential. A survey of knowledge, attitude, and practice of more than 300 registrants at the 2018 World Congress in Fetal Medicine by the authors of the TOTAL trial found that overall knowledge of CDH and FETO was high.[29] Overall, 43% of maternal–fetal medicine specialists refer families for FETO only within the context of a randomized clinical trial, whereas 32% offer FETO upon parent request. This study highlighted that many fetal clinicians face significant personal and practical dilemmas when counseling families with a prenatal diagnosis of CDH.

Technical advances may help improve FETO by decrease known adverse events. The "Smart-TO"-balloon (BS Medical Tech Industry, Niederroedern, France) has a magnetic valve that opens by exposure to a strong magnetic field such as an MRI scanner, and after deflation is swallowed by the fetus or exits the fetal mouth into the amniotic fluid.[44] After successful large animal studies,[52,53] Deprest and colleagues are now pursuing a first-in-human trial.

An additional consideration is whether fetal intervention should be expanded to fetuses with CDH and additional anomalies. Up to 25% of patients with CDH have associated structural anomalies such as cardiac defects, excluding cases with an identified genetic syndrome or karyotype abnormality.[54] Yet, the TOTAL trials and most centers define other structural anomalies as exclusion criteria for fetal intervention. Only a handful of case series reporting patients with associated cardiac and lung anomalies that underwent FETO are published to this date.[55,56] Finally, there is a need for multicenter collaborations and database sharing, given the relatively small number of patients at each center. There has been a call for prospective registration of cases treated with FETO, to improve our understanding of the appropriate duration of balloon occlusion as well as the impact of preterm delivery.[44]

Best practices

- What is the current practice for patients with CDH: Fetal therapy is an option for patients with a fetus diagnosed with severe CDH.
- What changes in current practice are likely to improve outcomes? Improved methods for early diagnosis and disease stratification of fetuses with CDH.
- Is there a Clinical Algorithm? No clinical algorithms currently exist.

CLINICS CARE POINTS

- Fetal ultrasound examination and MRI can be used to predict severity of disease with measurements of o/e LHR, o/e TFLV, and ratio of herniated liver volume to the thoracic cavity size.
- In the largest clinical trial to date, FETO has been shown to improve survival for fetuses with severe CDH. However, no significant improvement was seen in fetuses with moderate CDH.
- FETO and future fetal interventions for CDH should only be performed in high volume fetal treatment centers with expertise in perinatal management of CDH.

DISCLOSURE

None of the authors have any commercial or financial conflicts of interest. There were no funding sources.

REFERENCES

1. Politis MD, Bermejo-Sanchez E, Canfield MA, et al. Prevalence and mortality in children with congenital diaphragmatic hernia: a multicountry study. Ann Epidemiol 2021;56:61–69 e3.
2. Shanmugam H, Brunelli L, Botto LD, et al. Epidemiology and prognosis of congenital diaphragmatic hernia: a population-based cohort study in Utah. Birth Defects Res 2017;109(18):1451–9.
3. Chiu PP. New insights into congenital diaphragmatic hernia - a surgeon's introduction to CDH Animal models. Front Pediatr 2014;2:36.
4. Kammoun M, Souche E, Brady P, et al. Genetic profile of isolated congenital diaphragmatic hernia revealed by targeted next-generation sequencing. Prenat Diagn 2018;38(9):654–63.
5. Slavotinek AM. The genetics of common disorders - congenital diaphragmatic hernia. Eur J Med Genet 2014;57(8):418–23.
6. Yu L, Sawle AD, Wynn J, et al. Increased burden of de novo predicted deleterious variants in complex congenital diaphragmatic hernia. Hum Mol Genet 2015;24(16):4764–73.
7. Zalla JM, Stoddard GJ, Yoder BA. Improved mortality rate for congenital diaphragmatic hernia in the modern era of management: 15 year experience in a single institution. J Pediatr Surg 2015;50(4):524–7.

8. Coughlin MA, Werner NL, Gajarski R, et al. Prenatally diagnosed severe CDH: mortality and morbidity remain high. J Pediatr Surg 2016;51(7):1091–5.

9. Harrison MR, Bjordal RI, Langmark F, et al. Congenital diaphragmatic hernia: the hidden mortality. J Pediatr Surg 1978;13(3):227–30.

10. Mah VK, Chiu P, Kim PC. Are we making a real difference? Update on 'hidden mortality' in the management of congenital diaphragmatic hernia. Fetal Diagn Ther 2011;29(1):40–5.

11. Harrison MR, Adzick NS, Longaker MT, et al. Successful repair in utero of a fetal diaphragmatic hernia after removal of herniated viscera from the left thorax. N Engl J Med 1990;322(22):1582–4.

12. Harrison MR, Adzick NS, Flake AW, et al. Correction of congenital diaphragmatic hernia in utero: VI. Hard-earned lessons. J Pediatr Surg 1993;28(10):1411–7 [discussion: 7-8].

13. Carmichael SL, Ma C, Lee HC, et al. Survival of infants with congenital diaphragmatic hernia in California: impact of hospital, clinical, and sociodemographic factors. J Perinatol 2020;40(6):943–51.

14. Kovler ML, Jelin EB. Fetal intervention for congenital diaphragmatic hernia. Semin Pediatr Surg 2019;28(4):150818.

15. Canadian Congenital Diaphragmatic Hernia C, Puligandla PS, Skarsgard ED, et al. Diagnosis and management of congenital diaphragmatic hernia: a clinical practice guideline. CMAJ 2018;190(4):E103–12.

16. Russo FM, Cordier AG, De Catte L, et al. Proposal for standardized prenatal ultrasound assessment of the fetus with congenital diaphragmatic hernia by the European reference network on rare inherited and congenital anomalies (ERNICA). Prenat Diagn 2018;38(9):629–37.

17. Oluyomi-Obi T, Van Mieghem T, Ryan G. Fetal imaging and therapy for CDH-Current status. Semin Pediatr Surg 2017;26(3):140–6.

18. Mehollin-Ray AR, Cassady CI, Cass DL, et al. Fetal MR imaging of congenital diaphragmatic hernia. Radiographics 2012;32(4):1067–84.

19. Oluyomi-Obi T, Kuret V, Puligandla P, et al. Antenatal predictors of outcome in prenatally diagnosed congenital diaphragmatic hernia (CDH). J Pediatr Surg 2017;52(5):881–8.

20. Yang SH, Nobuhara KK, Keller RL, et al. Reliability of the lung-to-head ratio as a predictor of outcome in fetuses with isolated left congenital diaphragmatic hernia at gestation outside 24-26 weeks. Am J Obstet Gynecol 2007;197(1):30 e1–7.

21. Petroze RT, Caminsky NG, Trebichavsky J, et al. Prenatal prediction of survival in congenital diaphragmatic hernia: an audit of postnatal outcomes. J Pediatr Surg 2019;54(5):925–31.

22. Deprest JA, Benachi A, Gratacos E, et al. Randomized trial of fetal surgery for moderate left diaphragmatic hernia. N Engl J Med 2021;385(2):119–29.

23. Deprest JA, Nicolaides KH, Benachi A, et al. Randomized trial of fetal surgery for severe left diaphragmatic hernia. N Engl J Med 2021;385(2):107–18.

24. Kim AG, Norwitz G, Karmakar M, et al. Discordant prenatal ultrasound and fetal MRI in CDH: wherein lies the truth? J Pediatr Surg 2020;55(9):1879–84.

25. Perrone EE, Abbasi N, Cortes MS, et al. Prenatal assessment of congenital diaphragmatic hernia at north American Fetal Therapy Network Centers: a continued plea for standardization. Prenat Diagn 2021;41(2):200–6.

26. Oliver ER, DeBari SE, Adams SE, et al. Congenital diaphragmatic hernia sacs: prenatal imaging and associated postnatal outcomes. Pediatr Radiol 2019;49(5):593–9.

27. Didier RA, Oliver ER, Rungsiprakarn P, et al. Decreased neonatal morbidity in 'stomach-down' left congenital diaphragmatic hernia: implications of prenatal ultrasound diagnosis for counseling and postnatal management. Ultrasound Obstet Gynecol 2021;58(5):744–9.
28. Verla MA, Style CC, Mehollin-Ray AR, et al. Prenatal imaging features and postnatal factors associated with gastrointestinal morbidity in congenital diaphragmatic hernia. Fetal Diagn Ther 2020;47(4):252–60.
29. Vergote S, Pizzolato D, Russo F, et al. The TOTAL trial dilemma: a survey among professionals on equipoise regarding fetal therapy for severe congenital diaphragmatic hernia. Prenat Diagn 2021;41(2):179–89.
30. Adzick NS, Outwater KM, Harrison MR, et al. Correction of congenital diaphragmatic hernia in utero. IV. An early gestational fetal lamb model for pulmonary vascular morphometric analysis. J Pediatr Surg 1985;20(6):673–80.
31. Harrison MR, Adzick NS, Bullard KM, et al. Correction of congenital diaphragmatic hernia in utero VII: a prospective trial. J Pediatr Surg 1997;32(11):1637–42.
32. Alcorn D, Adamson TM, Lambert TF, et al. Morphological effects of chronic tracheal ligation and drainage in the fetal lamb lung. J Anat 1977;123(Pt 3):649–60.
33. Hedrick MH, Ferro MM, Filly RA, et al. Congenital high airway obstruction syndrome (CHAOS): a potential for perinatal intervention. J Pediatr Surg 1994;29(2):271–4.
34. Bealer JF, Skarsgard ED, Hedrick MH, et al. The 'PLUG' odyssey: adventures in experimental fetal tracheal occlusion. J Pediatr Surg 1995;30(2):361–4 [discussion: 4–5].
35. DiFiore JW, Fauza DO, Slavin R, et al. Experimental fetal tracheal ligation reverses the structural and physiological effects of pulmonary hypoplasia in congenital diaphragmatic hernia. J Pediatr Surg 1994;29(2):248–56 [discussion: 56-7].
36. Hedrick MH, Estes JM, Sullivan KM, et al. Plug the lung until it grows (PLUG): a new method to treat congenital diaphragmatic hernia in utero. J Pediatr Surg 1994;29(5):612–7.
37. Harrison MR, Adzick NS, Flake AW, et al. Correction of congenital diaphragmatic hernia in utero VIII: response of the hypoplastic lung to tracheal occlusion. J Pediatr Surg 1996;31(10):1339–48.
38. VanderWall KJ, Skarsgard ED, Filly RA, et al. Fetendo-clip: a fetal endoscopic tracheal clip procedure in a human fetus. J Pediatr Surg 1997;32(7):970–2.
39. Harrison MR, Albanese CT, Hawgood SB, et al. Fetoscopic temporary tracheal occlusion by means of detachable balloon for congenital diaphragmatic hernia. Am J Obstet Gynecol 2001;185(3):730–3.
40. Harrison MR, Keller RL, Hawgood SB, et al. A randomized trial of fetal endoscopic tracheal occlusion for severe fetal congenital diaphragmatic hernia. N Engl J Med 2003;349(20):1916–24.
41. Deprest J, Jani J, Gratacos E, et al. Fetal intervention for congenital diaphragmatic hernia: the European experience. Semin perinatology 2005;29(2):94–103.
42. Perrone EE, Deprest JA. Fetal endoscopic tracheal occlusion for congenital diaphragmatic hernia: a narrative review of the history, current practice, and future directions. Transl Pediatr 2021;10(5):1448–60.
43. Deprest J, Flake A. How should fetal surgery for congenital diaphragmatic hernia be implemented in the post-TOTAL trial era: a discussion. Prenat Diagn 2022;42(3):301–9.
44. Russo F, Benachi A, Gratacos E, et al. Antenatal management of congenital diaphragmatic hernia: what's next. Prenat Diagn 2022;42(3):291–300.

45. Van Calster B, Benachi A, Nicolaides KH, et al. The randomized Tracheal Occlusion to Accelerate Lung growth (TOTAL)-trials on fetal surgery for congenital diaphragmatic hernia: reanalysis using pooled data. Am J Obstet Gynecol 2022; 226(4):560 e1–e24.
46. Russo FM, De Bie F, Hodges R, et al. Sildenafil for antenatal treatment of congenital diaphragmatic hernia: from bench to bedside. Curr Pharm Des 2019;25(5): 601–8.
47. Russo FM, Da Cunha M, Jimenez J, et al. Complementary effect of maternal sildenafil and fetal tracheal occlusion improves lung development in the rabbit model of congenital diaphragmatic hernia. Ann Surg 2022;275(3):e586–95.
48. Figueira RL, Antounians L, Zani-Ruttenstock E, et al. Fetal lung regeneration using stem cell-derived extracellular vesicles: a new frontier for pulmonary hypoplasia secondary to congenital diaphragmatic hernia. Prenat Diagn 2022;42(3): 364–72.
49. Antounians L, Catania VD, Montalva L, et al. Fetal lung underdevelopment is rescued by administration of amniotic fluid stem cell extracellular vesicles in rodents. Sci Transl Med 2021;13(590):1–12.
50. Chalphin AV, Lazow SP, Labuz DF, et al. Transamniotic stem cell therapy for experimental congenital diaphragmatic hernia: structural, transcriptional, and cell kinetics analyses in the nitrogen model. Fetal Diagn Ther 2021;48(5):381–91.
51. Hendriks S, Grady C, Wasserman D, et al. A new ethical framework for assessing the unique challenges of fetal therapy trials. Am J Bioeth 2022;22(3):45–61.
52. Basurto D, Sananes N, Bleeser T, et al. Safety and efficacy of smart tracheal occlusion device in diaphragmatic hernia lamb model. Ultrasound Obstet Gynecol 2021;57(1):105–12.
53. Sananes N, Regnard P, Mottet N, et al. Evaluation of a new balloon for fetal endoscopic tracheal occlusion in the nonhuman primate model. Prenat Diagn 2019; 39(5):403–8.
54. Ruano R, Ali RA, Patel P, et al. Fetal endoscopic tracheal occlusion for congenital diaphragmatic hernia: indications, outcomes, and future directions. Obstet Gynecol Surv 2014;69(3):147–58.
55. Jani JC, Nicolaides KH, Gratacos E, et al. Severe diaphragmatic hernia treated by fetal endoscopic tracheal occlusion. Ultrasound Obstet Gynecol 2009;34(3): 304–10.
56. Seravalli V, Jelin EB, Miller JL, et al. Fetoscopic tracheal occlusion for treatment of non-isolated congenital diaphragmatic hernia. Prenat Diagn 2017;37(10):1046–9.

Updates in Neonatal Extracorporeal Membrane Oxygenation and the Artificial Placenta

Brianna L. Spencer, MD[a], George B. Mychaliska, MD[b],*

KEYWORDS

- ECLS • Neonatal ECMO • Preemie ECMO • Artificial placenta

KEY POINTS

- Extracorporeal life support is a lifesaving technique for neonates with respiratory and/or cardiac failure.
- Technological and medical advances have paved the way for applying the benefits of ECMO to support premature infants.
- Recreation of the fetal environment with an artificial placenta/womb is promising for improving morbidity and mortality of extremely premature infants.

INTRODUCTION

Extracorporeal life support (ECLS), initially performed in neonates, is now commonly used for both pediatric and adult patients requiring pulmonary and/or cardiac support.[1] ECLS can provide hemodynamic stability and gas exchange. Although it is not curative, it serves as a bridge to organ recovery or definitive therapy. Originally developed for term and near-term infants, there is experience with "preemie ECMO" (29–33 weeks estimated gestational age [EGA]) that demonstrates clinical feasibility.[2] For extremely premature infants less than 28 weeks EGA, an artificial placenta (AP) has been developed, which recreates the fetal environment, preserves fetal circulation, and provides protection and the milieu for normal organ development. This approach is currently investigational but clinical translation is promising. In this article, we discuss the status and advances in neonatal and "preemie ECMO" and the development of an AP and its potential use in extremely premature infants.

[a] Department of Surgery, University of Michigan, Michigan Medicine, Ann Arbor, MI, USA;
[b] Section of Pediatric Surgery, Department of Surgery, Fetal Diagnosis and Treatment Center, University of Michigan Medical School, C.S. Mott Children's Hospital, Ann Arbor, MI, USA
* Corresponding author. Department of Surgery, Pediatric Surgery, 2101 Taubman Center, 1500 E. Medical Center Drive, Ann Arbor, MI 48109
E-mail address: mychalis@med.umich.edu

Clin Perinatol 49 (2022) 873–891
https://doi.org/10.1016/j.clp.2022.07.002
0095-5108/22/© 2022 Elsevier Inc. All rights reserved.

NEONATAL EXTRACORPOREAL LIFE SUPPORT
Indications

ECLS has specific indications in the neonatal population, and this review focuses on neonatal patients with respiratory and combined respiratory/cardiac failure. Patients with congenital heart disease are beyond the scope of this review. Patients with severe respiratory and/or cardiac failure with high likelihood of mortality, as well as an etiology that is reversible are considered for neonatal ECMO.[3] Common neonatal indications for ECMO include congenital diaphragmatic hernia (CDH), meconium aspiration syndrome, pulmonary hypertension, and sepsis. CDH, meconium aspiration, and persistent pulmonary hypertension encompass approximately 75% of respiratory ECMO cases.[3] Neonates typically meet the following criteria: (1) inadequate oxygen delivery to tissues with maximal therapy, (2) severe hypoxic respiratory failure, (3) elevated oxygenation index (OI), and/or (4) severe pulmonary hypertension.[3] For patients in respiratory failure, the most common metric is OI.[4] An OI greater than 40 correlates with an 80% mortality and ECMO should be considered for neonates with an OI greater than 25.[5,6] Additionally, neonates with hypercapnic respiratory failure, sustaining a pH from 7 to 7.25 may benefit from ECMO (**Table 1**).[7] It should be noted that sudden hypercapnic respiratory failure with preserved oxygenation should prompt consideration of a distal ETT mucous occlusion that behaves physiologically like a one-way valve.

Contraindications

Contraindications to neonatal ECMO include the following: (1) no expectation of recovery from organ failure, (2) chromosomal abnormality not compatible with life, (3) uncontrolled bleeding, (4) vessel size too small for cannulation, and (5) severe brain bleeding/damage. Relative contraindications include EGA less than 34 weeks and weight less than 2.0 kg given early clinical experience with poor outcomes[8] (see **Table 1**). More recent advances have established the feasibility of "preemie ECMO" for infants 29 to 33 weeks EGA.[2] Typically, patients requiring ECLS need prolonged high ventilator settings, which can be associated with ventilator-induced lung injury and mortality. Extended ventilation greater than 7 days was initially a contraindication to ECLS but this has been extended to 14 days with no change in survival rates.[9–12] These guidelines may be further modified depending on specific ventilatory strategies used. Many infants treated by "gentle ventilation" strategies for longer than 2 weeks should still be considered for ECLS on a case-by-case basis selecting patients anticipated to have lung recovery.

Table 1
Indications and contraindications of neonatal ECMO

Indications	Contraindications
Oxygenation index >25	Lethal chromosomes or another anomaly
Pao_2 to Fio_2 ration <60	Poor predicted neurologic outcome/irreversible brain injury
pH < 7.25	Uncontrolled bleeding
Shock	ICH > Grade III
A-a DO2 > 500 mm Hg	Advanced multiorgan system failure
Pplat > 30 cm H_2O	Ventilation > 40 d
	Weight < 1.5 kg
	EGA < 29 wk

Adapted from Fallon BP, Gadepalli SK, Hirschl RB. Pediatric and neonatal extracorporeal life support: current state and continuing evolution. Pediatr Surg Int. 2021 Jan;37(1):17-35.

ECMO Outcomes

In the 2020 ELSO registry, the overall survival for neonatal patients who received ECMO for respiratory disease is 73%.[3] However, survival rates vary by diagnosis as follows: meconium aspiration (92%), persistent pulmonary hypertension (73%), sepsis (60%), CDH (50%), and prematurity (50%).[3]

Neonates who survive ECMO are at risk for several long-term health issues

Neurologic complications are common secondary to preexisting risk of bleeding, systemic anticoagulation, carotid and/or internal jugular (IJ) ligation, and physiologic perturbations.[13] Twenty-five percent of neonates requiring ECMO develop neurophysiologic deficits.[14] Not surprisingly, patients with neurologic complications have an increased mortality rate.[13] At 7 years of age, half of the neonatal ECMO survivors sustained some form of disability that persisted over time. One study of 135 patients found that although the patients' intelligence level fell within the normal range, they had increased behavioral problems in school.[15] Neonates requiring ECMO for CDH experience a spectrum of long-term health problems including respiratory, gastrointestinal, and neurologic complications. These complications correlate with the severity of CDH and duration of critical illness in the newborn period.

Mode of Support

Veno-arterial ECMO

The earliest mode of ECLS support was veno-arterial (VA) ECMO. VA ECMO was performed by open cut-down cannulation of the carotid artery and the IJ vein,[16,17] and it remains the most common method of cannulation for neonatal patients (**Fig. 1**). VA-ECMO provides both cardiac and pulmonary support and offloads the right side of the heart, which is particularly beneficial in patients with severe pulmonary hypertension. A major concern with VA ECMO is related to stroke risk and neurologic complications due to carotid artery ligation. Interestingly, differences in rates of neurologic complications and stroke related to age or cannulation site were not apparent after adjusting for other factors such as age, support type, severity of illness, in a study by Johnson and colleagues.[18] In a large study of 140 patients, Duggan found no difference in neurologic outcomes comparing carotid artery reconstruction versus ligation at the time of decannulation.[19] In a review of the ELSO registry in 2014, 21% neonates cannulated with VA ECMO sustained neurologic injuries. It is unclear if cerebral venous hypertension contributes to this neurologic injury after jugular cannulation.[20] In a retrospective review of 81 neonates treated with ECLS, 46% sustained frontal and temporoparietal white matter injury based on MRI.[21] Although the pattern of injury was similar between VA and VV modes, the frequency may be higher with VA ECMO. Finally, it should be noted that not all patients with MRI abnormalities develop significant clinical sequelae.

Veno-venous ECMO

Veno-venous (VV) ECMO provides respiratory support but does not provide direct cardiac support. Potential advantages to this cannulation method include preservation of the carotid artery, pulsatile blood flow and oxygenated coronary blood flow. There is a neurologic complication rate of 20% with neonatal VA ECMO, and these rates have been found to be lower with VV ECMO.[22] Ligation of the right carotid artery and jugular vein in VA ECMO may increase the risk of stroke.[23] Loss of pulsatile cerebral blood flow, decreased cerebral autoregulation, and circuit-associated emboli, or severe cardiorespiratory dysfunction during VA ECMO may explain the increased neurologic

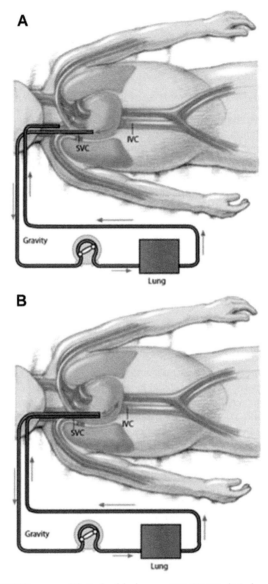

Fig. 1. (*A*) A VA ECMO versus (*B*) B double-lumen VV ECMO. (Frischer J.S., Stolar C.J.H., Hirschl R.B. (2020) Extracorporeal Membrane Oxygenation for Neonatal Respiratory Failure. In: Puri P. (eds) Pediatric Surgery. Springer, Berlin, Heidelberg. https://doi.org/10.1007/978-3-662-43588-5_58.)

complications compared with VV ECMO neonatal patients. In general, VV ECMO cannulation can be performed with 1 double-lumen cannula or 2 single-lumen cannulae (see **Fig. 1**). In neonates, dual-site cannulation was abandoned in the 1980s due to the small size of the femoral vein and concerns about limb morbidity. Placement of a right IJ double-lumen cannula avoids a second vessel access, and because the oxygenated blood enters the pulmonary vasculature, pulmonary artery vascular resistance is decreased.[24–26] The Origen double-lumen cannula was initially developed for

VV ECMO in the neonatal population. The Origen cannula was simple to insert via the right IJ cut-down technique without the need for fluoroscopy or echocardiography. However, a postoperative echocardiography was recommended to confirm position in the mid-right atrium with flow directed toward the tricuspid valve. Although effective, problems with this cannula included recirculation related, in part, to cannula design. In 2019, the Origen right atrial cannula was no longer produced.

Catheter Advances

In 2008, the Avalon dual-lumen bicaval cannula was developed as a single-site VV ECMO cannula. This cannula effectively drains blood from the inferior vena cava and superior vena cava and delivers oxygenated blood into the right atrium (**Fig. 2**B). This wire-reinforced cannula ranges in size from 13 to 31 French.[27] Because the distal catheter needs to land in the IVC, real-time imaging with fluoroscopy and echocardiography is required for safe and effective insertion. The Crescent cannula is a wire-enforced, bicaval cannula. The insertion site for the Crescent cannula is also in the RIJ (**Fig. 2**A). There are titanium markers along the cannula to allow for visualization with imaging. This is placed under fluoroscopy as well.[28] This catheter shows promise in the continued development of double-lumen cannulae for ECMO.[29]

Initial enthusiasm for the 13F Avalon catheter in neonates waned in light of safety and efficacy concerns. There is a short distance between the ICV/SVC holes and the right atrial infusion hole. As such, small changes in catheter position affect performance.[30] Although successfully performed in neonates by several groups,[31] several investigators expressed safety concerns, which eventually limited widespread adoption for neonates.[32]

Given safety concerns about the 13F Avalon cannula and the unavailability of the Origen cannula, ECMO centers transitioned to VA cannulation for most neonates in 2019. Due to this shift, there was resurgence in interest in the 2-cannula approach. This approach was studied in 11 patients from 2015 to 2019 with femoral vein and jugular access points. Because the femoral vein is small and ECMO flow rates are largely dependent on adequate drainage, they used the femoral vein for inflow and the jugular for drainage, which could accommodate a larger cannula. Nine out of 11 patients survived to home discharge, and although there was common femoral vein

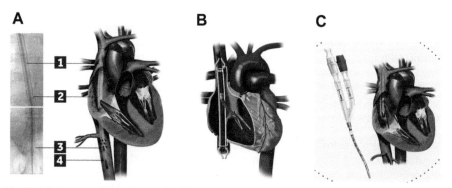

Fig. 2. (A) Crescent bicaval cannula. (B) Avalon cannula. (C) Crescent atrial cannula. ([A] Reproduced with permission of Medtronic, Inc., Minneapolis, MN; [B] *From* Hirose H, Yamane K, Marhefka G, Cavarocchi N. Right ventricular rupture and tamponade caused by malposition of the Avalon cannula for venovenous extracorporeal membrane oxygenation. J Cardiothorac Surg. 2012 Apr 20;7:36; and [C] *Courtesy of* MC3 Cardiopulmonary, Dexter, MI.)

occlusion, no clinical or functional deficit was noted in the cannulated limb at follow-up.[33]

In 2021, the Crescent* right atrial, jugular dual-lumen (13, 15, and 19 Fr) catheter was launched for clinical application (**Fig. 2**C). The 13 Fr catheter was designed for neonatal VV ECMO and is supplied with an introducer to facilitate wire-guided placement via Seldinger technique or cut down with an obturator. The design features include radiopaque markers to aid in positioning and axial orientation. The reinfusion port size, shape, and location were designed to optimize flow performance and minimize recirculation. Given the recent launch of this catheter, published data on safety and efficacy are not available but it is anticipated to increase the application of VV ECMO in neonates.

Anticoagulation: Monitoring and Treatment

Bleeding and thrombosis remain unsolved problems in the management of ECLS patients. The most common method of anticoagulation for neonatal ECMO remains continuous heparin infusion. There are many institutional protocols for regulating heparin levels in this population.[34] ATIII is required for heparin functionality, and in some institutions, it is monitored and replaced but should be used judiciously.[35] The main methods for monitoring anticoagulation are activated clotting time (ACT), prothrombin time (PTT) anti-Xa levels, and thromboelastography. ACT is most commonly used and can be performed at the bedside but there remain concerns about the accuracy and reliability of ACT in many clinical scenarios. As such, there has been an interest in other monitoring approaches. PTT measures intrinsic coagulation pathway and is a more specific measurement of heparin effect on the patient. Anti-Xa is the most specific, measuring the inhibition of Xa by heparin ATIII complexes. A retrospective review comparing ACT versus anti-Xa levels did not demonstrate any major differences between 2 groups or any increased complications.[36] Our center and others have adopted a hybrid approach adding anti-Xa measurements to routine ACT measurements in patients with complex coagulation scenarios. Although anti-Xa measurements seem promising, there is currently no consensus on which measurement is best.[37]

Alternative anticoagulants to heparin are currently being evaluated, including bivalirudin and argatroban. Because they are direct thrombin inhibitors, do not depend on ATIII and do not have the risk of HIT, they may provide more stable anticoagulation compared with heparin.[38] A literature review comparing bivalirudin to heparin overall demonstrated more stable coagulation profiles with similar thromboembolic events.[39-41] In one of the largest series of neonatal and pediatric patients on ECLS studying with bivalirudin, it was found to be a feasible anticoagulation option for patients who could not receive heparin.[42] Current data, primarily in the pediatric population, support the safety of bivalirudin, and many centers are adopting this approach.[43] Preliminary data in neonatal CDH patients suggest safety and efficacy[44] but further data are required in the neonatal population in order to make a definitive transition in practice.

Although there are new advances in improving anticoagulation with ECMO, all anticoagulation poses a bleeding risk especially in neonatal and "preemie" ECMO. The ECLS laboratory at the University of Michigan (UM) has developed a nitric oxide surface-based anticoagulation system to obviate systemic anticoagulation while on ECMO. The surface coating is based on S-nitroso-N-acetyl-l, L-penicillamine (SNAP). Nitric oxide is released from the SNAP-based polymer coatings for as long as 20 days and has been shown to prevent thrombosis.[45-48] Additionally, we found that adding argatroban to the coating reduces fibrin formation.[49] This technology will be essential for providing extracorporeal support to extremely premature infants for whom the risk of systemic anticoagulation is prohibitive.

Preemie ECMO

The application of ECMO in premature infants is limited by the increased risk for intracranial hemorrhage (ICH). The risk of ICH in premature infants on ECMO is high given the baseline ICH risks and requirement for systemic anticoagulation. Early studies with premature infants on ECMO found the risk of morbidity and mortality to be high[8]; however, recent experience demonstrates lower risks and clinical feasibility.[2,50,51] It was initially thought that neonates with weight less than 2 kg had significantly decreased survival due in part because of prematurity and size constraints to maintain adequate flows with small cannulas. Multiple studies have shown reasonable survival, as high as 40% in infants as small as 1.6 kg.[52,53]

The outcomes of all neonates with gestational ages 29 to 34 weeks on ECMO from 1976 to 2008 were evaluated by Church and colleagues. The survival of the 29 to 33-week EGA cohort was 48% compared with the clinically established 34-week EGA cohort at 58%. There was no significant difference in ICH rate but a statistically significant difference in the incidence of cerebral infarct (22% vs 16%). Although the rates of survival and cerebral infarction were worse for the more premature cohort, these differences were modest and clinically acceptable.[2]

Clinical Outcomes for Extremely Low Gestational Age Newborns

One in 10 infants in the United States is born prematurely (defined by less than 37 weeks EGA).[54] There is increasing risk of morbidity and mortality with extremely low gestational age newborns (ELGANs) defined as neonates born at less than 28 weeks EGA. This mortality risk is up to 38.4% for ELGANs, compared with 0.2% for full-term infants.[54] Prematurity remains an unsolved problem and a great opportunity exists to improve outcomes in this vulnerable population.

The poor outcomes for this patient population stem from 2 interrelated factors: organ immaturity and the unintended iatrogenic consequences of conventional medical treatments. The positive-pressure ventilation required by many of these infants has been associated with negative physiologic effects on the lung, including decreased surfactant production,[55] increased pulmonary vascular resistance, and activation of local and systemic inflammatory responses.[55] Cardiac output is also negatively affected due to the decreased pulmonary blood flow.[56] The associated elevation in intrathoracic and thus intracranial pressure has been associated with an increased risk of intraventricular hemorrhage.[57] Finally, the high fraction of inspired oxygen (Fio_2) that these patients require is a major contributor to retinopathy of prematurity (ROP).[58] Other predictable complications of ELGANs include sepsis and necrotizing enterocolitis (NEC).

A greater appreciation for the deleterious effects of these supportive measures has stimulated many clinical advances and improved survival of premature neonates. Understanding that premature lungs are in the canalicular stage of development and that positive pressure ventilation is deleterious, the ventilatory approach has shifted to less invasive and gentler respiratory strategies. This approach has resulted in improvements in overall and BPD-specific outcomes. This strategy avoids endotracheal intubation in favor of nasal continuous positive airway pressure to the extent possible.[59–61] The use of nasal intermittent positive pressure ventilation may further help prevent intubation, although effects of this ventilation strategy on overall survival and long-term outcomes are not yet known.[62] When endotracheal intubation is necessary, gentler ventilation strategies have been associated with improved outcomes. These include using the lowest possible ventilator settings, permissive hypercapnia ($Paco_2$ 45–60 mm Hg), and early extubation when possible.[63–68] A restrictive oxygen strategy has been associated with lower rates of ROP[69,70] and lower need for supplemental oxygen at 36 weeks postconceptual age.[70] This is counterbalanced by evidence of higher rates of mortality,[69–71] NEC, and patent ductus arteriosus requiring surgical ligation with the restrictive oxygen target.

A variety of ventilation modes has been evaluated to limit ventilator-induced lung injury for ELGANs. Volume targeted ventilation, which may limit the overdistension of the lung (volutrauma), has been associated with a lower incidence of BPD and decreased mortality compared with pressure-limited ventilation.[72] High-frequency oscillatory ventilation (HFOV) has been frequently studied as an alternative to conventional ventilation for premature neonates with respiratory distress syndrome. These trials consistently show no benefit of HFOV over conventional ventilation in terms of mortality or neurologic outcomes.[73] However, some trials have shown a decrease in the rate of chronic lung disease in those patients managed with HFOV.[74]

Artificial Placenta

Despite advances and refinements in the care of ELGANs, the mortality and morbidity remain high especially at the earliest gestational ages compatible with life. A radical paradigm shift in the treatment of prematurity would be to recreate the intrauterine environment using an AP or artificial womb. This pioneering approach was initiated more than 50 years ago,[75] and several investigators refined the approach as technology improved and our understanding of fetal physiology matured. In the past 15 years, there has been a renewed interest by several research groups, which have accelerated the technology to the point of clinical translation. Two similar but distinct approaches have emerged: the transumbilical AV-ECLS "artificial womb" and the VV-ECLS "artificial placenta" approach. Both approaches maintain fetal circulation, a low oxygen fetal environment with no mechanical ventilation and fluid filled lungs. In addition, both approaches have demonstrated multiorgan protection and ongoing development during extracorporeal support. We will highlight the similarities/differences, recent advances, and remaining milestones necessary for clinical translation.

Pumpless Arteriovenous-Extracorporeal Life Support

The ECLS Laboratory at the UM began study on the development of an AP in the early 2000s with an evaluation of the relationship between flow through an AV circuit and gas exchange in a rabbit model.[76] This paved the way for the development of an AP using pumpless AV ECLS with a custom low-resistance oxygenator using transumbilical cannulation. Five of 7 near-term lambs survived the 4-hour study period.[77] However, all animals developed progressive decline in cardiac function that resulted in hypotension, hypoxia, and a decrease in flows by 54% during the study period. This led the authors to conclude that a pumpless system, even when used with a low-resistance oxygenator, would be limited by cannula resistance and umbilical arterial spasm resulting in diminished flows and cardiac failure. Although a pumpless transumbilical AV mode is simple and attractive, it is in series with the systemic circulation, which puts additional strain on the heart that worsens in the presence of any degree of vasospasm.

More recently, significant advances have been made in the pumpless AV-ECLS AP approach by the research team at Children's Hospital of Philadelphia. They have developed the Extra-uterine Environment for Neonatal Development (EXTEND) system using a pumpless AV circuit. They found that the UA/UV approach resulted in successful placement of larger cannulae, longer circuit runs, higher weight-adjusted circuit flows, and fewer flow interruptions.[78] A subsequent study used echocardiography to identify increased heart strain in the first 2 weeks of support on EXTEND with return to baseline by the third week.[79] They demonstrated 4 weeks of support with hemodynamic stability, maintenance of fetal circulation, adequate gas exchange, and evidence of fetal growth.[80] They have made significant progress in mitigating umbilical vessel spasm by topical papaverine administration, atraumatic operative technique during cannulation, maintaining warmth, physiologic oxygen saturation of the umbilical venous inflow when initiating circuit flow and immediate transfer from the womb to their Biobag device. Although an advance, the potential for vascular spasm was not entirely ameliorated and one study demonstrated 30% of animals died due to vascular spasm limiting flows.[79]

A collaborative Western Australian-based program involving researchers from the Women and Infants Research Foundation, the University of Western Australia, and Tohoku University Hospital in Japan have developed a similar pumpless AV-ECLS AP platform called the ex vivo intrauterine environment (EVE) system. This system began development with the goal of addressing 2 problems that hampered previous attempts at a pumpless AP. First, they decreased the volume and resistance of the circuit by including a smaller, lower-resistance oxygenator. Second, they administered vasodilators to the fetus to maintain adequate organ circulation. With this system, they were able to support 5 premature lambs for 18.2 ± 3.2 hours.[81] Placing a second oxygenator in parallel reduced circuit resistance and prolonged survival to 60 hours.[82] The EVE system includes a "biobag" filled with artificial amniotic fluid, which had early issues with bacteremia.[83] They have subsequently achieved support up to 1 week in 5 of 6 preterm lambs without bacteremia.[84] Pumpless support using AV-ECLS (EXTEND and EVE platforms) requires 8 to 12 Fr cannulas and the absence of umbilical vessel spasm to maintain adequate flows (**Fig. 3**). Therefore, this approach is predicated on immediate transfer of the fetus from the womb to an "artificial womb."

Pump-Driven Veno-Venous Extracorporeal Life Support

We hypothesized that VV ECLS with right atrial drainage and umbilical vein reinfusion would surmount the challenges of an AV approach while still maintaining fetal circulation, hemodynamic stability, and adequate gas exchange. Using VV-ECLS with a pump, right atrial drainage, and umbilical vein reinfusion places the circuit in parallel with the systemic circulation, thereby adding little to no increased afterload on the patient's heart. With the goal of clinical translation for a premature infant after delivery,

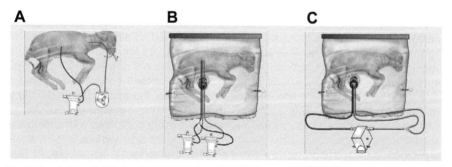

Fig. 3. Depiction of AP circuit. (*A*) AP University of Michigan. (*B*) Artificial womb (Perth, Aus, Japan). (*C*) Artificial womb (Philadelphia, PA). (*Adapted from* De Bie FR, Davey MG, Larson AC, Deprest J, Flake AW. Artificial placenta and womb technology: Past, current, and future challenges towards clinical translation. Prenat Diagn. 2021 Jan;41(1):145-158.)

we posited this cannulation strategy would allow for an adequately sized drainage cannula in the right atrium via the IJ vein and a smaller but acceptably sized umbilical vein cannula without limiting flows. White and colleagues supported 3 premature infants with VV-ECLS using the umbilical vein for reinfusion.[85] These babies lived for 10, 3, and 2 days with good gas-exchange parameters but all died of bleeding complications. Subsequently, this approach has been used clinically in 4-term or near-term neonates with good outcomes substantiating the feasibility of this approach.[86]

We developed a large animal model for an AP based on pump-driven VV-ECLS in 2012.[87] We supported 5 premature lambs (EGA 130–135 days; term = 145) using jugular vein drainage and umbilical vein reinfusion for more than 24 hours with stable hemodynamics and appropriate fetal gas exchange. Mean AP flow was 94 ± 20 mL/kg/min. Necropsy revealed a patent ductus arteriosus, foramen ovale, and sinus venosus. There was no difference in lung histology between the AP animals and controls, and there was no gross or microscopic ICH.

After establishing feasibility of VV-ECLS support, we sought to extend the duration of AP support and determine if premature lambs could be rescued by the AP and fetal circulation reinitiated, thus recreating a likely clinical scenario. To test this hypothesis, 7 premature sheep were delivered, intubated, and started on pressure-control ventilation. All sheep failed (persistent Po_2 or $Pco_2 < 60$ mm Hg and >100 mm Hg or hemodynamic instability) within 80 minutes and were transitioned to VV-ECLS AP support. Within an hour, arterial Po_2 and Pco_2 returned to target range; lactate normalized within 13 hours. Necropsy after 70 hours of support revealed a patent ductus arteriosus, foramen ovale, and sinus venosus in all sheep.[88] This study demonstrated that the AP can serve as a rescue therapy after failure of mechanical ventilation and fetal circulation can be reinitiated.

Airway Management

Although all AP systems maintain fluid-filled lungs and avoid gas ventilation, there are 2 distinct approaches based in part on the vascular access strategy. The pumpless AV ECLS EXTEND and EVE systems both use a fluid-filled Biobag as an "artificial womb." This is a closed environment with continuous fluid exchange. They have made substantial advances in reducing the infections that had previously plagued this approach.[84,89] This approach is necessary, in part, to prevent the umbilical vasospasm in a transumbilical AV-ECLS system. Proponents of this approach point out that it recreates the intrauterine environment and allows for normal glottic resistance required for maintenance of normal airway pressures and lung growth (**Table 2**).

An alternative approach is to recreate critical fetal physiology, and not necessarily replicate the entire womb. Our laboratory has developed an alternative approach to lung management (see **Fig. 3**). After delivery, we intubate the fetal lamb and fill its lungs with liquid perfluorocarbon—an inert liquid that is not absorbed by the lungs and thus will not cause tissue edema or fluid and electrolyte shifts—to a level of 5 to 8 cmH$_2$O which allows for fetal breathing movements. We then maintain the baby in a standard incubator. This approach resulted in lung development similar to gestational-age-matched controls and reduced lung injury compared with alternative management strategies.[90] This has become our standard airway-management strategy and has continued to provide evidence of lung development in later studies.[91] This strategy could be modified to accelerate lung growth,[92] and transition from the AP to liquid ventilation before air breathing.[93]

Some of the potential benefits of our approach include relative simplicity of implementation and easier access to the infant by the care team and family members.

Table 2
Artificial placenta/artificial womb at different institutions

	Artificial Placenta Model	Artificial Womb Model	
Model Name	AP	EVE	EXTEND
Year of most recent update	2022	2017	2022
Species	Lamb	Lamb	Lamb
Configuration	VV	VA	VA
Pump	Yes	No	No
Cannulation	JV/UV (10–12Fr)	UV/UA (10/8)	UV/UA (12/12)
Amniotic fluid management	Fluid filled ETT	Sterile, complete sunmersion (6L)	Sterile, complete sunmersion (2–4L)
Issues leading to mortality	• Cannula related • Arythmia • Tamponade • Arrest	• Equipment failure • Thrombo-embolism • Cannula	• Equipment failure • Cannula related • Umbilical spasm • Circuit clotting
Clinical issues	Newborn at predicted high risk of mortality, rescue therapy	Continuation of physiologic environment of fetus, could delay birth	Continuation of physiologic environment of fetus, could delay birth
Advantages	Recreates essential fetal physiology Enhanced newborn risk stratification	Mimic natural feta physiology Avoids barotrauma	Mimic natural fetal physiology Avoids barotrauma
Disadvantages	• Varying degrees of barotrauma before clinical application • Fetal circulation may not be reinitiated if applied late as rescue therapy	• Need for EXIT procedure for cannulation/maternal risks • Limited fetal risk stratification • Complicated fetal care with placental barrier • Corticosteroid use	• Need for EXIT procedure for cannulation/maternal risks • Limited fetal risk stratification • Complicated fetal care with placental barrier

Adapted from De Bie FR, Davey MG, Larson AC, Deprest J, Flake AW. Artificial placenta and womb technology: Past, current, and future challenges towards clinical translation. Prenat Diagn. 2021 Jan;41(1):145-158.

Cannulation Challenges and Miniaturization

Current versions of the AP use some form of umbilical access. Cannulation of these vessels is straightforward in animal models in which access can be secured in a controlled fashion while the animal is still connected to the mother's placenta, before the onset of vasospasm or desiccation of the cord. Translation of this technique to clinical use would require an ex utero intrapartum treatment (EXIT) procedure or modified cesarean delivery with the AV-ECLS approach. Alternatively, cannulation can be performed after delivery but spasm of the umbilical vessels could limit cannula size with the VV-ECLS approach.

To address this challenge, surgeons must develop techniques for limiting postdelivery vasospasm of the umbilical vessels or identify an alternative cannulation strategy. Peng and colleagues performed ex vivo dilation of segments of umbilical vessels immediately after delivery to determine the extent to which these vessels could be dilated postdelivery to facilitate cannulation. They found a dilation threshold of 7 mm for the umbilical vein and 6 mm for the umbilical artery,[94] suggesting that large-bore cannulation of these vessels may be feasible.

Another approach is the use of a single cannula in the IJ vein, obviating umbilical access altogether. This cannulation strategy is commonly used in ECMO through a dual-lumen cannula; however, a dual-lumen cannula would not provide adequate flows when miniaturized to 5 to 6 Fr. An alternative single-vessel, trans-jugular approach was developed more than 30 years ago at the University of Michigan.[95] This system uses tidal flow perfusion through a single-lumen cannula. It is currently being evaluated as a potential perfusion strategy for the AP. A major benefit of this system is that it allows for maximization of the diameter of the drainage cannula—the limiting variable in extracorporeal support. The primary limitation of this system is recirculation—occurring with each transition between drainage and reinfusion—which decreases the efficiency of the oxygen delivery. Longer occluder cycle times reduce the degree of recirculation but are also associated with larger volume and pressure fluctuations for the patient, which can result in hemodynamic instability and hemolysis. In our most recent study on the tidal-flow system, we have supported 3 premature sheep (EGA 118–124 days) for 24 hours, maintaining adequate gas exchange and hemodynamics.[96]

Premature infants born at 23 to 27 weeks typically weigh 500 to 800 grams. Most premature sheep models used for AP development use 110 to 120 days EGA sheep because they are equivalent to the lung development of 23 to 24 weeks human infants. However, they weigh 2 to 4 kg, which greatly exceeds the weight of the target patient population. Preliminary studies using a sheep model at 115 days gestation (1.8 kg) demonstrated adequacy of support for 18 hours with 6 Fr infusion and drainage catheters (unpublished results). Future research will focus on smaller lambs and longer duration of support.

Technical and physiologic feasibility of miniaturizing the pumpless AV-ECLS approach has been reported. In the animal models, 8 to 12 F cannulas were placed during an EXIT procedure obviating size limitations from umbilical vessel spasm. Using EXTEND, 5 extremely preterm (EGA 85–96 days) lambs weighing 480 to 850 grams were cannulated via the umbilical artery and umbilical vein and supported for 4 to 7 days with mean circuit flows of 213 mL/kg/min and stable gas exchange and hemodynamics.[78] However, all lambs developed hydrops leading to demise. The researchers speculate this was due to cardiac immaturity and inability to accommodate high postmembrane pressures. In a similar miniaturization study using the EVE platform, 7 out of 8 lambs (EGA 95 days) survived for 5 days on support with good gas exchange, stable hemodynamics, and normal echocardiographic parameters. Interestingly, despite circuit flows well above 200 mL/kg/min in all animals, there was no evidence of high output cardiac failure or hydrops.[84]

In the last decade, the AP has progressed into a well-developed technology poised for clinical translation in the near future. Several key milestones including miniaturization and development of nonthrombogenic circuits must be accomplished before it can be trialed in humans.

Clinical Application

Although the pumpless AV-ECLS platforms more closely recreate intrauterine physiology, clinical application may require an EXIT procedure or a modified cesarean section with a classic incision. The incidence of maternal intraoperative adverse events associated with cesarean deliveries at 24 to 25 weeks was 63.5% compared with 30.8% at 26 to 27 weeks[97]; an emergent EXIT procedure would likely further increase these risks. Because it relates to the fetus, this approach would lack any risk stratification for the infant apart from gestational age and thus would limit initial clinical application to the patients on the cusp of viability. Further research is required to mitigate these potential maternal risks and refine patient selection.

The approach to patient selection for a postnatal VV-ECLS AP is 2-fold. Similar to inclusion criteria for ECMO, it could be applied to critically ill premature infants after failing maximal medical therapy (see **Table 2**). This cohort would be expected to have suffered significant barotrauma and may not reap all the lung protective and developmental benefits of an AP. It could also be applied before respiratory failure in a cohort of ELGANs anticipated to have high mortality and morbidity according to risk stratification metrics. The Score of Neonatal Acute Physiology Perinatal Extension and the Clinical Risk Index for Babies II have been developed to estimate mortality risk in premature neonates. Recent studies suggest these markers may be useful in predicting high mortality in premature infants in the early newborn period.[98–100] This will serve as good starting points but will need to be validated for their use as predictive models to identify the best candidates for AP support. In order to have the greatest impact on morbidity and mortality of premature infants, the AP should be widely available and easily implemented at any neonatal ECMO center. When patient selection criteria are refined, there may be a hybrid approach to clinical application based on careful consideration of risks and benefits. Fetuses at the border of viability may benefit from a preemptive AV-ECLS approach, whereas fetuses precipitously delivered or older ELGANs may benefit from a postnatal VV-ECLS approach after risk stratification.

SUMMARY

ECLS remains an effective lifesaving technique for neonates with respiratory and/or cardiac failure. Technological and medical advances have paved the way for applying the benefits of extracorporeal support to premature infants. Recreation of the fetal environment with an AP/womb holds the promise of improving the mortality and morbidity of extremely premature infants.

DISCLOSURE

The authors do not have any commercial or financial conflicts of interest to disclose.

REFERENCES

1. Bartlett RH, Gazzaniga A, Fong S, et al. Prolonged extracorporeal cardiopulmonary support in man. J Thorac Cardiovasc Surg 1974;68(6):918–32.

2. Church JT, Kim AC, Erickson KM, et al. Pushing the boundaries of ECLS: outcomes in <34 week EGA neonates. J Pediatr Surg 2017;52(11):1810–5.

3. Wild KT, Rintoul N, Kattan J, et al. Extracorporeal life support organization (ELSO): guidelines for neonatal respiratory failure. Asaio j 2020;66(5):463–70.

4. Fallon BP, Gadepalli SK, Hirschl RB. Pediatric and neonatal extracorporeal life support: current state and continuing evolution. Pediatr Surg Int 2021;37(1): 17–35.

5. Baumgart S, Hirschl RB, Butler SZ, et al. Diagnosis-related criteria in the consideration of extracorporeal membrane oxygenation in neonates previously treated with high-frequency jet ventilation. Pediatrics 1992;89(3):491–4.

6. Smith DW, Frankel LR, Derish MT, et al. High-frequency jet ventilation in children with the adult respiratory distress syndrome complicated by pulmonary barotrauma. Pediatr Pulmonol 1993;15(5):279–86.

7. Swaniker F, Kolla S, Moler F, et al. Extracorporeal life support outcome for 128 pediatric patients with respiratory failure. J Pediatr Surg 2000;35(2):197–202.

8. Cilley RE, Zwischenberger JB, Andrews AF, et al. Intracranial hemorrhage during extracorporeal membrane oxygenation in neonates. Pediatrics 1986;78(4): 699–704.

9. Jobe AH. Mechanisms of lung injury and bronchopulmonary dysplasia. Am J Perinatol 2016;33(11):1076–8.

10. Lewis DA, Gauger P, Delosh TN, et al. The effect of pre-ECLS ventilation time on survival and respiratory morbidity in the neonatal population. J Pediatr Surg 1996;31(8):1110–4 [discussion: 1114-5].

11. Zabrocki LA, Brogan TV, Statler K, et al. Extracorporeal membrane oxygenation for pediatric respiratory failure: survival and predictors of mortality. Crit Care Med 2011;39(2):364–70.

12. Domico MB, Ridout DA, Bronicki R, et al. The impact of mechanical ventilation time before initiation of extracorporeal life support on survival in pediatric respiratory failure: a review of the Extracorporeal Life Support Registry. Pediatr Crit Care Med 2012;13(1):16–21.

13. Mok YH, Lee JH, Cheifetz IM. Neonatal extracorporeal membrane oxygenation: Update on management strategies and long-term outcomes. Adv Neonatal Care 2016;16(1):26–36.

14. Ijsselstijn H, Schiller RM, Holder C, et al. Extracorporeal life support organization (ELSO) guidelines for follow-up after neonatal and pediatric extracorporeal membrane oxygenation. Asaio j 2021;67(9):955–63.

15. Madderom MJ, Reuser JJ, Utens EM, et al. Neurodevelopmental, educational and behavioral outcome at 8 years after neonatal ECMO: a nationwide multicenter study. Intensive Care Med 2013;39(9):1584–93.

16. Bartlett RH. Esperanza: the first neonatal ECMO patient. Asaio j 2017;63(6): 832–43.

17. Bartlett RH, Andrews AF, Toomasian JM, et al. Extracorporeal membrane oxygenation for newborn respiratory failure: forty-five cases. Surgery 1982; 92(2):425–33.

18. Johnson K, Jarobe MD, Mychaliska GB, et al. Is there a best approach for extracorporeal life support cannulation: a review of the extracorporeal life support organization. J Pediatr Surg 2018;53(7):1301–4.

19. Duggan EM, Maitre N, Zhai A, et al. Neonatal carotid repair at ECMO decannulation: patency rates and early neurologic outcomes. J Pediatr Surg 2015; 50(1):64–8.

20. Teele SA, Salvin JW, Barrett CS, et al. The association of carotid artery cannulation and neurologic injury in pediatric patients supported with venoarterial extracorporeal membrane oxygenation*. Pediatr Crit Care Med 2014;15(4):355–61.
21. Wien MA, Witehead MT, Bulas D, et al. Patterns of brain injury in newborns treated with extracorporeal membrane oxygenation. AJNR Am J Neuroradiol 2017;38(4):820–6.
22. Rollins MD, Hubbard A, Zabrocki L, et al. Extracorporeal membrane oxygenation cannulation trends for pediatric respiratory failure and central nervous system injury. J Pediatr Surg 2012;47(1):68–75.
23. Jsselstijn HI, Hunfeld M, Schiller R, et al. Improving long-term outcomes after extracorporeal membrane oxygenation: from Observational follow-up programs toward risk stratification. Front Pediatr 2018;6:177.
24. Drucker NA, Wang SK, Markel TA, et al. Practice patterns in imaging guidance for ECMO cannulation: a survey of the American Pediatric Surgical Association. J Pediatr Surg 2020;55(8):1457–62.
25. Klein MD, Andrews AF, Wesley JR, et al. Venovenous perfusion in ECMO for newborn respiratory insufficiency. A clinical comparison with venoarterial perfusion. Ann Surg 1985;201(4):520–6.
26. Bunge JJH, Caliskan K, Gommers D, et al. Right ventricular dysfunction during acute respiratory distress syndrome and veno-venous extracorporeal membrane oxygenation. J Thorac Dis 2018;10(Suppl 5):S674–82.
27. Berdajs D. Bicaval dual-lumen cannula for venovenous extracorporeal membrane oxygenation: Avalon© cannula in childhood disease. Perfusion 2015; 30(3):182–6.
28. Cavayas YA, Sampson C, Yusuff H, et al. Use of a tracheal dilator for percutaneous insertion of 27F and 31F Avalon(©) dual-lumen cannulae for veno-venous extracorporeal membrane oxygenation in adults. Perfusion 2018;33(7):509–11.
29. Fleet D, Morris I, Faulkner G, et al. Experience with the Crescent(®) cannula for adult respiratory VV ECMO: a case series. Perfusion 2021;Ahead of print. 2676591211031462.
30. Muhammad J, Rezaeimoghaddam M, Cakmak B, et al. Patient-specific atrial hemodynamics of a double lumen neonatal cannula in Correct caval position. Artif Organs 2018;42(4):401–9.
31. Lazar DA, Cass DL, Olutoye OO, et al. Venovenous cannulation for extracorporeal membrane oxygenation using a bicaval dual-lumen catheter in neonates. J Pediatr Surg 2012;47(2):430–4.
32. Speggiorin S, Robinson SG, Harvey C, et al. Experience with the Avalon® bicaval double-lumen veno-venous cannula for neonatal respiratory ECMO. Perfusion 2015;30(3):250–4.
33. Lillie J, Pienaar A, Budd J, et al. Multisite veno-venous cannulation for neonates and Nonambulatory children. Pediatr Crit Care Med 2021;22(8):692–700.
34. Barton R, Ignjatovic V, Monagle P. Anticoagulation during ECMO in neonatal and paediatric patients. Thromb Res 2019;173:172–7.
35. Wong TE, Huang YS, Weiser J, et al. Antithrombin concentrate use in children: a multicenter cohort study. J Pediatr 2013;163(5):1329–13234.e1.
36. Rama G, Middlesworth W, Neunert C, et al. Antifactor Xa monitoring and Hematologic complications of pediatric extracorporeal membrane oxygenation. Asaio j 2021;67(1):91–5.
37. Padhya DR, Prutsky GJ, Nemergut ME, et al. Routine laboratory measures of heparin anticoagulation for children on extracorporeal membrane oxygenation: systematic review and meta-analysis. Thromb Res 2019;179:132–9.

38. Sanfilippo F, Asmussen S, Maybauer D, et al. Bivalirudin for alternative anticoagulation in extracorporeal membrane oxygenation: a systematic review. J Intensive Care Med 2017;32(5):312–9.
39. Kaseer H, Soto M, Sanghavi D, et al. Heparin vs bivalirudin anticoagulation for extracorporeal membrane oxygenation. J Card Surg 2020;35(4):779–86.
40. Hamzah M, Jarden AM, Ezetendu C, et al. Evaluation of bivalirudin as an alternative to heparin for systemic anticoagulation in pediatric extracorporeal membrane oxygenation. Pediatr Crit Care Med 2020;21(9):827–34.
41. Ranucci M. Bivalirudin and post-cardiotomy ECMO: a word of caution. Crit Care 2012;16(3):427.
42. Nagle EL, Dager WE, Duby JJ, et al. Bivalirudin in pediatric patients maintained on extracorporeal life support. Pediatr Crit Care Med 2013;14(4):e182–8.
43. Seelhammer TG, Bohman JK, Schulte PJ, et al. Comparison of bivalirudin versus heparin for maintenance systemic anticoagulation during adult and pediatric extracorporeal membrane oxygenation. Crit Care Med 2021;49(9):1481–92.
44. Snyder CW, Goldenberg NA, Nguyen AT, et al. A perioperative bivalirudin anticoagulation protocol for neonates with congenital diaphragmatic hernia on extracorporeal membrane oxygenation. Thromb Res 2020;193:198–203.
45. Brisbois EJ, Handa H, Major TC, et al. Long-term nitric oxide release and elevated temperature stability with S-nitroso-N-acetylpenicillamine (SNAP)-doped Elast-eon E2As polymer. Biomaterials 2013;34(28):6957–66.
46. Major TC, Brant DO, Reynolds MM, et al. The attenuation of platelet and monocyte activation in a rabbit model of extracorporeal circulation by a nitric oxide releasing polymer. Biomaterials 2010;31(10):2736–45.
47. Wo Y, Brisbois EJ, Colletta A, et al. Origin of long-term Storage stability and nitric oxide release behavior of CarboSil polymer doped with S-nitroso-N-acetyl-D-penicillamine. ACS Appl Mater Inter 2015;7(40):22218–27.
48. Bellomo TR, Jeakle MA, Meyerhoff ME, et al. The effects of the combined argatroban/nitric oxide-releasing polymer on platelet Microparticle-induced Thrombogenicity in coated extracorporeal circuits. Asaio j 2021;67(5):573–82.
49. Major TC, Brisbois EJ, Jones AM, et al. The effect of a polyurethane coating incorporating both a thrombin inhibitor and nitric oxide on hemocompatibility in extracorporeal circulation. Biomaterials 2014;35(26):7271–85.
50. Wild KT, Hedrick HL, Rintoul NE. Reconsidering ECMO in premature neonates. Fetal Diagn Ther 2020;47(12):927–32.
51. Burgos CM, Frenckner B, Broman LM. Premature and extracorporeal life support: is it time? A Systematic review. ASAIO J 2021;68(5):633–45.
52. Rozmiarek AJ, Qureshi FG, Cassidy L, et al. How low can you go? Effectiveness and safety of extracorporeal membrane oxygenation in low-birth-weight neonates. J Pediatr Surg 2004;39(6):845–7.
53. Gadepalli SK, Hirschl RB. Extracorporeal life support: updates and controversies. Semin Pediatr Surg 2015;24(1):8–11.
54. Ely DM, Driscoll AK. Infant mortality in the United States, 2019:data from the period Linked birth/infant death file. Natl Vital Stat Rep 2021;70(14):1–18.
55. Dreyfuss D, Saumon G. Ventilator-induced lung injury: lessons from experimental studies. Am J Respir Crit Care Med 1998;157(1):294–323.
56. Biondi JW, Schulman DS, Soufer R, et al. The effect of incremental positive end-expiratory pressure on right ventricular hemodynamics and ejection fraction. Anesth Analg 1988;67(2):144–51.
57. Aly H, Hammad TA, Essers J, et al. Is mechanical ventilation associated with intraventricular hemorrhage in preterm infants? Brain Dev 2012;34(3):201–5.

58. Cayabyab R, Ramanathan R. Retinopathy of prematurity: Therapeutic strategies based on Pathophysiology. Neonatology 2016;109(4):369–76.
59. Fischer HS, Bührer C. Avoiding endotracheal ventilation to prevent bronchopulmonary dysplasia: a meta-analysis. Pediatrics 2013;132(5):e1351–60.
60. Schmölzer GM, Kumar M, Pichler G, et al. Non-invasive versus invasive respiratory support in preterm infants at birth: systematic review and meta-analysis. Bmj 2013;347:f5980.
61. Subramaniam P, Ho JJ, Davis PG. Prophylactic nasal continuous positive airway pressure for preventing morbidity and mortality in very preterm infants. Cochrane Database Syst Rev 2016;(6):Cd001243.
62. Lemyre B, Laughon M, Bose C, et al. Early nasal intermittent positive pressure ventilation (NIPPV) versus early nasal continuous positive airway pressure (NCPAP) for preterm infants. Cochrane Database Syst Rev 2016;12(12):Cd005384.
63. Supplemental Therapeutic oxygen for Prethreshold retinopathy of prematurity (STOP-ROP), a randomized, controlled trial. I: primary outcomes. Pediatrics 2000;105(2):295–310.
64. Carlo WA, Stark AR, Wright LL, et al. Minimal ventilation to prevent bronchopulmonary dysplasia in extremely-low-birth-weight infants. J Pediatr 2002;141(3):370–4.
65. Mariani G, Cifuentes J, Carlo WA. Randomized trial of permissive hypercapnia in preterm infants. Pediatrics 1999;104(5 Pt 1):1082–8.
66. Woodgate PG, Davies MW. Permissive hypercapnia for the prevention of morbidity and mortality in mechanically ventilated newborn infants. Cochrane Database Syst Rev 2001;2001(2):Cd002061.
67. Robbins M, Trittmann J, Martin E, et al. Early extubation attempts reduce length of stay in extremely preterm infants even if re-intubation is necessary. J Neonatal Perinatal Med 2015;8(2):91–7.
68. Al Faleh K, Liew K, Anabrees K, et al. Success rate and neonatal morbidities associated with early extubation in extremely low birth weight infants. Ann Saudi Med 2011;31(6):577–80.
69. Askie LM, Darlow BA, Davis PG, et al. Effects of targeting lower versus higher arterial oxygen saturations on death or disability in preterm infants. Cochrane Database Syst Rev 2017;4(4):Cd011190.
70. Askie LM, Darlow BA, Finer N, et al. Association between oxygen saturation targeting and death or disability in extremely preterm infants in the neonatal oxygenation prospective meta-analysis collaboration. Jama 2018;319(21):2190–201.
71. Manja V, Saugstad OD, Lakshminrusimha S. Oxygen saturation targets in preterm infants and outcomes at 18-24 Months: a systematic review. Pediatrics 2017;139(1).
72. Klingenberg C, Wheeler KI, McCallion N, et al. Volume-targeted versus pressure-limited ventilation in neonates. Cochrane Database Syst Rev 2017;10(10):Cd003666.
73. Cools F, Askie LM, Offringa M, et al. Elective high-frequency oscillatory versus conventional ventilation in preterm infants: a systematic review and meta-analysis of individual patients' data. Lancet 2010;375(9731):2082–91.
74. Cools F, Offringa M, Askie LM. Elective high frequency oscillatory ventilation versus conventional ventilation for acute pulmonary dysfunction in preterm infants. Cochrane Database Syst Rev 2015;(3):Cd000104.

75. Zapol WM, Kolobow T, Pierce GG, et al. Artificial placenta: two days of total extrauterine support of the isolated premature lamb fetus. Science 1969; 166(905):617–8.

76. Ivascu FA, Somand DM, Skrzypchak AM, et al. Development of an artificial placenta: CO2 elimination and hemodynamics as a function of arteriovenous blood flow. J Pediatr Surg 2005;40(6):1034–7.

77. Reoma J, Rojas A, Kim AC, et al. Development of an artificial placenta I: pumpless arterio-venous extracorporeal life support in a neonatal sheep model. J Pediatr Surg 2009;44(1):53–9.

78. Hornick MA, Davey MG, Partridge EA, et al. Umbilical cannulation optimizes circuit flows in premature lambs supported by the EXTra-uterine Environment for Neonatal Development (EXTEND). J Physiol 2018;596(9):1575–85.

79. Ozawa K, Davey MG, Tian Z, et al. Fetal echocardiographic assessment of cardiovascular impact of prolonged support on EXTrauterine Environment for Neonatal Development (EXTEND) system. Ultrasound Obstet Gynecol 2020; 55(4):516–22.

80. Partridge EA, Davey MG, Hornick MA, et al. An Extrauterine environment for neonatal development: Extending fetal physiology beyond the womb. Semin Fetal Neonatal Med 2017;(Epub).

81. Miura Y, Matsuda T, Funakubo A, et al. Novel modification of an artificial placenta: pumpless arteriovenous extracorporeal life support in a premature lamb model. Pediatr Res 2012;72(5):490–4.

82. Miura Y, Matsuda T, Usuda H, et al. A Parallelized pumpless artificial placenta system significantly prolonged survival time in a preterm lamb model. Artif Organs 2016;40(5):E61–8.

83. Miura Y, Usuda H, Watanabe S, et al. Stable control of physiological parameters, but not infection, in preterm lambs maintained on ex vivo uterine environment therapy. Artif Organs 2017;41(10):959–68.

84. Usuda H, Watanabe S, Miura Y, et al. Successful maintenance of key physiological parameters in preterm lambs treated with ex vivo uterine environment therapy for a period of 1 week. Am J Obstet Gynecol 2017;217(4):457.e1–13.

85. White JJ, Andrews HG, Risemberg H, et al. Prolonged respiratory support in newborn infants with a membrane oxygenator. Surgery 1971;70(2):288–96.

86. Kato J, Nagaya M, Niimi N, et al. Venovenous extracorporeal membrane oxygenation in newborn infants using the umbilical vein as a reinfusion route. J Pediatr Surg 1998;33:1446–8.

87. Gray BW, Sabbagh A, Rojas A, et al. Development of an artificial placenta IV: 24 hour venovenous extracorporeal life support in premature lambs. Asaio j 2012; 58(2):148–54.

88. Gray BW, Sabbagh A, Zakem SJ, et al. Development of an artificial placenta V: 70 h veno-venous extracorporeal life support after ventilatory failure in premature lambs. J Pediatr Surg 2013;48(1):145–53.

89. Partridge EA, Davey MG, Hornick MA, et al. An extra-uterine system to physiologically support the extreme premature lamb. Nat Commun 2017;8:15112.

90. Church JT, Perkins EM, Coughlin MA, et al. Perfluorocarbons prevent lung injury and Promote development during artificial placenta support in extremely premature lambs. Neonatology 2018;113(4):313–21.

91. Coughlin MA, Werner NL, Church JT, et al. An artificial placenta protects against lung injury and promotes continued lung development in extremely premature lambs. ASAIO J 2018;65(7):690–7.

92. Mychaliska G, Bryner B, Dechert R, et al. Safety and efficacy of perflubron-induced lung growth in neonates with congenital diaphragmatic hernia: Results of a prospective randomized trial. J Pediatr Surg 2015;50(7):1083–7.
93. Hirschl RB. Current experience with liquid ventilation. Paediatr Respir Rev 2004; 5(Suppl A):S339–45.
94. Peng J, Rochow N, Dabaghi M, et al. Postnatal dilatation of umbilical cord vessels and its impact on wall integrity: Prerequisite for the artificial placenta. Int J Artif Organs 2018;41(7):393–9.
95. Zwischenberger JB, Toomasian JM, Drake K, et al. Total respiratory support with single cannula venovenous ECMO: double lumen continuous flow vs. single lumen tidal flow. Trans Am Soc Artif Intern Organs 1985;31:610–5.
96. Kading JC, Langley MW, Lautner G, et al. Tidal flow perfusion for the artificial placenta: a paradigm shift. ASAIO J 2019;66(7):796–802.
97. Bertholdt C, Menard S, Delorme P, et al. Intraoperative adverse events associated with extremely preterm cesarean deliveries. Acta Obstet Gynecol Scand 2018;97(5):608–14.
98. McLeod JS, Menon Anitha, Matsuko Niki, et al. Comparing mortality risk models in VLBW and preterm infants: systematic review and meta-analysis. J Perinatol 2020;40(5):695–703.
99. Sotodate G, Oyama K, Matsumoto A, et al. Predictive ability of neonatal illness severity scores for early death in extremely premature infants. J Matern Fetal Neonatal Med 2022;35(5):846–51.
100. De Bie FR, Davey MG, Larson AC, et al. Artificial placenta and womb technology: past, current, and future challenges towards clinical translation. Prenatal Diagn 2021;41:p145–58. https://doi.org/10.1002/pd.5821.

Surgical Management of Congenital Diaphragmatic Hernia

Matthew T. Harting, MD, MS[a], Tim Jancelewicz, MD, MA, MS[b],*

KEYWORDS

- Congenital diaphragmatic hernia • CDH • Surgery • Diaphragm • ECLS • ECMO

KEY POINTS

- Congenital diaphragmatic hernia (CDH) is a surgical disease with survival dependent on diaphragm repair.
- Postnatal preoperative care is complex, includes defined therapeutic targets/clinical thresholds, and diaphragmatic repair should occur following clinical stabilization.
- Principles regarding the use of extracorporeal life support (ECLS) in CDH include proper patient selection, minimization of delay to ECLS if deemed necessary, and proper decision-making regarding operative timing and procedure if unrepaired once cannulated.
- Key operative principles include the use of a dome-shaped patch, a tension-free repair, and monitoring of peak inspiratory pressure with temporary abdominal closure if necessary to prevent abdominal compartment syndrome.
- The incidence of long-term adverse surgical outcomes in CDH is directly related to the size of the CDH defect, and surveillance for complications is necessary into adulthood.

INTRODUCTION

Although a great number of refinements in treatment approaches and new therapeutic modalities have emerged in the management of newborns with a congenital diaphragmatic hernia (CDH), a fundamental principal remains unchanged: survival of every patient depends on successful surgical repair of the diaphragmatic defect. In other words, failure to reduce the hernia and achieve repair (ie, non-repair) is associated with 100% mortality. The whole course of CDH care is therefore fundamentally dependent on the decision regarding the optimal timing of repair and the best approach. This decision influences every component of care including preoperative stabilization,

[a] Department of Pediatric Surgery, Children's Memorial Hermann Hospital, University of Texas McGovern Medical School, 6431 Fannin Street, MSB: 5.233, Houston, TX 77030, USA; [b] Division of Pediatric Surgery, Le Bonheur Children's Hospital, University of Tennessee Health Science Center, 49 North Dunlap Street Second Floor, Memphis, TN 38105, USA
* Corresponding author.
E-mail address: tjancele@uthsc.edu

Clin Perinatol 49 (2022) 893–906
https://doi.org/10.1016/j.clp.2022.08.004
0095-5108/22/© 2022 Elsevier Inc. All rights reserved.
perinatology.theclinics.com

prevention of lung injury while optimizing pulmonary function until the surgical reduction of herniated contents and correction of the defect, and enabling both tolerance of and recovery from the procedure. Decision-making can be challenging given the myriad of possible clinical courses and the broad range of CDH severity. The purpose of this report is to summarize the postnatal surgical management of CDH including the use of extracorporeal life support (ECLS) with attention to new principles and recent trends, and to address relevant ongoing controversies.

POSTNATAL AND PREOPERATIVE MANAGEMENT

Risk prediction begins long before birth. Prenatal risk prediction (eg, lung-to-head ratio and lung volumes) allows the multidisciplinary care team to anticipate the severity of pulmonary hypoplasia and hypertension as well as informs the resuscitation process at delivery while also facilitating critical prenatal education and counseling.[1] At birth, care must involve rapid assessment and intervention. At some centers, infants with adequate respiratory function may be initially managed with supplemental oxygen only. Patients with respiratory distress require immediate intubation with avoidance of hand bagging. Conventional ventilation is typically initiated as a first-line strategy, with transition to other modalities when acceptable parameters are exceeded (see below).[2] Intravenous and arterial access, along with gastric decompression, are established. Ideally, the infant is maintained in a minimal stimulation environment. Important initial variables to be measured or monitored include:

- Preductal and postductal oxygen saturation (SaO_2)
- Arterial blood gas (ABG) after 30 min of life
- Chest radiography to confirm diagnosis and ensure proper endotracheal and orogastric tube position
- Echocardiogram (ECHO) between 4 and 12 h of life to assess cardiac anatomy and function
- Intracranial ultrasound (US) as a baseline for high-risk neonates before ECLS

Resuscitation proceeds using *therapeutic targets* and *clinical thresholds/limits* to guide decision-making such as operative timing and transitions in care. Suggested targets and thresholds, derived from European[3] and North American[4,5] clinical practice guidelines, include:

- Preductal blood SaO2 > 85% (during the first few hours of life, an initial, transient SaO2 > 70% may be tolerated, as long as it is improving)
- Adequate tissue oxygen delivery and perfusion [assessed by physical examination, urine output (UOP) > 1-2 cc/kg/h, and lactate < 3 mmol/L]
- Blood gas: partial pressure of carbon dioxide ($PaCO_2$): 45 to 70 mm Hg, pH 7.2 to 7.4
- Conventional ventilator settings: maximum peak inspiratory pressure (PIP) 26, maximum rate 50 to 60 (adjust I-time appropriately), maximum positive end-expiratory pressure (PEEP) 5–6

Inability to remain within these clinical ranges due to inadequate oxygenation and/or ventilation indicates failure of conventional ventilation and need for escalation of support, such as use of high-frequency oscillatory ventilation (HFOV). Suggested HFOV settings are mean airway pressure (MAP) 2 above conventional ventilation MAP (maximum 14–15), amplitude twice that of MAP or higher to achieve optimal shake (to level of the umbilicus), and frequency of 8 to 10 Hz (optimized to the last CO_2). With the failure of HFOV, the next transition is to ECLS.

TIMING OF REPAIR

If escalation of care to HFOV or ECLS is avoided, readiness for surgical repair may be determined. Resuscitation before a repair will usually last between 36 h and 7 days, and stability of the patient is more important than any specific number of days of resuscitation before repair.[6,7] General features of a "stable" patient with CDH who is ready for operative intervention are shown in **Table 1**.

Although most of the targets listed in **Table 1** are straightforward to evaluate, pulmonary hypertension (PH) assessment, and the subsequent use of this information to inform clinical decision-making regarding optimal timing of repair, is an enigmatic process. The degree of PH (along with cardiac anatomy and cardiac function) is likely best assessed via ECHO following the postnatal circulatory transition (5–10-fold decrease in pulmonary vascular resistance in the first few hours of life[9]) and after the initial, stimulating, immediate postnatal interventions which include intubation, gastric decompression, vascular access, and transport.[10,11] Yet, it cannot be delayed for too long, given the importance of assessment of cardiac anatomy and function, along with the estimation of PH, hence the 4 to 12 h of life window, depending on clinical situation. Assessment of ventricular function, along with right ventricular systolic pressures, right ventricular size, septal position, and ductal/atrial shunting all inform fluid resuscitation, use of inotropic, lusitropic, or vasopressor pharmacology, risk assessment, and transition to ECLS or operative intervention.[12–14] Before progressing to surgery, which is a highly stimulating and physiology-altering event, PH should be stable (ie, consecutive ECHOs without significant increase, absence of significant pre–post ductal oxygenation gradient, and/or optimal blood gases), occasionally requiring PH-directed pharmacotherapy.[15] In the event of large changes in right-sided pressures, additional time may allow the highly reactive pulmonary vasculature to be stabilized, mitigating rapid decompensation during or immediately following diaphragmatic repair.

As moving into the current era of delayed repair first advocated by Nakayama and Grosfeld 30 years ago,[16,17] some caveats to this blanket approach to CDH have been elucidated, though there is still no universal consensus regarding optimal timing, likely due to the heterogeneity of the disease. At CDH study group (CDHSG) centers, among patients who do not receive ECLS treatment, over 90% of infants are repaired within 2 weeks and two-thirds are repaired between days 2 and 5 of life.[7] This unadjusted

Table 1
Initial resuscitation targets and criteria indicating readiness (stability) for surgical repair of the CDH

Initial Targets	Preoperative Targets
Preductal oxygen saturation 85–95%[a]	Resolution of hypoxia (FiO$_2 \leq$50%)
Adequate tissue oxygen delivery[b]	Blood pressure normalization
Adequate tissue perfusion[b]	Adequate tissue oxygen delivery[b]
PaCO$_2$: 45–70 mm Hg	Adequate tissue perfusion[b]
pH: 7.2–7.4	Stabilization of pulmonary hypertension[c]

[a] May allow 70% to 85% for brief periods.
[b] Assessed by physical examination, urine output (>1-2 cc/kg/h), and lactate (<5 mmol/L).
[c] Defined by a stable pre-ductal oxygen saturation and repeat echocardiography with stable or improving measures of pulmonary hypertension (tricuspid regurgitation and/or right ventricular septal position); ideally, the calculated right ventricular systolic pressures would be at or near systemic, systolic blood pressures.
Data from Refs.[3,6,8]

analysis showed that mortality was significantly higher among those that underwent repair on day of life (DOL) 4 to 7 (6.6%) and DOL ≥8 (12.3%), compared with DOL 0 to 3 (3.9%). Not surprisingly, a protracted delay to repair was associated with low birthweight and Apgar scores, cardiac abnormalities, larger defects, patch repair, and intrathoracic liver, confirming that physiologic stabilization requires more time among infants with more severe CDH. When these factors were controlled for, there was no difference in survival based on timing of repair. A Cochrane review identified two small randomized trials comparing early (<24 h) to late (>24 h) surgical intervention.[18] Although one trial showed a trend toward increased mortality in the early surgery group (54% mortality in the early group versus 43% in the late group),[19] there was no statistically significant difference in survival. No difference in length of stay was identified. Numerous additional papers seem to suggest that there is no real benefit from any particular repair timing.[20]

It is possible that these results are strongly influenced by patients with less severe CDH (CDHSG classification A and B defect[21]) who have an overall survival >95% and could tolerate surgery well, irrespective of timing. More severe CDH (C and D defect) patients may be more susceptible to increased stress, pulmonary edema, PH exacerbation, and ventilatory fluctuation potentially associated with operative diaphragmatic repair. However, it is also possible that severe CDH phenotypes may benefit from an *early* repair approach to avoid the situation of non-repair or need for repair while on ECLS, though repair before optimal stabilization may result in an increased risk of postoperative ECLS use.[22] At the center level, a policy of aggressive surgical management with an effort to prioritize repair even in the sickest infants is associated with 2.7 additional survivors for every 100 patients with CDH, though high center volume and experience are clearly essential components of this strategy.[23]

Use of Extracorporeal Life Support

Treatment with ECLS is associated with improved survival only for the most severe CDH patients, and only at centers with the highest CDH volume and ECLS experience.[24] Thus, proper patient selection and avoidance of ECLS in low-risk patients are paramount considerations. That said, once the clinical thresholds listed above have been exceeded despite appropriate support with pre-specified limits (eg, HFOV), ECLS should be initiated without delay so as to minimize the risk of iatrogenic lung injury while also minimizing exposure to hypoxia and acidosis. Specific indications for ECLS use are listed in **Table 2**. Relative contraindications to ELCS include gestational age ≤32 weeks, weight ≤1.7–2 kg, intracranial hemorrhage, and major (lethal) genetic syndromes.[25,26] Concomitant severe congenital heart disease may be considered a relative contraindication for ECLS based on severity of the cardiac defect, ability to stabilize the individual patient, and center ability/expertise. Either venoarterial (VA) or venovenous (VV) ECLS support may be used, and the data do not support a strong recommendation for either approach.

A detailed review of ECLS management is out of the scope of this article and can be found elsewhere,[25] but some key elements are fundamental to the discussion of surgical management of CDH, as patients treated with ECLS necessitate unique consideration in preoperative preparation before diaphragmatic repair. First, timing of repair in relation to ECLS cannulation [usually early (<72 h) versus late (after several weeks) on ECLS, or after ECLS] must be decided given the need for preoperative optimization, which may require several days. Second, repair on ECLS may occur at the bedside in the intensive care unit or in the operating room, and this requires special pre- and perioperative care of the patient and the circuit.

Timing of repair remains controversial. Options include early repair on ECLS, delayed repair on ECLS, and attempting to wean off before repair (repair after or off

Table 2
Indications for ECLS use in CDH

ECLS Indications	Considerations
Hypoxic/hypercapnic respiratory failure	1. Continuous mandatory ventilation (CMV) settings PIP > 26–28 cm H2O, PEEP > 6 cm H2O, RR > 50 2. HFOV settings MAP > 14, frequency <7 Hz, amplitude >40 3. Inability to achieve or maintain preductal SpO2 > 85% 4. Persistent severe respiratory acidosis (PCO2 > 70 mm Hg) with pH < 7.20
Circulatory failure	1. Inadequate oxygen delivery (DO2) with metabolic acidosis 2. Inadequate end-organ perfusion, lactate >3, oliguria 3. Refractory systemic hypotension nonresponsive to fluid and vasoactive medications 4. Pulmonary hypertension ± right ventricular dysfunction 5. Left ventricular failure
Acute clinical deterioration	1. Preductal desaturation <70% with inability to recover with ventilator optimization 2. Hemodynamic instability recalcitrant to inotrope and chronotrope initiation/titration

From Guner Y, Jancelewicz T, Di Nardo M, Yu P, Brindle M, Vogel AM, Gowda SH, Grover TR, Johnston L, Mahmood B, Gray B, Chapman R, Keene S, Rintoul N, Cleary J, Ashrafi AH, Harting MT; ELSO CDH Interest Group. Management of Congenital Diaphragmatic Hernia Treated With Extracorporeal Life Support: Interim Guidelines Consensus Statement From the Extracorporeal Life Support Organization. ASAIO J. 2021 Feb 1;67(2):113-120.

ECLS) and, if liberation from ECLS is unsuccessful, repairing late on ECLS. Decisions regarding timing must balance disparate challenges including dramatic changes in fluid status, risk of hemorrhage while anticoagulated, potential inability to wean from ECLS, and the potential advantage of relieving intrathoracic compression early and restoring more physiologic anatomy. Previous studies comparing on-ECLS to after-ECLS repair have significant limitations, particularly due to the exclusion of non-repaired patients within the analysis.[27,28] However, recent work addressed these limitations with a propensity-matched, intention-to-treat analysis, and the authors show convincingly that early surgical repair on ECLS is superior to late on- or off-ECLS approaches when the risk of non-repair is taken into consideration.[29] In response to these data and to general improvements in ECLS management overall, many centers are now converting or have already converted to an early-on-ECLS repair approach for most CDH patients who arrive to ECLS unrepaired (personal correspondence).

When repair is undertaken on ECLS, numerous perioperative concerns exist regarding tissue edema, the ECLS circuit, and optimal anticoagulation (**Table 3**). Patients that progress to pre-repair ECLS support can become edematous as significant fluid shifts are likely. Tissue edema can make operative dissection challenging, render tissue more friable, and prolong postoperative recovery; this is one of the major reasons for advocation of early repair on ECLS, before significant edema occurs. Minimization of fluid and product administration, along with diuresis, should be optimized with a goal of even-to-negative fluid balance in the period preceding diaphragmatic repair. This must be

Table 3
Perioperative management for CDH repair during ECLS treatment

	Considerations for CDH Repair on ECLS
Circuit	Minimize clots within ECLS circuit • The circuit should be largely free from clots before surgery to limit disseminated intravascular coagulopathy (DIC) from overwhelming consumption of clotting factors by existing circuit thrombi
Anemia	Goal hematocrit ~35%–45%
Platelets	Goal platelet count >100,000/uL
Clotting factors	Goals during repair • Fibrinogen >150 mg/dL • PTT ≤ 60 s • Thromboelastography/rotational thromboelastometry (TEG/ROTEM) be used as adjuncts to evaluate the whole coagulation cascade. Consider these adjuncts to optimize the patient preoperatively and replete specific factors postoperatively
Anticoagulation	Lowering anticoagulation targets during perioperative period • Many centers initiate a high-risk bleeding protocol with decreased ACT, Anti-Xa, TEG/ROTEM, or aPTT goals, whereas some centers hold anticoagulation entirely
Antifibrinolytics	Aminocaproic acid (Amicar) or tranexamic acid (TXA) infusion may be used to reduce bleeding risk by inhibiting fibrinolysis thus limiting clot breakdown • Start with a preoperative bolus, followed by an infusion that continues through the operation and up to 48 h postoperative • Amicar—100 mg/kg bolus 6 h preop, then 30 mg/kg/h infusion for 24–48 h • TXA—4–10 mg/kg bolus prep, then 1–4 mg/kg/h infusion for 24–48 h

Adjuncts	• Fibrin sealants—consider application to the operative field to limit surface oozing
	• Chest tube(s)
	• Temporary abdominal closure
	  ○ Silo or patch for skin
	  ○ Prevents abdominal compartment syndrome in the case of postoperative bleeding and edema
	  ○ Allows placement of surgical packs in case of surface oozing

From Guner Y, Jancelewicz T, Di Nardo M, Yu P, Brindle M, Vogel AM, Gowda SH, Grover TR, Johnston L, Mahmood B, Gray B, Chapman R, Keene S, Rintoul N, Cleary J, Ashrafi AH, Harting MT; ELSO CDH Interest Group. Management of Congenital Diaphragmatic Hernia Treated With Extracorporeal Life Support: Interim Guidelines Consensus Statement From the Extracorporeal Life Support Organization. ASAIO J. 2021 Feb 1;67(2):113-120.

balanced with hemodynamic status and product needs to maintain low but acceptable ECLS parameters. The overarching goal of preoperative anticoagulation management for CDH infants undergoing diaphragmatic repair on ECLS is to minimize anticoagulation while simultaneously maintaining circuit flow and preventing major clotting complications.[30,31] During surgery, meticulous hemostasis and tissue handling are essential, and techniques to reduce the chances of bleeding complications include minimal dissection of the posterior rim of diaphragm and generous use of electrocautery and hemostatic agents. A chest tube and temporary abdominal closure with a patch will allow early identification and rapid treatment of postoperative bleeding respectively.

OPERATIVE REPAIR OF THE CONGENITAL DIAPHRAGMATIC HERNIA

After stabilization and the decision to repair the CDH has been made according to the criteria outlined above, the operation may proceed using one of several approaches: ipsilateral subcostal incision, thoracotomy, or thoracoscopy. Subcostal laparotomy is by far the most common approach[32] as it provides excellent visualization of the defect, facilitates organ reduction, enables adequate exposure to identify and address intraoperative complications, and allows the use of an abdominal wall patch if there is insufficient domain after reduction. This approach is well-tolerated postoperatively. The subcostal laparotomy approach has been used reliably over time, has a predictable postoperative course/complication profile, and can be used for all CDH severities.

The operation proceeds with reduction of hernia contents from the chest with careful attention to the spleen, which can be easily lacerated. A true hernia sac, which is present less than 20% of the time, should be excised. The thoracic and abdominal cavities should be inspected for associated anomalies including pulmonary sequestration. The diaphragm edges are freed and unrolled, and a decision regarding closure is then made.

Closure of the defect may occur with a primary repair or with a patch that substitutes the missing diaphragm. Although a primary diaphragmatic re-approximation/repair is possible for many A defects and some B defects, a patch is necessary for more than 50% of all patients with CDH and 100% of high-risk, C and D defects.[33] If a prosthetic is used, a large, dome-shaped patch is a technical imperative, as it optimizes intraabdominal space, allowing diaphragmatic movement and patient growth, and reduces the risk of recurrence.[34] Options for patch material include synthetic, biologic, and autologous. Patch options and considerations are shown in **Table 4**. A combination patch, such as a polytetrafluoroethylene (PTFE or GoreTex)/Marlex, may provide the strengths of each including minimizing adhesion formation while incorporating into the available diaphragm/chest wall, and decreasing recurrence.[35] Moreover, a patch overlay on a primary repair (particularly with an minimally invasive surgical [MIS] repair, as noted below), may provide additional strength against recurrence.

After repair, incisional closure is addressed. With reduction of the hernia and closure of the fascia, respiratory compliance can be significantly compromised due to a tight abdominal wall closure.[41,42] Attention should thus be paid to the PIP during closure, and a large patch that bows into the hemithorax may also help prevent this problem.[43] If respiratory compromise occurs, a temporary abdominal closure is an option (fascial patch/prosthetic silo, vacuum-assisted closure, or skin-only closure, with delayed closure after resolution of edema or improved abdominal domain). Such an approach is used in roughly 10% of cases and is more common with repair on ECLS and with right-sided lesions.[44,45]

Because of the potential for rapid mediastinal shifting and lung injury, routine chest tube use has become uncommon unless repair occurs during ECLS.[46,47] Without drainage, the thoracic space typically fills with fluid, and the lung grows to fill the space over time. However, chest tube placement may be associated with fewer pleural complications than cases that require postoperative drain placement; minimally invasive approaches may need a tube to treat a pneumothorax, whereas open techniques may require drainage of an effusion.[48] Chest tubes should always be placed to water seal and not to suction. Symptomatic pleural fluid can be treated with repeated thoracentesis. If used, chest tubes should be removed expeditiously to avoid contamination and infection of the thoracic space, especially in the presence of a prosthetic patch.

Table 4
Diaphragmatic replacement options

Type	Examples	Strengths & Weaknesses
Nonabsorbable (synthetic)	• Polytetrafluoroethylene (PTFE, Gore-Tex) • PTFE and polypropylene (Marlex)	• Durable, available • Does not grow • Challenging if infected • Recurrence and skeletal deformity
Absorbable (biologic)	• Porcine intestinal submucosa • Porcine dermal collagen (Permacol) • Human cadaveric dermis (AlloDerm) • Fetal bovine dermal collage (Surgimend) • Polylactic co-glycolic acid (PLGA) • Porcine dermis (Strattice)	• Significantly increased risk of recurrence[36] • Decreased infectious risk • May allow tissue ingrowth (theoretical)
Autologous (muscle) flap	• Reverse latissimus dorsi muscle • Serratus anterior muscle • Internal oblique/transversus abdominis muscle	• May grow with patient • Lower recurrence rate reported[37] • Potential option for repair of recurrent CDH or infected prosthetic
Tissue-engineered patches[38-40]	• Amniotic fluid stem cell-derived • Mesenchymal stem cell-derived • Umbilical cord-derived	• May grow and could function • Improved mechanical and functional outcomes compared with biologics • Remains investigational

MINIMALLY INVASIVE THORACOSCOPIC REPAIR

The MIS approach to CDH is now used in 10-20% of repairs and has a unique set of advantages and disadvantages.[32] This approach is usually reserved for low-risk CDH, given the increased risk intraoperative hypercarbia and acidosis which, even over brief periods, may have critical neurologic consequences.[49] Therefore, even in low-risk CDH, the thoracoscopic approach demands a minute-by-minute critical care approach by the anesthesia team. Further, the nuanced technical demands for this approach require experience and expertise, as evidenced by the increased rate of recurrence.[50–53] Despite these challenges, the MIS approach offers several advantages, the most notable of which is a significant fivefold reduction in the rate of reoperation for a bowel obstruction secondary to adhesive disease.[32] Further, reduction in postoperative pain, decreased narcotic use, decreased ventilator days, decreased length of stay, and improved cosmesis also highlight strengths, both extrapolated and directly evidence-based.

POSTOPERATIVE MANAGEMENT

Maintained vigilance is required in the postoperative period, as significant physiologic changes must be expected in response to surgery. Unfortunately, there is little agreement or quality data to guide how patients are best managed after repair. Minimization of lung injury should remain the main goal (permissive hypercapnia). Acceptable ventilator parameters and criteria for care escalation should remain the same as preoperatively. A pulmonary hypertensive crisis may occur after surgery, especially in the context of inadequate analgesia or sedation, and should be treated accordingly. The overarching pathway is stabilization, followed by weaning of ventilatory support and optimization of nutrition with transition to oral feeds as soon as tolerated.

LONG-TERM SURGICAL OUTCOMES

Multisystem adverse outcomes, either as a surgical complication or as a result of high-risk disease, are common, primarily in severe CDH. There are excellent reviews and recommendations regarding long-term surveillance.[54–58] With regards to surgical outcomes, consequences to CDH repair must be monitored both acutely postoperatively and over the long term, into adulthood. Hernia recurrence is most common within the first year and is more likely with large defects and after patch repair.[33] It is, however, possible to have a recurrence late in childhood or adolescence and after a primary repair. Recurrence may not be associated with symptoms, thus necessitating surveillance imaging to look for changes in the diaphragmatic contour.[59] Additional postoperative complications and associated timing of occurrence are shown in **Table 5**.

As the child grows, the prosthetic patch does not, and there is resultant tension on the chest wall, leading to significant chest deformity in more than half of patients with C or D defects.[60] A similar rate is observed after muscular flap repair. Primary repair patients are much less likely to have chest deformity (<10%).

Table 5		
Postoperative surgical complications directly related to diaphragm repair		
Early/Acute (<7 d)	**Short-Term (1–6 wk)**	**Long-Term (≥2 mo)**
Hemorrhage	Infection	Adhesions
Abdominal compartment syndrome	Re-herniation/patch failure	Re-herniation/patch failure
Re-herniation/patch failure		Bowel obstruction
Pleural effusion/chylothorax		

Thoracic scoliosis occurs in 15% and is less common but not unusual after primary repair, suggesting that scoliosis may be part of the congenital disease spectrum rather than solely due to tension from a patch.[57] Early screening is necessary to enable prompt referral to an orthopedic specialist for management.[61]

Other complications such as incisional hernias and bowel obstruction may also occur. Because of prenatal herniation of abdominal contents into the thoracic cavity, the bowel is nonrotated, and rare cases of midgut volvulus have been reported; however, this is not meaningfully preventable, and the risk is much lower than with classic malrotation.

SUMMARY

The surgical care of patients with CDH is complex but may be optimized with a management plan that employs well-defined criteria for transitions in care. Delay of diaphragm repair until stabilization has been achieved remains the fundamental principle guiding initial care of these patients, but it is also important to focus on avoidance of non-repair. This philosophy may require operation before optimal stabilization with anticipated postoperative use of ECLS; if ECLS is needed before repair is achieved, early repair after cannulation is becoming an accepted approach that may be associated with higher survival. Improvements and refinements in risk-stratification will influence the ongoing evolution in management, optimizing outcomes while mitigating intervention-related complications.

CLINICS CARE POINTS

- Congenital diaphragmatic hernia (CDH) is a surgical disease withsurvival dependent on diaphragmatic defect repair
- Postnatal preoperative care is complex but can be simplified with the use of *therapeutic targets/ranges* and defined *clinical thresholds* for transitions in care
- Diaphragmatic repair should occur after clinical stabilization (36 h to 7 days) and not after an arbitrary number of days
- Principles regarding the use of extracorporeal life support (ECLS) in CDH include proper patient selection, minimization of delay to ECLS if deemed necessary, and proper decision-making regarding operative timing if unrepaired once cannulated
- Repair on ECLS requires careful preoperative and intraoperative management of patient and circuit, as well as meticulous surgical technique to minimize the risk of complications
- Key operative principles include the use of a dome-shaped patch, a tension-free repair, and monitoring of PIP with temporary abdominal closure if necessary to prevent abdominal compartment syndrome
- Thoracoscopic minimally invasive surgical repair of the CDH is associated with specific advantages and disadvantages, and requires the proper patient selection and intraoperative management to optimize outcomes
- The incidence of long-term adverse surgical outcomes in CDH is directly related to the size of the CDH defect, and surveillance for complications is necessary in adulthood

DISCLOSURE

The authors have no commercial or financial conflicts of interest or any funding sources to disclose.

REFERENCES

1. Jancelewicz T, Brindle ME. Prediction tools in congenital diaphragmatic hernia. Semin Perinatol 2020;44(1):151165.
2. Snoek KG, Capolupo I, van Rosmalen J, et al. Conventional mechanical ventilation versus high-frequency oscillatory ventilation for congenital diaphragmatic hernia: a randomized clinical trial (The VICI-trial). Ann Surg 2016;263(5):867–74.
3. Snoek KG, Reiss IK, Greenough A, et al. Standardized postnatal management of infants with congenital diaphragmatic hernia in europe: the CDH EURO consortium consensus - 2015 Update. Neonatology 2016;110(1):66–74.
4. Canadian Congenital Diaphragmatic Hernia C, Puligandla PS, Skarsgard ED, et al. Diagnosis and management of congenital diaphragmatic hernia: a clinical practice guideline. CMAJ 2018;190(4):E103–12.
5. Jancelewicz T, Brindle ME, Guner YS, et al. Toward standardized management of congenital diaphragmatic hernia: an analysis of practice guidelines. J Surg Res 2019;243:229–35.
6. Gentili A, Pasini L, Iannella E, et al. Predictive outcome indexes in neonatal congenital diaphragmatic hernia. J Matern Fetal Neonatal Med 2015;28(13):1602–7.
7. Hollinger LE, Lally PA, Tsao K, et al, Congenital Diaphragmatic Hernia Study G. A risk-stratified analysis of delayed congenital diaphragmatic hernia repair: does timing of operation matter? Surgery 2014;156(2):475–82.
8. Logan JW, Rice HE, Goldberg RN, et al. Congenital diaphragmatic hernia: a systematic review and summary of best-evidence practice strategies. J Perinatol 2007;27(9):535–49.
9. Singh Y, Tissot C. Echocardiographic evaluation of transitional circulation for the neonatologists. Front Pediatr 2018;6:140.
10. Ferguson DM, Gupta VS, Lally PA, et al. Early, Postnatal pulmonary hypertension severity predicts inpatient outcomes in congenital diaphragmatic hernia. Neonatology 2021;118(2):147–54.
11. Gupta VS, Harting MT. Congenital diaphragmatic hernia-associated pulmonary hypertension. Semin Perinatol 2020;44(1):151167.
12. Patel N, Massolo AC, Kipfmueller F. Congenital diaphragmatic hernia-associated cardiac dysfunction. Semin Perinatol 2020;44(1):151168.
13. Gien J, Kinsella JP. Management of pulmonary hypertension in infants with congenital diaphragmatic hernia. J Perinatol 2016;36(Suppl 2):S28–31.
14. Jain A, Giesinger RE, Dakshinamurti S, et al. Care of the critically ill neonate with hypoxemic respiratory failure and acute pulmonary hypertension: framework for practice based on consensus opinion of neonatal hemodynamics working group. J Perinatol 2022;42(1):3–13.
15. Abman SH, Hansmann G, Archer SL, et al. Pediatric pulmonary hypertension: guidelines from the american heart association and american thoracic society. Circulation 2015;132(21):2037–99.
16. Nakayama DK, Motoyama EK, Tagge EM. Effect of preoperative stabilization on respiratory system compliance and outcome in newborn infants with congenital diaphragmatic hernia. J Pediatr 1991;118(5):793–9.
17. West KW, Bengston K, Rescorla FJ, et al. Delayed surgical repair and ECMO improves survival in congenital diaphragmatic hernia. Ann Surg 1992;216(4):454–60 [discussion: 460-452].

18. Moyer V, Moya F, Tibboel R, et al. Late versus early surgical correction for congenital diaphragmatic hernia in newborn infants. Cochrane Database Syst Rev 2002;(3):CD001695.

19. de la Hunt MN, Madden N, Scott JE, et al. Is delayed surgery really better for congenital diaphragmatic hernia?: a prospective randomized clinical trial. J Pediatr Surg 1996;31(11):1554–6.

20. Puligandla PS, Grabowski J, Austin M, et al. Management of congenital diaphragmatic hernia: a systematic review from the APSA outcomes and evidence based practice committee. J Pediatr Surg 2015;50(11):1958–70.

21. Congenital Diaphragmatic Hernia Study G, Lally KP, Lally PA, et al. Defect size determines survival in infants with congenital diaphragmatic hernia. Pediatrics 2007;120(3). e651–657.

22. Kays DW, Talbert JL, Islam S, et al. Improved survival in left liver-up congenital diaphragmatic hernia by early repair before extracorporeal membrane oxygenation: optimization of patient selection by multivariate risk modeling. J Am Coll Surg 2016;222(4):459–70.

23. Harting MT, Hollinger L, Tsao K, et al. Aggressive surgical management of congenital diaphragmatic hernia: worth the effort?: a multicenter, prospective, cohort study. Ann Surg 2018;267(5):977–82.

24. Jancelewicz T, Langham MR Jr, Brindle ME, et al. Survival benefit associated with the use of extracorporeal life support for neonates with congenital diaphragmatic hernia. Ann Surg 2022;275(1):e256–63.

25. Guner Y, Jancelewicz T, Di Nardo M, et al. Management of congenital diaphragmatic hernia treated with extracorporeal life support: interim guidelines consensus statement from the extracorporeal life support organization. ASAIO J 2021;67(2):113–20.

26. Church JT, Kim AC, Erickson KM, et al. Pushing the boundaries of ECLS: outcomes in <34 week EGA neonates. J Pediatr Surg 2017;52(11):1810–5.

27. Delaplain PT, Harting MT, Jancelewicz T, et al. Potential survival benefit with repair of congenital diaphragmatic hernia (CDH) after extracorporeal membrane oxygenation (ECMO) in select patients: study by ELSO CDH Interest Group. J Pediatr Surg 2019;54(6):1132–7. In Press.

28. Congenital Diaphragmatic Hernia Study Group, Bryner BS, West BT, et al. Congenital diaphragmatic hernia requiring extracorporeal membrane oxygenation: does timing of repair matter? J Pediatr Surg 2009;44(6):1165–71 [discussion: 1171-1162].

29. Dao DT, Burgos CM, Harting MT, et al. Surgical repair of congenital diaphragmatic hernia after extracorporeal membrane oxygenation cannulation: early repair improves survival. Ann Surg 2019;274(1):186–94.

30. Bembea MM, Annich G, Rycus P, et al. Variability in anticoagulation management of patients on extracorporeal membrane oxygenation: an international survey. Pediatr Crit Care Med 2013;14(2). e77–84.

31. Ozment CP, Scott BL, Bembea MM, et al. Anticoagulation and transfusion management during neonatal and pediatric extracorporeal membrane oxygenation: a survey of medical directors in the United States. Pediatr Crit Care Med 2021; 22(6):530–41.

32. Putnam LR, Tsao K, Lally KP, et al. Minimally invasive vs open congenital diaphragmatic hernia repair: is there a superior approach? J Am Coll Surg 2017; 224(4):416–22.

33. Putnam LR, Gupta V, Tsao K, et al. Factors associated with early recurrence after congenital diaphragmatic hernia repair. J Pediatr Surg 2017;52(6):928–32.

34. Verla MA, Style CC, Lee TC, et al. Does creating a dome reduce recurrence in congenital diaphragmatic hernia following patch repair? J Pediatr Surg 2022; 57(4):637–42.
35. Riehle KJ, Magnuson DK, Waldhausen JH. Low recurrence rate after Gore-Tex/ Marlex composite patch repair for posterolateral congenital diaphragmatic hernia. J Pediatr Surg 2007;42(11):1841–4.
36. Jancelewicz T, Vu LT, Keller RL, et al. Long-term surgical outcomes in congenital diaphragmatic hernia: observations from a single institution. J Pediatr Surg 2010; 45(1):155–60 [discussion: 160].
37. Dewberry L, Hilton S, Gien J, et al. Flap repair in congenital diaphragmatic hernia leads to lower rates of recurrence. J Pediatr Surg 2019;54(12):2487–91.
38. Kunisaki SM, Fuchs JR, Kaviani A, et al. Diaphragmatic repair through fetal tissue engineering: a comparison between mesenchymal amniocyte- and myoblast-based constructs. J Pediatr Surg 2006;41(1):34–9 [discussion: 34-39].
39. Fauza DO. Tissue engineering in congenital diaphragmatic hernia. Semin Pediatr Surg 2014;23(3):135–40.
40. Deprest J, Gucciardo L, Eastwood P, et al. Medical and regenerative solutions for congenital diaphragmatic hernia: a perinatal perspective. Eur J Pediatr Surg 2014;24(3):270–7.
41. Harting MT, Lally KP. Surgical management of neonates with congenital diaphragmatic hernia. Semin Pediatr Surg 2007;16(2):109–14.
42. Rana AR, Khouri JS, Teitelbaum DH, et al. Salvaging the severe congenital diaphragmatic hernia patient: is a silo the solution? J Pediatr Surg 2008;43(5): 788–91.
43. Loff S, Wirth H, Jester I, et al. Implantation of a cone-shaped double-fixed patch increases abdominal space and prevents recurrence of large defects in congenital diaphragmatic hernia. J Pediatr Surg 2005;40(11):1701–5.
44. Waag KL, Loff S, Zahn K, et al. Congenital diaphragmatic hernia: a modern day approach. Semin Pediatr Surg 2008;17(4):244–54.
45. Maxwell D, Baird R, Puligandla P. Abdominal wall closure in neonates after congenital diaphragmatic hernia repair. J Pediatr Surg 2013;48(5):930–4.
46. Ponsky TA, Rothenberg SS, Tsao K, et al. Thoracoscopy in children: is a chest tube necessary? J Laparoendosc Adv Surg Tech A 2009;19(Suppl 1):S23–5.
47. Morini F, Lally KP, Lally PA, et al. Treatment strategies for congenital diaphragmatic hernia: change sometimes comes bearing gifts. Front Pediatr 2017;5:195.
48. Schlager A, Arps K, Siddharthan R, et al. Tube Thoracostomy at the time of congenital diaphragmatic hernia repair: reassessing the risks and benefits. J Laparoendoscopic Adv Surg Tech Part A 2017;27(3):311–7.
49. Bishay M, Giacomello L, Retrosi G, et al. Hypercapnia and acidosis during open and thoracoscopic repair of congenital diaphragmatic hernia and esophageal atresia: results of a pilot randomized controlled trial. Ann Surg 2013;258(6): 895–900.
50. Jancelewicz T, Langer JC, Chiang M, et al. Thoracoscopic repair of neonatal congenital diaphragmatic hernia (CDH): outcomes after a systematic quality improvement process. J Pediatr Surg 2013;48(2):321–5 [discussion: 325].
51. Gander JW, Fisher JC, Gross ER, et al. Early recurrence of congenital diaphragmatic hernia is higher after thoracoscopic than open repair: a single institutional study. J Pediatr Surg 2011;46(7):1303–8.
52. Kamran A, Zendejas B, Demehri FR, et al. Risk factors for recurrence after thoracoscopic repair of congenital diaphragmatic hernia (CDH). J Pediatr Surg 2018; 53(11):2087–91.

53. Criss CN, Coughlin MA, Matusko N, et al. Outcomes for thoracoscopic versus open repair of small to moderate congenital diaphragmatic hernias. J Pediatr Surg 2018;53(4):635–9.
54. American Academy of Pediatrics Section on S, American Academy of Pediatrics Committee on F, Newborn Lally KP, Engle W. Postdischarge follow-up of infants with congenital diaphragmatic hernia. Pediatrics 2008;121(3):627–32.
55. IJsselstijn H, Breatnach C, Hoskote A, et al. Defining outcomes following congenital diaphragmatic hernia using standardised clinical assessment and management plan (SCAMP) methodology within the CDH EURO consortium. Pediatr Res 2018;84(2):181–9.
56. Chiu PP, Ijsselstijn H. Morbidity and long-term follow-up in CDH patients. Eur J Pediatr Surg 2012;22(5):384–92.
57. Hollinger LE, Buchmiller TL. Long term follow-up in congenital diaphragmatic hernia. Semin Perinatol 2020;44(1):151171.
58. Morini F, Valfre L, Bagolan P. Long-term morbidity of congenital diaphragmatic hernia: a plea for standardization. Semin Pediatr Surg 2017;26(5):301–10.
59. Jancelewicz T, Chiang M, Oliveira C, et al. Late surgical outcomes among congenital diaphragmatic hernia (CDH) patients: why long-term follow-up with surgeons is recommended. J Pediatr Surg 2013;48(5):935–41.
60. Russell KW, Barnhart DC, Rollins MD, et al. Musculoskeletal deformities following repair of large congenital diaphragmatic hernias. J Pediatr Surg 2014;49(6):886–9.
61. Eby SF, Hilaire TS, Glotzbecker M, et al. Thoracogenic spinal deformity: a rare cause of early-onset scoliosis. J Neurosurg Spine 2018;29(6):674–9.

Management of Congenital Lung Malformations

Brittany N. Hegde, MD[a,b], KuoJen Tsao, MD[a,b], Shinjiro Hirose, MD[c,*]

KEYWORDS

- Congenital lung malformations • Bronchopulmonary sequestrations
- Congenital pulmonary airway malformation • Congenital lobar emphysema
- Bronchogenic cyst

KEY POINTS

- Congenital lung lesions have intricacies involved in diagnosis, prenatal, and postnatal management.
- This article has focused on a current review of the literature and evidenced-based recommendations for various aspects of caring for patients with congenital lung lesions.
- Long-term studies are needed to gain a true understanding of the natural history of these diseases and to develop consensus, evidenced-based management guidelines.

INTRODUCTION

Congenital lung malformations (CLMs) represent a spectrum of lesions, and all have a unique cause that often coincides with a distinctive clinical approach.[1] Due to improvements in access to prenatal care and use of prenatal ultrasound, the incidence of these lesions is increasing and estimated to be around 1 in 2500 to 8000 live births.[1] Because fetal interventions continue to improve, prenatal and postnatal management strategies continue to evolve to provide the best care possible for neonates with these underlying lung abnormalities. Previously lethal lung malformations are now able to be managed in the prenatal period successfully with fewer adverse effects.[1] The overall survival for those with CLMs has increased significantly from 60% to currently more than 95% with the aforementioned improvements in prenatal diagnosis and treatment to minimize the development of pulmonary hypoplasia leading to cardiovascular failure and eventual death.[1]

[a] Department of Pediatric Surgery, McGovern Medical School at the University of Texas Health Science Center at Houston, 6431 Fannin Street, MSB 5.256, Houston, TX 77030, USA; [b] Center for Surgical Trials and Evidence-Based Practice (C-STEP), McGovern Medical School at the University of Texas Health Science Center at Houston, 6431 Fannin Street, MSB 5.256, Houston, TX 77030, USA; [c] Division of Pediatric, Thoracic, and Fetal Surgery, University of California-Davis Medical Center, 2335 Stockton Boulevard, Sacramento, CA 95817, USA
* Corresponding author.
E-mail address: shirose@ucdavis.edu

Clin Perinatol 49 (2022) 907–926
https://doi.org/10.1016/j.clp.2022.08.003
0095-5108/22/© 2022 Elsevier Inc. All rights reserved.
perinatology.theclinics.com

This article will focus on the following CLMs: congenital pulmonary airway malformations (CPAMs), formally known as congenital cystic adenomatoid malformations, bronchopulmonary sequestration (BPS), congenital lobar emphysema (CLE), and bronchogenic cyst (BCs). Each of these malformations will be further defined and examined from an embryologic, pathophysiologic, and clinical management perspective unique to that specific lesion. A review of current recommendations in both medical and surgical management of these lesions will be discussed as well as widely accepted treatment algorithms.

Fetal Lung Embryology

To understand the cause and natural history of CLMs, it is imperative to understand the embryology of the lung. Fetal lung development is an intricately coordinated progression directed by mesenchymal–epithelial interactions and various regulatory factors[2] (**Fig. 1**). Embryologic lung development begins at 3 to 4 weeks gestation and is divided into 5 different stages. The embryonic stage (3–7 weeks) is when the lung bud is created from endoderm and divides into the right and left bronchi around gestational day 28. Further division of the secondary bronchial buds occurs during this time as well as development of the pulmonary vasculature.[3] The pseudoglandular stage (5–17 weeks) is when rapid growth occurs and all bronchial dividing is completed by week 16 as well as development of cilia and supportive cartilage. Abnormal development during this stage is thought to lead to the development of BPS and CPAMs (types I, II, III).[2,3] The canalicular stage (16–26 weeks) is when development of areas of gas exchange occur, as well as differentiation of type 1 and type 2 pneumocytes and lamellar bodies that

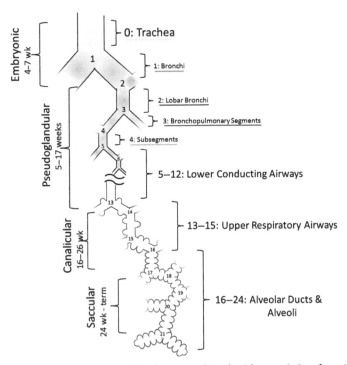

Fig. 1. Stages of embryologic lung development. (*Used with permission from* Woods JC, Schittny JC. Lung Structure at Preterm and Term Birth. *Fetal Neonatal Lung Dev.* Published online April 5, 2016:126-140.)

produce surfactant. Abnormalities in development in this stage greatly affect the ability to perform gas exchange. The saccular stage (24–38 weeks) is when alveolar saccules form and the alveolocapillary membrane is thin enough to perform gas exchange by 24 weeks.[2] Abnormalities in development in this stage are thought to lead to the development of type IV CPAMs.[3] Finally, the alveolar stage (36 weeks to 8 years) is when alveoli are formed and the interface for gas exchange and the capillary network continues to mature. Alveoli creation is completed by 8 years of age. Abnormalities in development in this stage are thought to lead to the development of CLE.[2,3]

Congenital Lung Malformations

Congenital pulmonary airway malformation etiology
CPAMs are CLMs that involve overproliferation and enlargement of terminal respiratory bronchioles that do not contain standard alveoli. These lesions do preserve a usual blood supply from the pulmonary arteries and continued communication with the normal respiratory tree. CPAMs are usually unilateral and involve only one lobe of the lung.[4] Incidence of these are reported to be around 1 in 10,000 live births.[5] In 1977, Stocker introduced a classification of CPAMs based other anatomy and embryological origins[6] (**Table 1**).

Bronchopulmonary sequestration etiology
BPSs are lesions noted to be nonfunctional and not connected to normal tracheobronchial tree. These lesions are often noted to be supplied by an aberrant systemic artery from the aorta, origin of which is quite variable. BPS develops in 2 ways: intralobar or extralobar sequestrations. It is hypothesized that during embryologic development, a supernumerary lung bud is formed posterior to the normal lung bud eventually becoming aberrant lung tissue. The interlobar versus extralobar distinction of BPS depends on the timing of the supernumerary lung bud development in relation to pleura. If lung bud develops before the pleura then the BPS will become intralobar, and if after the pleura, then it will become extralobar and develop its own pleura.[6] Additionally, hybrid lesions may develop that share characteristics with CPAMs and BPSs. They are often cystic but blood supply is often from the aorta similar to BPS lesions.[7]

Congenital lobar emphysema etiology
CLE is used to describe lung tissue that is distended, hyperlucent on X-rays and has increased echogenicity on ultrasound. CLE is thought to originate from alterations in interactions between the endoderm and mesoderm of embryologic lung tissue that

Table 1
Stocker classification of congenital pulmonary airway malformation lesions

Type	Location	Characterization	%	Prognosis
Type 0	Trachea Bronchus	Whole lung Lungs small, solid, firm	1–3%	Fatal
Type 1	Distal bronchi Proximal bronchioles	One large dominant cyst Late presentations Most common	50–65%	Good
Type 2	Bronchiolar	Multiple small cysts Other anomalies	10–40%	Poor
Type 3	Alveolar	Cystic with solid Solid appearance	5–10%	Severe
Type 4	Acinar	Thin wall, fluid filled small cysts	10–15%	Good

can cause increasing hyperinflation. Incidence of CLE is thought to be around 1 per 20,000 to 30,000 births and is usually diagnosed in the postnatal period due to imaging characteristics being understated and difficult to differentiate on prenatal ultrasound. Associated anomalies can occur including cardiovascular abnormalities in 14% of cases. Less commonly renal, gastrointestinal, musculoskeletal, and cutaneous abnormalities may also exist.[2] CLE can be asymptomatic or present with respiratory distress, tension pneumothorax, wheezing, or atelectasis due to lung compression.[4]

Bronchogenic cyst etiology

BC occurs because of abnormal development of foregut. They are known as foregut duplication cysts that contain cartilage, smooth muscle, and glands. BC do not communicate with tracheobronchial tree and are often filled with fluid or mucous. Most are found within the mediastinum near the trachea but can be located throughout the peripheral lung tissue. The differentiation between types of foregut duplication cysts is predicated on pathologic analysis with BC being lined with ciliated epithelium. BC can cause a variety of symptoms including compression on trachea/bronchus, dysphagia, infections, and hemorrhage leading to the possible development of hemothorax.[2]

Prenatal Management

Prenatal diagnosis of fetal abnormalities has greatly improved because imaging techniques continue to improve. About congenital pulmonary lesions, advances in ultrasound techniques have increased the ability for prenatal diagnosis of these abnormalities.[6]

Ultrasound characteristics

Prenatal diagnosis of CLMs most commonly occurs via abnormalities seen on routine fetal ultrasound generally in the second trimester.[6] The increase in the detection on fetal ultrasound has led to a better understanding of these lesions and allowed for further planning as to how to manage delivery and postnatal care.[8]

Ultrasound is widely used during pregnancy to monitor the growing fetus. Fetal lung tissue on routine ultrasound seems similar in echogenicity to that of the liver or spleen. Congenital pulmonary abnormalities can have variable echogenicity, either increased or decreased, depending on specific lesion characteristics. Mass effect may also be noted on ultrasound depending on the size of the lesion. Large lesions can cause compression of various thoracic structures, including the esophagus, which can result in polyhydramnios due to impaired swallowing. These large abnormalities can also cause compression on adjacent areas of the lung resulting in the underdevelopment of normal lung tissue as well as shift of mediastinal structures due to mass effect. This mediastinal shift can not only cause lung compression but also affect cardiac function and decrease the amount of blood return due to venous compression. This venous compression leading to cardiac failure can progress to an entity referred to as nonimmune fetal hydrops, a poor prognostic indicator.[8,9] Large lesions do not always maintain their size as the fetus progresses in gestational age. Many are known to decrease in size or even resolve on recurrent ultrasound surveillance. CPAM lesions on ultrasound are commonly noted to be unilateral and to seem more echogenic than the surrounding lung tissue. To differentiate CPAMS from other congenital lesions on ultrasound, evaluating if the lesions contain a cystic component often leads to the diagnosis of CPAM if all other imaging criteria are met.[8] CPAMs can be categorized as microcystic (no visible cystic element) or macrocytic (cystic structures greater than 1 cm in diameter) depending on imaging characteristics.[10] Most of the prenatal imaging evidence is based on CPAMs due their most common prevalence.

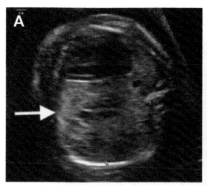
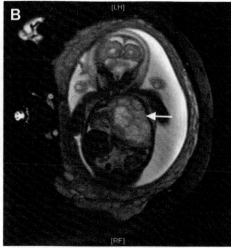

Fig. 2. CPAM prenatal ultrasound and MR image. A 32-year-old G3P2 female with a fetus at 28 2/7 weeks diagnosed with CPAM. Noted on ultrasound (*A*) to have a CPAM (designated by *arrow*) measuring 6.9 × 5.1 × 5.3 with a CVR 3.9 and evidence of hydrops/polyhydramnios. MRI findings (*B*) with evidence of large left-sided CPAM hyperintense on T2-weighted imaging.

Ultrasounds while useful in identifying abnormal pulmonary lesions are sometimes not able to provide a clear diagnosis with certainty[8] (**Fig. 2A**).

Various measurements are performed on ultrasound imaging to aid in monitoring CPAMs diagnosed during prenatal period. Size of the lesion is often measured and serially monitored. Large lesions are often defined as occupying two-thirds of volume of thorax as well as contributing to mediastinal shift. Shift of mediastinal structures can be measured as well as mass effect on the diaphragm, monitoring if it is flat or everted. Lesions can also be characterized depending on whether they involve a cystic or solid component, and both aspects can be measured and serially followed on further ultrasounds.[11] Measurement of CPAM volume to head circumference ratio (CVR) has been used as a prognostic indictor when CPAMs are diagnosed during the prenatal period. CVR is calculated using the volume formula for an ellipse to calculate volume of mass (height × width × length × 0.52) and dividing that volume by head circumference to allow correction for gestational age. Various studies have shown that a CVR of greater than 1.6 was associated with increased risk for the development of fetal hydrops and that those with CVR of less than 1.6 have a less than 3% risk of developing hydrops.[4,6,12] The CVR has been used as a measurement by physicians to follow CPAMs throughout the prenatal period and to establish an objective measurement to prompt potential fetal intervention.

The other CLMs are also easily identified with prenatal ultrasound although their differentiation may be challenging. The prognostic measurements associated with CPAMs should not be used to extrapolate outcomes for these other CLMs. Often in cases of ambiguity, further imaging may be necessary. Using ultrasound to confirm a diagnosis of BPS often requires use of Color Doppler to identify feeding vessels, which are pathognomonic for BPS.[6,13] On ultrasound, BPS lesions seem hyperechoic, solid, well-defined lung mass.[4,14] However, despite the ability to identify abnormal blood supply of BPS lesions, ultrasound is not able to define parenchymal abnormalities that may be located around the sequestration (**Fig. 3**A, B). MRI or computed

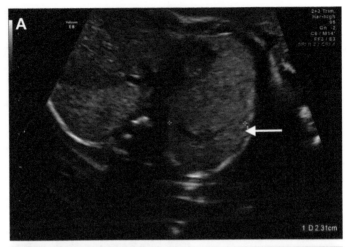

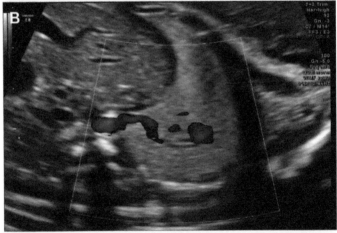

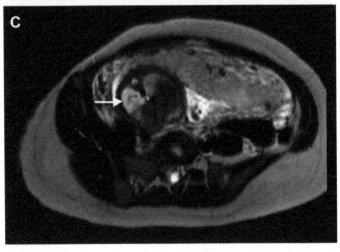

tomography (CT) scans can be used to further delineate the lung lesion. BPS seems hyperintense on T2-weighted images, and MRI is useful to fully define the abnormal blood supply of BPS lesion and surrounding parenchymal abnormalities without exposure to radiation[15] (**Fig. 3**C). CT scans can be helpful in identifying parenchymal abnormalities but may be inferior to MRI in fully defining BPS blood supply and are generally avoided during gestation.[4,8,14] It is very difficult to characterize a BPS as intralobar versus extralobar from prenatal ultrasound. Often the presence of a surrounding pleural effusion or abdominal location is the only distinguishing feature that points toward an extralobar BPS compared with intralobar BPS.[6,16]

MRI characteristics. MRI is sometimes used to assist in diagnosis when ultrasound is found to be limited in assisting with diagnosis of abnormal pulmonary lesions in the fetus. MRI is usually avoided in first trimester but further development of fast MRI has allowed for the ability to obtain high-quality images despite fetal movements and maternal breathing patterns. MRI has the ability to accurately display fetal thorax anatomy, establish the size of the lung lesion, and demonstrate a special relationship to other structures in the fetal thorax. MRI can also be helpful in determining lung volume, which is a useful prognostic indicator.[8]

MRI characteristics of normal lung tissue include high signal on T2-weighted imaging, and the signal intensity is higher than compared with the chest wall but lower than amniotic fluid. Lung lesions frequently exhibit even further increased intensity on MRI than compared with normal lung tissue.[8]

In a systematic review by Downard and colleagues, they evaluated the literature on the comparison of ultrasound imaging versus MRI in the diagnosis of congenital pulmonary lesions. In this review, the authors found that fetal MRI could sometimes alter the initial ultrasound diagnosis. However, this change in diagnosis did not always lead to a change in management but did often alter the appropriate prenatal parental counseling. Fetal MRI is beneficial when the diagnosis is not completely straightforward via ultrasound, or when further characterization of the lesion is necessary when management requires fetal intervention as the most accurate, detailed information about the lesion is then required[12,14] (**Fig. 2**B).

Congenital pulmonary airway malformation prenatal treatment strategies

Understanding imaging characteristics of CPAMs and their potential sequela can lead to risk stratification of patients to assist in developing appropriate management strategies. High-risk features noted on ultrasound or MRI include CVR greater than 1.6, placentomegaly, abnormal fetal echocardiography, diaphragmatic eversion, mediastinal shift, and lung hypoplasia. The American Pediatric Surgical Association recommends that these conditions warrant close monitoring with serial ultrasounds and referral to a fetal treatment center for optimal surveillance and management.[12]

CVR calculations have shown in multiple studies to correlate with the development of fetal hydrops and substantial increased risk of fetal demise. Microcystic CPAMs are thought to reach their maximal growth potential around 28 weeks. Therefore, it is recommended that serial surveillance ultrasounds occur at least weekly for fetuses less than 28 weeks with microcystic CPAMs with CVRs greater than 1.6, sometimes twice

◀―――――――――――――――――――――――――――――――――――――

Fig. 3. BPS prenatal MRI and ultrasound. A 19-year-old female patient with fetus at 28 3/7 weeks gestation noted to have BPS lesion on ultrasound (*A*), with evidence of systemic arterial supply on Doppler ultrasound (*B*) consistent with BPS diagnosis. MRI showed a T2-hyperintense lesion measuring 3.6 × 2.4 × 2.1 in the left lower lobe with systemic blood supply from thoracic aorta at level of hiatus (*C*). MTR of 37%.

weekly depending on individual fetal characteristics. Those with CVRs less than 1.6 can be monitored either weekly or every other week unless concerning features develop.[16] Those that remain without evidence of hydrops can often be managed expectantly after birth. Those that develop hydrops often require fetal intervention, medical and/or surgical, for a chance at survival.

The use of maternal steroids has been a highly debated in the management of pre-natally diagnosed CPAMs with high-risk features. A study by Tsao and colleagues was the first to demonstrate benefit of maternal administration of steroids for CPAMs with hydrops. The authors demonstrated resolution of hydrops in 3 patients given steroids and subsequently were able to deliver at term without respiratory complications.[17] Subsequent studies have found that administering maternal betamethasone, 12 mg, in 2 doses separated by 24 hours have had a beneficial effect on those with microcys-tic CPAMs, with the majority having resolution of hydrops and surviving to discharge.[12,18,19] Therefore, prenatal steroid administration should be considered in fetuses with microcytic CPAM lesions with high-risk factors and potentially could avoid the need for surgery for macrocystic disease.[12]

Macrocytic CPAMs have additional management options for fetuses that develop the high-risk features and concerning signs of hydrops. The growth pattern for macro-cystic CPAMs is less predictable than that for microcystic ones. Macrocystic CPAMs can undergo enlargement of a dominant cyst throughout gestation. As a result, macro-cytic CPAMs can undergo transamniotic needle decompression or have a thora-coamniotic shunt placed if cyst enlargement causes fetal hydrops.[16,18,20,21] Studies have been performed to examine if decompression of macrocytic CPAMs by these methods improve fetal survival and have shown an association with increased fetal survival, despite a lack of consensus guidelines and high-quality evidence. Therefore, these methods should be considered as a management strategy in fetuses with macrocytic CPAMs.[12,18] Macrocystic lesions generally do not respond well to ste-roids; therefore, are usually managed with transamniotic needle decompression or with a thoraco-amniotic shunt. Microcystic lesions will often respond to steroids but depending on risk factors may require potential fetal intervention.

CPAMs with hydropic features that are less than 32 weeks gestation that do not improve or are not candidates for the above measures can be considered for fetal sur-gery. Fetal surgery requires that patients have a normal karyotype and no other asso-ciated anomalies detected by ultrasound or fetal echocardiography. During open fetal surgery, an open thoracotomy is performed via the fifth intercostal space and appro-priate lobectomy or partial resection is performed. Benefits seen from resection in sur-viving patients included hydrops resolution in 1 to 2 weeks, resolution of mediastinal shift by 3 weeks, and in utero lung growth after resection.[16] Fetal lobectomy is offered less commonly today due to success of maternal steroid use and close serial imaging follow-up of patients with CPAMs. Despite this, open fetal surgery remains a valid op-tion for those unresponsive to maternal steroid administration.[12]

In fetuses where there is a concern for significant respiratory difficulties at birth and a persistently high CVR after 32 weeks gestation, a controlled ex-utero intrapartum treat-ment (EXIT) procedure may be considered. During an EXIT procedure, a controlled hys-terotomy is performed with a fetal lobectomy while the fetus remains on placental support. Maternal general anesthesia is used with inhaled anesthetics as well as intra-venous magnesium and nitrates are used to promote continued uterine relaxation to allow optimal utero-placental circulation and gas exchange for continued fetal support. After the operation is complete, the fetus is delivered, and the airway is managed as required by fetal response to delivery. Rarely extracorporeal membrane oxygenation (ECMO) support after EXIT procedure is required due to persistent pulmonary hypertension. Studies performed examining the use of the EXIT procedure have lacked randomization and long-term follow-up; therefore, consensus guidelines for this procedure have not been made. However, in specialized fetal centers fetuses with concerning features after 32 weeks gestation, the EXIT procedure can be considered.[12,16,22,23]

Treatment and management. Fetal centers are specialized treatment facilities where those with prenatally diagnosed lung lesions are referred for monitoring and possible treatment. Most fetal centers have developed their own protocols and algorithms for the treatment of various fetal disorders. This algorithm is an example of one fetal center's approach to the prenatally diagnosed fetal lung lesion. First, CVR measurements are used to direct monitoring and possible treatment. Then, determining if the fetus has hydropic features versus no hydrops determines whether fetal intervention is considered. What type of fetal intervention considered depends on the type of lesion in question. As always, gestational age of the fetus is an important consideration when choosing a treatment plan (**Fig. 4**).

Bronchopulmonary sequestration prenatal management. Many BPS lesions will decrease in size during the prenatal period. Therefore, most BPS lesions often do not require fetal intervention and allow for observation and close serial monitoring for the potential development of concerning features.[6,16]

Large lesions can develop mass effect and cause hydrops in similar fashion to CPAMs. However, more commonly, hydrops develops due to the production of excess fluid leading to a large hydrothorax. Management of these lesions often requires serial thoracentesis or a thoracoamniotic shunt to resolve these symptoms.[1,16]

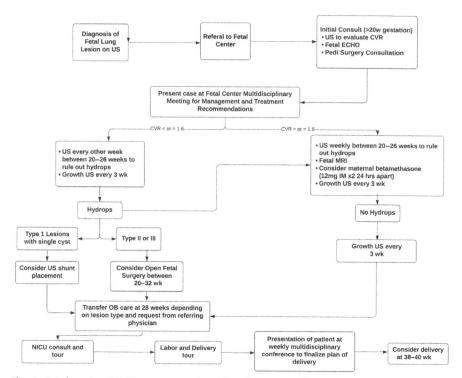

Fig. 4. Fetal center CPAM treatment algorithm. (*Courtesy of* K. Tsao, MD, Houston, Texas.)

Additionally, hydrops associated with BPS lesions may develop secondary to their blood supply. Their abnormal systemic arterial blood supply with venous drainage via the pulmonary veins leads to "left-to-left" shunting that results in high-output cardiac failure and development of hydrops. BPS lesions that subsequently develop hydrops are almost universally fatal without treatment interventions.[6]

The use of maternal steroids in specific BPS lesions has not been studied as well as their use for CPAMs, and the benefit of such treatment requires further study to truly understand its effect.[10] Fetal surgery may be considered for BPS lesions that cause fetal hydrops without the element of hydrothorax, although this is rare. Only those diagnosed at less than 30 weeks gestation are considered for open fetal surgery. Those at or beyond 30 weeks gestation are considered for early delivery and postdelivery intervention.[6]

Additionally, various techniques have been described to terminate the blood supply of BPSs in those with high-risk features including hydrops. First, the use of intrafetal vascular laser ablation has been highly successful. Gottschalk and colleagues[24] demonstrated that out of 12 patients, 11 (97.1%) were successfully treated with vascular laser ablation that resulted in resolution or shrinkage of their BPS. Similarly, sclerosing agents to obliterate the blood supply to BPS lesions have been described as a minimally invasive approach for high-risk features including fetal hydrops. Bermudez and colleagues published a study where the authors used ultrasound guided fetal sclerotherapy as treatment of large BPS lesions associated with hydrops. Three fetuses underwent this therapy where the feeding vessel to each BPS was accessed percutaneously and sclerotherapy with polidocanol was performed. Each fetus demonstrated destruction of blood flow to the BPS lesion and subsequent ultrasound surveillance demonstrated resolution of hydropic features. Further investigation of this fetal sclerotherapy in comparison with other fetal interventions is needed before accepting its widespread use.[25]

Congenital lobar emphysema prenatal management. CLE diagnosis in the prenatal period is rare and frequently presents in the early postnatal period as respiratory distress in a newborn. However, there are some described cases in the literature but those lesions rarely require any fetal intervention.[26] The common ultrasound imaging characteristic of CLE is echogenic appearance with or without cystic inclusions.[16,26] These lesions can be differentiated from BPS by the absence of any systemic abnormal blood supply (**Fig. 5**). MRI may also be helpful to further define the abnormal lesion to further differentiate CLE from other lesions in the differential including CPAM and BPS.[27] CLE lesions may grow in size due to the accumulation of fluid within these lesions but most eventually decrease in size and some are even undistinguishable compared with normal lung tissue by the end of gestational period.[1,16] Despite the apparent "disappearance" of these lesions, they can still cause respiratory distress in the newborn period due to air trapping and call for continued close monitoring of the newborn.[26]

Bronchogenic cyst prenatal management. BC may be diagnosed prenatally via ultrasound. These lesions have the appearance of a well-defined, fluid-containing, unilocular, round mass on ultrasound (**Fig. 6**). BC may sometimes be confused for other CLMs; therefore, MRI may be a useful adjunct to assist in confirming diagnosis.[28] Diagnosis of BC prenatally can be important to identify those lesions that are at risk for causing compressive effects on normal lung parenchyma leading to potential hydrops and fatal fetal outcomes. A case report by Teresa and colleagues[29] demonstrated successful prenatal cyst aspiration at 23 weeks gestation to alleviate the

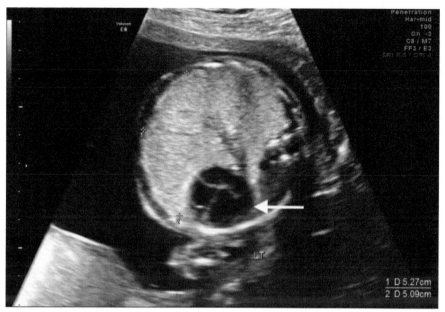

Fig. 5. CLE prenatal ultrasound. A 33-year-old female patient with a 23 3/7 week fetus found to have right lung lesion on ultrasound with cystic appearance consistent with CLE.

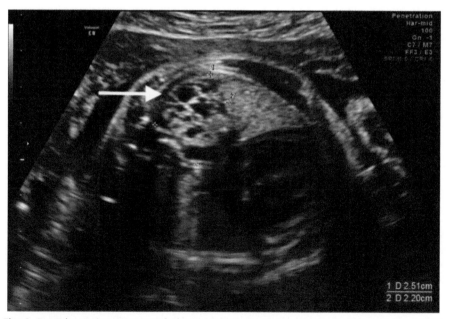

Fig. 6. Bronchogenic cyst prenatal ultrasound images. A 26-year-old female patient with 23 2/7 week fetus with evidence on ultrasound of cystic lesion concerning for bronchogenic cyst.

compressive effects of a large BC allowing for continued fetal growth and monitoring during gestational period. Further studies are needed to establish the true benefit and effect on fetal outcomes. Thoracoamniotic shunting may also be used to decrease the accumulation of fluid and decrease the compressive effects of large BC.[1] Few instances of fetal surgery have been described, including resection using the previously described EXIT procedure for large BC that cause airway obstruction. These cases are rare but should allow for these methods of intervention to be considered if fetal circumstances dictate urgent intervention. The majority of BC is managed successfully in the postnatal period.[1,29]

Pulmonary Lesions Delivery Management

Consensus guidelines on delivery management of prenatally diagnosed congenital pulmonary lesions have not been described. However, most can agree that fetuses with prenatally diagnosed CLMs should have thorough delivery planning. Most physicians recommend transport to a tertiary care facility with the abilities to provide essential postnatal care for these infants. The need for a multidisciplinary team involving neonatologists, pediatric surgeons, pediatric anesthesiologists, and pediatric radiologists is crucial for the successful delivery of these infants with the potential for severe respiratory distress at birth. The availability of this team also allows for early interventions if necessary. Facilities with the ability to provide ECMO as an adjunctive therapy for infants with severe respiratory distress and pulmonary hypertension would be also be ideal. Fetal centers around the country are often involved early due to the referrals they receive for prenatally diagnosed lung lesions. They may assist with delivery planning to optimize delivery of infants with these lesions because the wide spectrum of their presentation from asymptomatic to severe respiratory distress makes delivery predictions difficult.[16,29] Arshad and colleagues, aimed to evaluate if CVR could be used to predict which fetus might require early surgery. They evaluated a total of 53 patients and compared those who required early surgery to those that were able to be managed with later surgery. They found that a CVR threshold of greater than 0.9 had the best prediction for need for early surgery.[30] Further long-term studies are needed to validate these findings and show the potential use of CVR to direct delivery management.

Postnatal Management

The postnatal management of CLMs is a deeply debated topic without a consensus set of evidenced-based guidelines for clinicians to follow. Often recommendations are based less on evidence and more on physician preference or comfort level with the given management strategy. Frequently symptomatic lesions are imaged early and offered early surgical intervention. Asymptomatic lesions may be monitored with delayed imaging and surgically resected at a later date.

Postnatal imaging

X-ray images of CPAMs may visualize retained fluid within the lesion or increased aeration with visualization of air-filled cysts on imaging[6] (**Fig. 7**A). If symptomatic and deemed need for resection, further imaging is obtained to define the anatomy such as CT scan or MRI (**Fig. 7**B).

Postnatal imaging is crucial for surgical planning on symptomatic patients with BPS. BPSs have a systemic arterial/venous supply that helps to differentiate them from CPAMs. Doppler ultrasound can assist with mapping out the blood supply, as can CT scans with contrast. CT scans often provide more information about parenchymal

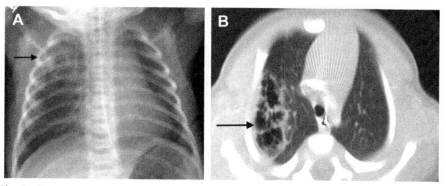

Fig. 7. CPAM postnatal X-ray and CT scan. (*A*) A postnatal X-ray image of a newborn with a right upper lobe lung lesion with cystic appearance consistent with CPAM. (*B*) A postnatal CT image of the same right upper lobe lung lesion with multiple cysts noted in the apex of right upper lobe.

lung abnormalities or intra-abdominal location of lesions (**Fig. 8**). MRIs may also be used to gain further information if needed.[8]

CLE can seem as hyperinflated lung on X-ray or a radio-opaque mass due to delayed clearance of fluid from the overdistended lobe (**Fig. 9**). If there are any diagnostic uncertainties, CT or ventilation/perfusion scans may be used to confirm the diagnosis. On CT scan, CLE lesions seem less attenuated or darker than normal lung tissue and will be visibly enlarged.[8]

BC may be visible on chest X-ray as an oval soft tissue density or with a visible air fluid level if located intraparenchymal. Chest CT often further delineates not only the cyst characteristics but also its relation to surrounding structures in the mediastinum. This imaging is important for operative planning[8,31] (**Fig. 10**).

Symptomatic lesions

Most clinicians agree that symptomatic lesions should be removed, regardless of lesion type. Surgical resection may involve an open thoracotomy or minimally invasive thoracoscopic approach, depending on physician familiarity and patient tolerance. For CPAMs lobectomy is the surgery of choice but there have been instances of

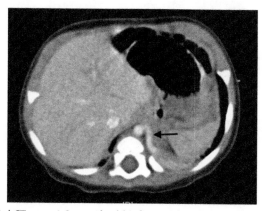

Fig. 8. BPS postnatal CT scan. A 3-month-old infant with CT scan imaging of lower lobe BPS lesion with systemic arterial blood supply from descending aorta (*arrow*).

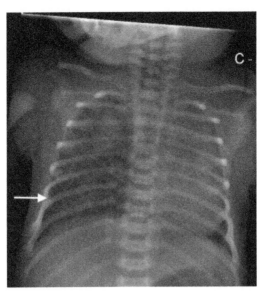

Fig. 9. CLE X-ray. X-ray of a newborn infant with hyperinflation of right lower lobe consistent with CLE.

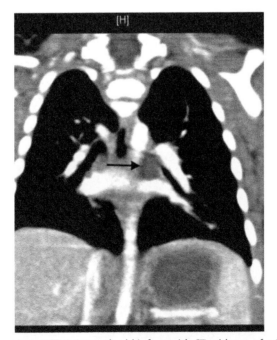

Fig. 10. Bronchogenic cyst CT. A 4-month-old infant with CT evidence of a 10.6 × 10.2 × 10.5 lesion (*arrow*) between descending aorta and left main pulmonary artery causing moderate narrowing of left mainstem bronchus consistent with bronchogenic cyst.

segmentectomies and other lung-preserving operations that have been performed. However, there has been no evidence that lung-preserving operations are superior to lobectomy.[4,12]

Removal of BPSs does require caution with ligation of their blood supply. Most arterial supply comes from the abdominal aorta and may cross the diaphragm. This makes careful ligation imperative due to concern that these vessels may retract into the abdominal cavity and lead to uncontrolled hemorrhage if not ligated adequately.[31] One alternative approach to resection for BPS is that of arterial embolization. This is performed percutaneously by either interventional radiology or cardiology. Studies have shown a variable response. A study by Cho and colleagues demonstrated 7% complete regression, 83% partial regression, with 9.5% having no response to embolization. About 9.5% had complications after procedure that included infection, pain, fever, and migration of substance used for embolization. This study concluded that surgical resection was the optimal treatment method but that embolization could be used in those patients that were high risk for operative intervention.[32]

Resection of CLE often includes lobectomy to remove affected portion of the lung and is often done via an open approach due to the size of these lesions and difficulty with mobilization thoracoscopically. Anesthetic management is crucial with severe cases requiring positioning and prepping and draping before the initiation of positive pressure ventilation to avoid massive overdistention of the abnormal lung tissue. Due to the variable association of CLE with cardiac abnormalities, some clinicians recommend obtaining an echocardiogram prior to surgical resection.[1,4,8,33]

As with other congenital pulmonary lesions, symptomatic BC should undergo resection. Resection may include enucleation of the cyst if located in the mediastinum, or wedge/anatomic resections if located intraparenchymal. Most clinicians recommend thoracoscopic approach for BC resection. If symptomatic infants are too unstable for surgery, an aspiration of the cyst may be performed to stabilize the infant before pursuing surgical resection.[1,31]

Asymptomatic lesions

Management of the asymptomatic patient is controversial, regardless of lesion type. Some physicians advocate for an observational approach, whereas other physicians opt for a resection strategy that is delayed until a few months of age once the anesthesia complications for newborns have lessened. Those that argue for an eventual resection often state that the risks of observation outweigh the benefit of elective resection, given the improvements in elective infant surgery. In a review of the literature by Downard and colleagues, they found that the reported rate of asymptomatic CPAM lesions becoming symptomatic varied from 3% to 86%. This inconsistency in reported evidence has led to physician preference and institutional protocols based on institutional experience to drive decisions on operative management of asymptomatic lesions.[12,34]

Infants with CLE without symptoms at birth require close monitoring. Air trapping may worsen due to positive pressure and cause tension-like physiology. Those infants who remain asymptomatic at birth are not recommended to undergo resection and may be observed clinically for progression of symptoms.[1,4,8,33]

For infants with BC, asymptomatic lesions are still recommended to undergo surgical resection due to risk of further infections, persistent exponential growth rate as children age, and the potential for malignant transformation.[4,28]

Malignant transformation. Malignant transformation of CPAMs is a concern and has been used as an argument for resection. This argument has been aided by the lack of evidence to assist clinicians in risk stratifying patients to define those that are low risk and could benefit from observation. A study by Feinberg and colleagues sought to define an algorithm to assist with surgical decision-making in reference to the malignant potential of these lesions. In this study, they defined certain unique characteristics that were closely associated with both pleuropulmonary blastoma and CPAMs to assist with developing an algorithm to assist with clinical decision-making. They found pleuropulmonary blastoma to be closely associated with symptoms such as pneumothorax, bilateral involvement. The DICER1 gene mutation was noted to be seen in two-thirds of pleuropulmonary blastoma cases. CPAMs were noted to be highly associated with a prenatal diagnosis, evidence of systemic feeding vessel, and lung hyperinflation. An algorithm was then developed to assist with risk stratification. According to this study, an observational management strategy for those infants with asymptomatic CPAM lesions without any high-risk features is feasible. These clinicians recommend careful close follow-up with any change in clinical status or growth in the lesion prompting resection[35] **(Fig. 11)**.

Malignant transformation, although rare, has been documented in children with BC with evidence of rhabdomyosarcoma, pulmonary blastoma, and malignant mesenchymal tumors present in resected pathologic condition.[4] These concerns demonstrate why surgical resection of asymptomatic BC is recommended.

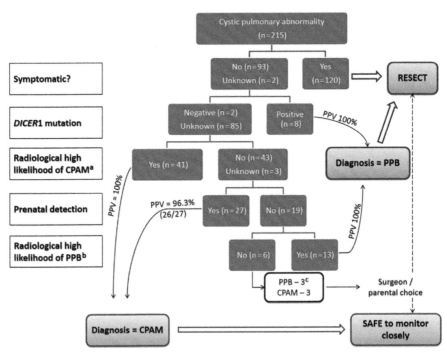

Fig. 11. Algorithm for malignant potential of CPAM. [a]CPAM high likelihood factors=any hyperinflated region or systemic feeding vessel. [b]PPB high likelihood factors=multilobar or bilateral abnormality, mediastinal shift or complex cyst. [c]Including 1 case in whom no CT was avaiable for review. (*From* Feinberg A, Hall NJ, Williams GM, Schultz KA, Miniati D, Hill DA, Dehner LP, Messinger YH, Langer JC. Can congenital pulmonary airway malformation be distinguished from Type I pleuropulmonary blastoma based on clinical and radiological features? J Pediatr Surg. 2016 Jan;51(1):33-7.)

OUTCOMES

The outcomes of CLMs have improved over time. Previous studies estimated perinatal mortality of those diagnosed with a fetal lung lesion anywhere from 9% to 49%. More recent studies have shown a trend of improvement in perinatal mortality rates from 49% in 1992 to 12% in 2005. This trend is likely related to improved ultrasound techniques to detect small lesions that would not have been detected earlier, and improvement in fetal management strategies over time.[36]

Asymptomatic infants at birth with lung lesions as described above are often managed conservatively with either scheduled elective resection or serial follow-up to monitor for the development of symptoms. Many studies have shown that a short hospital length of stay and low morbidity are associated with elective resection of these CLMs.[37] A study performed by Tsai and colleagues on morbidity and mortality after elective resection of asymptomatic lung lesions on 105 infants showed no evidence of mortality, and an overall morbidity of 6.7% due to the complications of postoperative blood transfusion and air leak. They demonstrated that the postoperative course for these infants was relatively uneventful, and that no infants had ongoing respiratory complications after resection.[38] These findings demonstrate that the surgical management of asymptomatic lesions is a well-tolerated intervention with few, if any, postoperative complications. Many investigators have attempted to determine outcome predictors of being asymptomatic at birth based on prenatal ultrasound characteristics. Some studies have shown that a low CVR of less than 1.0 and fetuses without hydrops have a greater than 95% likelihood to be asymptomatic at birth.[37]

Infants with symptomatic lesions after birth often undergo urgent or emergent resection. Many studies have confirmed that infants that require intervention after birth due to respiratory compromise have more complicated postoperative course. This includes requiring a prolonged neonatal intensive care unit stay, postoperative ventilator requirement for 1 to 2 weeks, and up to 25% may require ECMO to assist with management of pulmonary hypertension. A study by Johnson and colleagues demonstrated that infants with symptomatic lesions requiring intervention after birth had a median length of stay of 36.5 days, significantly longer than those infants who were asymptomatic and underwent elective resection. However, all infants survived to hospital discharge. They also found that both gestational age and infant birthweight correlate with length of hospitalization, with those infants with lower birth weights and younger gestational age requiring longer hospitalization. The infants in this study were followed postoperatively for median of 35.5 months. During this time period, all infants were able to be weaned from supplemental oxygen but 50% required bronchodilators to assist with chronic lung disease and asthma-related complications.[37] These investigators showed that symptomatic infants often require more support and longer hospital stays but that all infants survived the immediate postnatal period and were able to be weaned from respiratory support in the postnatal period.

Fetuses with large lung lesions and CVRs that subsequently develop hydrops are often considered for fetal surgical intervention. These operations occur at designated fetal centers that specialize in these type of operations. Outcomes are often stratified based on predictors of poor outcome in the fetus based on imaging characteristics of the lesion. Various studies have found that CVRs greater than 1.6, and the development of hydrops has been associated with worse fetal outcomes. A study by Cass and colleagues demonstrated that a lesion size of 5.2 cm and a CVR of 2 were the most significant predictors for poor fetal outcome after fetal surgery. They also demonstrated that patients with smaller lesions with a CVR less than 2 do very well, with a likelihood of survival around 100%.[38] Considering these observations, Kunisaki and colleagues[39] detailed that for fetuses with CVR greater than 1.6, 63% of those that underwent surgery survived in comparison to 100% of those with a CVR less than 1.6. Kuroda and colleagues[40] also reported similar survival of those with CVR greater than 1.6 with an estimated 56% survival. Cass and colleagues[41] reported a 76% survival in those patients with CVR greater than 1.6. Outcomes are worse if fetal hydrops is present; Adzick and colleagues[16] and Grethel and colleagues[42] reported a survival of 57% and 54%, respectively, in those patients. These data show that lesions with smaller CVRs have better outcomes than those with larger CVRs and hydropic fetal features. These specialized fetal centers should be involved in determining management strategies of those with prenatally diagnosed fetal lung lesions.

SUMMARY

CLMs have intricacies involved in diagnosis, prenatal, and postnatal management. As demonstrated throughout this review, further research including more overarching long-term studies are needed to gain a true understanding of the natural history of these diseases, and to develop consensus, evidenced-based management guidelines.

CLINICS CARE POINTS

- Prenatally diagnosed CPAMs may be serially monitored with ultrasounds and CVR calculations may be used to predict those that will develop hydrops.
- Microcystic CPAMs diagnosed prenatally that are large or develop hydrops should be treated with maternal steroids.
- All lung lesions diagnosed postnatally should undergo further evaluation and be considered for resection.
- Special consideration and imaging is needed to assist with surgical planning for resection of BPS lesions given their blood supply that frequently arises from the systemic blood supply and may retract into the abdomen and must be ligated carefully.
- Malignant transformation, although rare, is a concern with congenital lung lesions and certain risk stratification algorithms exist to assist providers with clinical decision making regarding asymptomatic lesions.

DISCLOSURE

The authors have nothing to disclose.

REFERENCES

1. Zobel M, Gologorsky R, Lee H, et al. Congenital lung lesions. Semin Pediatr Surg 2019;28(4):150821.
2. Correia-Pinto J, Gonzaga S, Huang Y, et al. Congenital lung lesions—underlying molecular mechanisms. Semin Pediatr Surg 2010;19(3):171–9.
3. Davis RP, Mychaliska GB. Neonatal pulmonary physiology. Semin Pediatr Surg 2013;22:179–84.
4. Durell J, Lakhoo K. Congenital cystic lesions of the lung. Early Hum Dev 2014; 90(12):935–9.
5. Boucherat O, Jeannotte L, Hadchouel A, et al. Pathomechanisms of congenital cystic lung diseases: focus on congenital cystic adenomatoid malformation and pleuropulmonary blastoma. Paediatr Respir Rev 2016;19:62–8.

6. Azizkhan RG, Crombleholme TM. Congenital cystic lung disease: contemporary antenatal and postnatal management. Pediatr Surg Int 2008;24(6):643–57, 2008 246.
7. Cruz-Martinez R, Martínez M, Martínez-Rodríguez M, et al. Fetal laser ablation of feeding artery of cystic lung lesions with systemic arterial blood supply. Ultrasound Obs Gynecol 2017;49:744–50.
8. Williams HJ, Johnson KJ. Imaging of congenital cystic lung lesions. Paediatr Respir Rev 2002;3(2):120–7.
9. Usui N, Kamata S, Sawai T, et al. Outcome predictors for infants with cystic lung disease. J Pediatr Surg 2004;39(4):603–6.
10. Peranteau WH, Boelig MM, Khalek N, et al. Effect of single and multiple courses of maternal betamethasone on prenatal congenital lung lesion growth and fetal survival. J Pediatr Surg 2016;51(1):28–32.
11. Vu L, Tsao K, Lee H, et al. Characteristics of congenital cystic adenomatoid malformations associated with nonimmune hydrops and outcome. J Pediatr Surg. 42(8):1351-1356 doi:10.1016/j.jpedsurg.2007.03.039.
12. Downard CD, Calkins CM, Williams RF, et al. Treatment of congenital pulmonary airway malformations: a systematic review from the APSA outcomes and evidence based practice committee. Pediatr Surg Int 2017. https://doi.org/10.1007/s00383-017-4098-z.
13. Hernanz-Schulman M, Stein SM, Neblett WW, et al. Pulmonary sequestration: diagnosis with color Doppler sonography and a new theory of associated hydrothorax. Radiology 1991;180(3):817–21.
14. Alamo L, Reinberg O, Vial Y, et al. Comparison of foetal US and MRI in the characterisation of congenital lung anomalies. Eur J Radiol 2013;82(12):e860–6.
15. Quinn TM, Hubbard AM, Adzick NS. Prenatal magnetic resonance imaging enhances fetal diagnosis. J Pediatr Surg 1998;33(4):553–8.
16. Adzick NS. Management of fetal lung lesions. Clin Perinatol 2009;36(2):363–76.
17. Tsao KJ, Hawgood S, Vu L, et al. Resolution of hydrops fetalis in congenital cystic adenomatoid malformation after prenatal steroid therapy. J Pediatr Surg 2003; 38(3):508–10.
18. Knox EM, Kilby MD, Martin WL, et al. In-utero pulmonary drainage in the management of primary hydrothorax and congenital cystic lung lesion: a systematic review. Ultrasound Obstet Gynecol 2006;28(5):726–34.
19. Curran PF, Jelin EB, Rand L, et al. Prenatal steroids for microcystic congenital cystic adenomatoid malformations. J Pediatr Surg 2010;45(1):145–50.
20. Brown MF, Lewis D, Brouillette RM, et al. Successful prenatal management of hydrops, caused by congenital cystic adenomatoid malformation, using serial aspirations. J Pediatr Surg 1995;30(7):1098–9.
21. Wilson RD. In Utero therapy for fetal thoracic abnormalities. Prenat Diagn 2008; 28(7):619–25.
22. Hedrick HL, Flake AW, Crombleholme TM, et al. The ex utero intrapartum therapy procedure for high-risk fetal lung lesions. J Pediatr Surg 2005;40(6):1038–44.
23. Cass DL, Olutoye OO, Cassady CI, et al. EXIT-to-resection for fetuses with large lung masses and persistent mediastinal compression near birth. J Pediatr Surg 2013;48(1):138–44.
24. Gottschalk I, Strizek B, Mallmann MR, et al. Outcome of Bronchopulmonary sequestration with massive pleural effusion after intrafetal vascular laser ablation. Fetal Diagn Ther 2018;44(2):149–55.
25. Bermudez C, P´Erez-Wulff J, Bufalino G, et al. Percutaneous ultrasound-guided sclerotherapy for complicated fetal intralobar bronchopulmonary sequestration. Ultrasound Obs Gynecol 2007;29:586–9.

26. Pariente G, Aviram M, Landau D, et al. Prenatal diagnosis of congenital lobar emphysema case report and review of the literature. J Ultrasound Med 2009; 28(8):1081–4.

27. Olutoye OO, Coleman BG, Hubbard AM, et al. Prenatal diagnosis and management of congenital lobar emphysema. J Pediatr Surg 2000;35(5):792–5.

28. Maurin S, Bourliere B, Potier A, et al. Bronchogenic cyst: clinical course from antenatal diagnosis to postnatal thoracoscopic resection. J Minim Access Surg 2013;9(1):25. Available at: https://go.gale.com/ps/i.do?p=HRCA&sw=w&issn= 09729941&v=2.1&it=r&id=GALE%7CA323901661&sid=googleScholar&linkaccess= fulltext. Accessed August 12, 2021.

29. Teresa L, Rios M, Júnior EA, et al. Prenatal diagnosis and postnatal findings of bronchogenic cyst. Case Rep Pulmonol 2013;2013. https://doi.org/10.1155/ 2013/483864.

30. Arshad SA; Garcia E, Ferguson D, et al. Prediction of Early Emergent/Urgent Surgery for Neonates with Prenatal Concern for Congenital Pulmonary Airway Malformation. Published online 2020.

31. Laje P, Liechty KW. Postnatal management and outcome of prenatally diagnosed lung lesions. Prenat Diagn 2008;28(7):612–8.

32. Jeng Cho M, Yeon Kim D, Chul Kim S, et al. Embolization versus surgical resection of pulmonary sequestration: clinical experiences with a thoracoscopic approach. J Pediatr Surg 2012;47:2228–33.

33. Mata JM, Castellote A. Pulmonary malformations beyond the neonatal period. p. 197-217. 2013. Pediatric Chest Imaging.

34. Laje P, Pearson EG, Simpao AF, et al. The first 100 infant thoracoscopic lobectomies: observations through the learning curve and comparison to open lobectomy. J Pediatr Surg 2015;50:1811–6.

35. Feinberg A, Hall NJ, Williams GM, et al. Can congenital pulmonary airway malformation be distinguished from Type I pleuropulmonary blastoma based on clinical and radiological features? ☆,☆☆. J Pediatr Surg 2016;51(1):33–7.

36. Ierullo AM, Ganapathy R, Crowley S, et al. Neonatal outcome of antenatally diagnosed congenital cystic adenomatoid malformations. Ultrasound Obs Gynecol 2005;26:150–3.

37. Johnson KN, Mon RA, Gadepalli SK, et al. Short-term respiratory outcomes of neonates with symptomatic congenital lung malformations ☆. J Pediatr Surg 2019; 54(9):1766–70.

38. Tsai AY, Liechty KW, Hedrick HL, et al. Outcomes after postnatal resection of prenatally diagnosed asymptomatic cystic lung lesions. J Pediatr Surg 2008;43(3): 513–7.

39. Kunisaki SM, Barnewolt CE, Estroff JA, et al. Large fetal congenital cystic adenomatoid malformations: growth trends and patient survival. J Pediatr Surg 2007; 42(2):404–10.

40. Kuroda T, Morikawa N, Kitano Y, et al. Clinicopathologic assessment of prenatally diagnosed lung diseases. J Pediatr Surg 2006;41(12):2028–31.

41. Cass DL, Olutoye OO, Cassady CI, et al. Prenatal diagnosis and outcome of fetal lung masses. J Pediatr Surg 2011;46(2):292–8.

42. Grethel EJ, Wagner AJ, Clifton MS, et al. Fetal intervention for mass lesions and hydrops improves outcome: a 15-year experience. J Pediatr Surg 2007;42(1): 117–23.

Advances in Complex Congenital Tracheoesophageal Anomalies

Somala Mohammed, MD, MPH[a], Thomas E. Hamilton, MD[b],*

KEYWORDS

- Esophageal atresia • Tracheoesophageal fistula • Tracheomalacia
- Tracheobronchomalacia • Esophageal leak • Esophageal strictures

KEY POINTS

- On diagnosis of EA/TEF, decompressing the esophageal pouch, minimizing positive pressure respiratory support, maintaining head of bed elevated, obtaining urgent echocardiogram, and preparing for surgical division of TEF with possible EA repair is essential.
- Various methods to achieve tension-induced esophageal lengthening exist but the ultimate approach to LGEA management should be tailored to the constellation of problems present in each individual patient.
- Incidence of tracheomalacia in patients with EA/TEF is high, for which patients benefit from preoperative dynamic tracheobronchoscopy and potential tracheopexy, if indicated. Separation of suture lines between the airway and esophagus helps reduce complications, such as recurrent or acquired TEF.
- Endoscopy has immense potential to assist in the management of esophageal leaks and strictures. Proactive endoscopic therapy may spare future esophageal stricture resections.
- Comprehensive longitudinal multidisciplinary care allows for durable patient outcomes in a highly complex subset of neonatal and pediatric patients.

INTRODUCTION

Esophageal atresia (EA) with or without tracheoesophageal fistula (TEF) (EA/TEF) is the most common anomaly of the esophagus (incidence 1/5000 births).[1] Due to significant advances in neonatal intensive care, anesthesia, nutrition, antimicrobial therapy, and surgical technique, survival associated with EA/TEF has improved to 91% to 98%,

Neither author has financial disclosures or conflicts of interest.
[a] Harvard Medical School, Boston Children's Hospital, 300 Longwood Avenue, Boston, MA 02115, USA; [b] Perelman School of Medicine at the University of Pennsylvania, Department of General, Thoracic and Fetal Surgery, Children's Hospital of Philadelphia, The Hub for Clinical Collaboration, 2nd Floor, 3500 Civic Center Boulevard, Philadelphia, PA 19104, USA
* Corresponding author.
E-mail address: hamiltonte@chop.edu

with mortality limited to cases involving coexisting life-threatening problems, such as extreme prematurity or complex congenital cardiac disease.[2–4] Because of improved survival, morbidity associated with EA/TEF warrants comprehensive, longitudinal multidisciplinary care.

Fig. 1 illustrates the most widely used EA/TEF classification scheme. Understanding the type of anomaly allows appropriate attention to relevant challenges and operative planning for the neonate.

DIAGNOSIS AND INITIAL MANAGEMENT

Although EA/TEF is usually diagnosed postnatally, it may be suspected on prenatal ultrasound or MRI (rates ranging from 16% to 36%).[5–7] Nonspecific signs, such as an absent or small stomach and polyhydramnios, raise prenatal suspicion. More specific findings include the presence of a blind-ending proximal esophageal pouch, which has been shown to have a high positive predictive value for EA and is seen in one-third of patients with prenatal diagnosis.[8,9] More recently, the presence of a dilated hypopharynx (DHP) has emerged as another sign suggesting EA.[10] Among 88 pregnant women who were evaluated prenatally for possible EA (of which 75 women had postnatal follow-up), DHP and/or dilated esophageal pouch was seen in 36% of those patients, 78% had postnatal EA diagnosis.[10] The authors of this study proposed an algorithm (**Table 1**) to predict EA risk based on a combination of prenatal findings. Accurately suspecting EA prenatally facilitates improved counseling regarding delivery plans, postnatal evaluation, and need for potential surgery; therefore, continued efforts to improve prenatal diagnosis remain essential.

Ultimately, EA/TEF remains a diagnosis made largely postnatally. Babies with prenatal suspicion or those with respiratory distress, increased oropharyngeal secretions, or feeding difficulties warrant further evaluation with attempt at passage of a naso/orogastric catheter. If unsuccessful, a plain radiograph is obtained to assess for coiling of the catheter in a blind ending upper esophagus (**Fig. 2**A). The presence of intestinal air suggests a TEF between the distal esophageal segment and the respiratory tract, consistent with a Gross Type C anomaly (**Fig. 2**B), whereas lack thereof corresponds to a Gross Type A anomaly (**Fig. 2**C).

On diagnosis, the proximal esophageal pouch is decompressed to avoid pooling of secretions or soiling of the respiratory tract from aspiration. Other important precautions include head of bed elevation, minimizing positive pressure respiratory support, and keeping the baby as calm as possible to avoid excessive swallowing of air. Although it may be tempting to acquire peripherally inserted central catheters in the Neonatal Intensive care unit in advance of anticipated surgery, we avoid this practice to minimize agitating the baby until the TEF is occluded or divided.

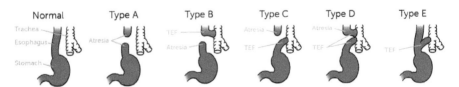

Fig. 1. Gross classification for EA/TEF. Type A: atresia only, no TEF (10% of cases); Type B: EA with TEF on proximal esophageal pouch (<1% of cases); Type C: EA with TEF on distal esophageal pouch (85% of cases); Type D: EA with TEFs on both upper and lower esophageal pouches (<1%); and Type E: TEF without EA (4%).

Table 1
Prediction algorithm for esophageal atresia based on presence or absence of primary and secondary signs

Condition	Percent Predicted to Have EA (95%)
No primary signs,[a] 1 or 0 secondary signs[b]	17 (7–35)
No primary signs,[a] Both secondary signs[b]	44 (22–69)
1 or both primary signs,[a] 1 or 0 secondary signs[b]	67 (42–85)
1 or both primary signs,[a] Both secondary signs[b]	89 (76–96)

[a] Primary signs: DHP, dilated proximal esophageal pouch.
[b] Secondary signs: polyhydramnios and small or absent stomach.
  Adapted from Tracy S, Buchmiller TL, Ben-Ishay O, Barnewolt CE, Connolly SA, Zurakowski D, Phelps A, Estroff JA. The Distended Fetal Hypopharynx: A Sensitive and Novel Sign for the Prenatal Diagnosis of Esophageal Atresia. J Pediatr Surg. 2018 Jun;53(6):1137-1141.

EA/TEF is often associated with other anomalies, specifically of the VACTERL complex or CHARGE syndrome. Therefore, coordination of subsequent studies is essential, particularly an echocardiogram to assess for cardiac or vascular anomalies and to determine the aortic arch sidedness. These findings have significant anesthetic and surgical implications.

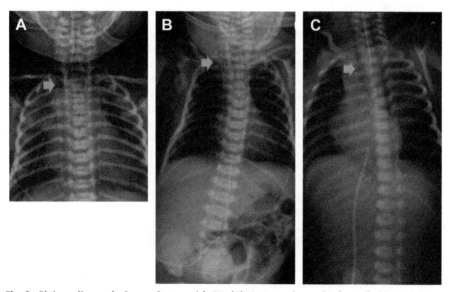

Fig. 2. Plain radiographs in newborns with EA. (*A*) Nasoesophageal tube coiled in atretic upper esophageal segment. (*B*) EA with distal TEF, as suggested by the presence of intraluminal intestinal air. (*C*) EA without distal TEF, as suggested by gasless abdomen. Arrows denotes nasoesophageal tube location.

SURGICAL REPAIR

We begin with rigid tracheobronchoscopy to aspirate airway secretions, assess associated tracheobronchomalacia (TBM), identify TEF location, and rule out any additional TEFs. After this, a Fogarty catheter is directed into the TEF with bronchoscopic visualization and then inflated to provide balloon occlusion. The patient is subsequently intubated over a rigid bronchoscope with the TEF in mind. If possible, the endotracheal tube (ETT) cuff is placed in the trachea beyond the TEF, thus providing an additional safety measure; not all TEFs are amenable to this strategy, however.

The anesthesia team places an arterial catheter. If the patient remains stable and successful temporizing control of the TEF (with balloon occlusion or cuffed ETT beyond TEF site) was achieved, we allow an attempt for central access. Otherwise, the case is performed with peripheral access only and central access is achieved on case conclusion. The patient's abdominal examination is monitored throughout. If the abdomen was distended preoperatively or if the patient would benefit from durable enteral access postoperatively (extremely premature patient, complex cardiac disease), then a gastrostomy is performed first with the gastric tube placed to water seal until the TEF can be surgically divided.

Depending on the aortic arch sidedness, a thoracotomy is performed. A thoracotomy is generally performed opposite the side of the aortic arch for improved exposure.We divide the azygous vein, except in cases where its caliber makes ligation prohibitive (eg, suspected interrupted inferior vena cava with azygous continuation). The distal esophagus is circumferentially dissected being mindful of the vagus nerves. A vessel loop is passed to control the TEF, at which point the balloon-based catheter is deflated and removed. The esophagus is dissected to its insertion into the airway, where the fistula is divided as flush with the airway as possible. Communication with the anesthesia team is essential because there is an open airway at this point.

The resultant tracheal wound is closed transversely using interrupted absorbable monofilament suture. This strategy results in essentially no tracheal diverticulum. If the patient's ETT can accommodate a flexible bronchoscope, the tracheal repair site is assessed endoscopically. Our practice has now evolved to include posterior tracheopexy at the time of newborn type C repair to separate tracheal and esophageal suture lines, support the otherwise-wide posterior membrane seen in EA/TEF patients, and preemptively address any future risk of dynamic airway collapse.

If the patient remains stable, we dissect the upper esophageal segment as far beyond the thoracic inlet as needed. The dissection is kept on the esophageal wall to minimize risk of injury to the recurrent laryngeal nerves (RLNs). We routinely use intraoperative nerve monitoring, even in newborns, to assess RLN function. Most newborn Type C EA/TEF procedures are amenable to primary esophago-esophageal anastomosis, which we perform with single-layer interrupted nonabsorbable monofilament sutures.

Once the anastomosis is complete, we perform a microvascular perfusion test using indocyanine green (ICG) SPY-PHY technology (Stryker, Kalamazoo, MI), even in newborns. A chest tube is placed. We do not use transanastomotic feeding tubes. The anesthesia team places a paravertebral catheter for analgesia. Postoperatively, patients are pharmacologically paralyzed for variable days based on the integrity, tension, blood supply, and overall assessment of the anastomosis. An esophagram is performed postoperative day 7 to 14, depending on the level of tension and overall clinical status. We have a proactive approach to esophageal stricture surveillance with most of our patients receiving endoscopy starting 1 month postoperatively if they are 3 kg or greater in size.

Indeed, many aspects of the procedure delineated above are innovative and evolve from within a high-volume referral-based practice encompassing various complex esophageal and airway disorders. Ultimately, surgeons and institutions should adapt the newborn EA/TEF repair in a manner that safely divides the fistula and adequately reconstructs the esophagus.

LONG GAP ESOPHAGEAL ATRESIA

The International Network of Esophageal Atresia defines long gap EA (LGEA) as "any esophageal atresia that lacks intra-abdominal air" or "all other types that technically prove difficult to repair."[11] This encompasses gap lengths ranging from one to many centimeters in length. Ultimately, LGEA management depends on various factors, such as surgeon experience, institutional resources, esophageal gap, associated airway symptoms, and more. Various techniques exist to achieve esophageal continuity. These include delayed primary anastomosis (after allowing natural growth), serial bougie dilation, esophageal myotomies, gastric pull-up, esophageal replacement, and tension-induced natural growth techniques (Foker process).

The authors' institution has been performing the Foker process since 2005, accumulating the world's largest experience. In a review comparing our historical cohort (2005–2013) of patients who underwent this technique to a more contemporary cohort (2014–2020), continued evolution of the procedure demonstrated improved outcomes, less morbidity, and increased esophageal preservation rates over time. Specifically, there were less leaks on traction, bone fractures, anastomotic leaks, or failed Foker procedures resulting in jejunal interposition in the contemporary cohort.[12] We also found that redo Foker procedures resulted in inferior outcomes compared with those initially performed at our institution.[12] This highlights the importance of appropriately planning the ideal LGEA operation or referring to a center with expertise when local resources and recently demonstrated experience are lacking.

With respect to our LGEA strategy, we comprehensively assess each patient and tailor the procedure to best address the constellation of problems present. This includes diagnostic laryngoscopy and rigid dynamic tracheobronchoscopy to assess for associated airway anomalies, such as laryngeal cleft, TBM, and TEF. We then perform contrast and endoscopic studies to assess the length and luminal quality of the upper and lower esophageal segments. A gap length is measured at rest and then again with pressure applied on each pouch (**Fig. 3**). These studies collectively guide operative strategy.

All patients undergo preoperative echocardiogram and contrast-enhanced chest computed tomography (CT) to evaluate aortic arch sidedness and great vessel anomalies. Preoperative vocal cord function is assessed with flexible nasolaryngoscopy (and is repeated postoperatively). Although we do not have an age threshold, we generally wait until size is 3.5 kg or greater before initiating surgical interventions for LGEA. In our experience, patients weighing less have had higher rate of traction system malfunction, including suture dislodgment.

At the time of LGEA repair, we explore the chest intending to achieve a primary anastomosis. We have a low threshold for cervical dissection to mobilize the upper esophagus. If a primary anastomosis cannot be achieved with acceptable tension and good tissue quality, the esophagus is placed on traction. If the patient has symptoms of severe TBM or bronchoscopy demonstrates greater than 50% tracheal collapse, a posterior tracheopexy is performed. For these patients, a right-sided approach is preferred in order to facilitate tracheobronchopexy.

If the patient has a short upper esophageal segment or a type B LGEA configuration, a cervical incision allows mobilization of the proximal esophagus and fistula division/

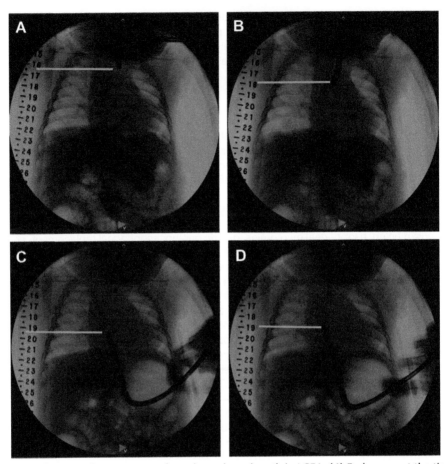

Fig. 3. Fluoroscopic assessment of esophageal gap length in LGEA. (*A*) Endoscope at the tip of upper esophageal pouch at rest and (*B*) with forward pressure. (*C*) Endoscope at tip of lower esophageal pouch at rest and (*D*) with forward pressure. In this patient, esophageal gap length at rest measured 3 cm and with forward pressure on each pouch reduced to 1 cm.

repair. Although others have approached proximal/cervical TEFs via minimally invasive surgery (MIS) (clipping/division strategies), we prefer the open approach. This allows full esophageal mobilization, identification/protection of RLNs, division of TEF as close to the airway with suture repair of the resultant tracheal wound, and placement of a silastic sleeve in the neck through which the esophagus passes thus minimizing its ability to adhere within the thoracic inlet.[12] The cervical incision does not preclude an MIS thoracic strategy, however. We consider MIS for patients without significant TBM and for those who have not previously had multiple thoracic operations. Either left-sided or right-sided MIS thoracic approach (regardless of sidedness of the aortic arch) is feasible. For example, patients with a large leftward upper esophageal pouch, minimal tracheomalacia, no TEF, and a history of previous right-sided surgeries could undergo a left-sided operation.[12]

The decision to pursue dynamic external versus static internal traction is based on esophageal gap length and patient comorbidities. If the gap is short, prolonged postoperative paralysis would be detrimental to the patient, or there is a high likelihood the patient could be extubated between serial traction adjustments, we favor static internal traction. For longer gaps, external traction with frequent bedside adjustments to the traction system or internal traction via serial thoracoscopic traction adjustments are considered.[12] Neuromuscular paralysis is used throughout the external traction process. Ultimately, the operative strategy is customized to each patient. Regardless of strategy—external or internal, open or MIS—the median daily rate of esophageal growth measured radiographically is 1.1 mm per esophageal segment.[13]

Whenever possible, intraoperative endoscopy is used to guide traction suture placement to assure that no suture is full-thickness or intraluminal. We also place silastic sleeves around the esophageal pouches in order to minimize adhesion formation. **Fig. 4** demonstrates our external traction setup. For the MIS traction system, endoscopy also guides suture placement, which are placed in a bucket-handle configuration through which additional suture (typically fiberwire) is passed (**Fig. 5**). This is brought around a rib with the knot tied in the subcutaneous tissues to maintain traction. The tails are untied and the fiberwire retied under thoracoscopic visualization with each traction adjustment.

We have learned many lessons in the process of refining this procedure. Although at the start of our experience, traction adjustments were performed every other day, we have realized that tension-induced lengthening responds to less frequent adjustments, too. This led to the increased use of internal traction and MIS approaches over time.[12] Patients undergoing MIS approach also had reduced duration of neuromuscular paralysis, shorter intensive care unit and hospital lengths of stay, and no greater risk of complications.[12] For patients who undergo rescue Foker procedure after failed LGEA repair elsewhere, however, the hospital course remains longer and more complicated. Consequently, some patients with prior failed LGEA repairs are best served with esophageal replacement instead of rescue lengthening procedures. The jejunal interposition (JI) is our preferred replacement when the native esophagus cannot be reconstructed but this operation is not performed in the neonatal period (deferred until patients are >10 kg in size).

ASSESSMENT OF ANASTOMOTIC INTEGRITY

Due to our institution's vast experience with complex esophageal and airway disorders, we now systematically evaluate every esophageal anastomosis with respect to blood supply, tension, and tissue quality because they each contribute to healing. Microvascular perfusion is assessed with ICG SPY-PHY technology, looking at speed and intensity of perfusion, and degree of hypoperfusion near the anastomosis. We note whether the anastomosis is in a reoperative field or involves a prior failed anastomosis. We gauge degree of tension by overall appearance (eg, sutures pulling through) and how much effort was required to achieve the anastomosis (eg, putting patient in flexed position). Altogether, our assessment guides postoperative management in that there is a low threshold to pharmacologically paralyze a patient if the anastomosis is on severe tension or involves poor tissue quality. This allows initial anastomotic healing without active swallowing or excessive movement and cervical extension. We have observed higher anastomotic complication rates in settings of poor integrity due to impaired perfusion, high tension, or poor tissue quality. Ongoing research is necessary to continue understanding factors that influence anastomotic outcomes to further refine operative technique and postoperative management.

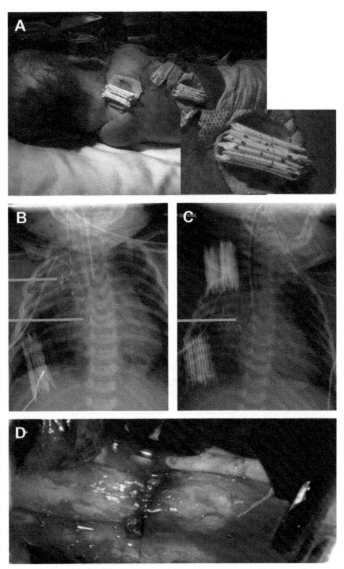

Fig. 4. External traction process for LGEA. (*A*) Traction sutures are brought out through the skin and tied to a silicone disk. Tension is transmitted to the esophageal segments by adding feeding tube fragments under the sutures. (*B*) Radiopaque clips on the traction system and the esophageal wall are tracked on plain radiographs until (*C*) the clips cluster together at which point esophago-esophageal anastomosis (*D*) is performed.

MANAGEMENT OF ESOPHAGEAL LEAKS AND STRICTURES

Although not standard practice within the field, we perform endoscopy on EA/TEF patients around 1 month postoperatively (if patients are >3 kg in size). Most LGEA patients receive a series of 3 planned dilations with intralesional steroid injections (ISI). Thereafter, stricture response to therapy and patient symptoms guide additional interventions, which typically include endoscopic incisional therapy (EIT) and/or stenting.

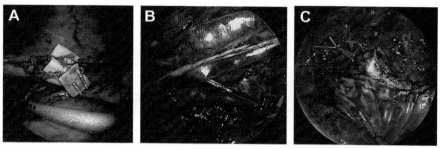

Fig. 5. Thoracoscopic internal traction process for LGEA. (*A*) Traction system sutures are placed on the esophageal pouches in mattress fashion with pericardial pledgets marked by radiopaque clips. Through the bucket-handle configuration, additional suture is passed. (*B, C*) Serial adjustments involve untying the knot and retying it under thoracoscopic visualization to set a new level of tension. In doing so, the esophageal pouches traverse the thoracic cavity.

We consider surgical resection for strictures refractory to endoscopic interventions. The point at which endoscopic therapy should be abandoned in favor of resection is unclear. In a retrospective study of 171 repaired EA patients who underwent serial endoscopies, factors associated with eventual need for stricture resection were discerned. The probability of remaining free from stricture resection decreased with increasing number of therapeutic endoscopies. A cutoff of 7 endoscopies discriminated between patients who needed stricture resection and those who did not.[14] Despite this, most patients remained free of stricture resection well beyond 7 therapeutic endoscopies.[14] Other predictors for needing stricture resection included esophageal leak, initial anastomotic diameter less than 3 mm, and need for advanced therapeutic endoscopic maneuvers (such as ISI, EIT, stenting).[15] Ultimately, we thought that proactive therapeutic endoscopies may spare stricture resections.

Patients who have undergone EA/TEF repair have a reported anastomotic leak rate of up to 38%.[16,17] Our institution routinely uses negative pressure wound therapy (also known as vacuum-assisted closure [VAC] therapy) for endoscopic management of esophageal leaks. This highly effective method helps close leak cavities and promote wound healing by stimulating angiogenesis, removing excess debris, and allowing granulation tissue formation.[18,19] Early experience with endoscopic VAC (e-VAC) therapy demonstrates technical feasibility, safety, and effectiveness in managing esophageal anastomotic leaks.[18] Additional centers have also reported on use of e-VAC therapy for esophageal leaks.[20–22] When institutional experience with advanced endoscopy is lacking, antibiotics and chest drainage or operative washout with tacking of esophageal segments to the prevertebral fascia should be considered.

MANAGEMENT OF RECURRENT OR ACQUIRED TRACHEOESOPHAGEAL FISTULA

Recurrent TEF (recTEF) complicates 5% to 10% of EA/TEF repairs.[23–27] Postoperative acquired TEF (acqTEF) can occur in addition to or even in the absence of prior congenital TEFs in the setting of esophageal anastomotic complications. These TEF variants rarely close spontaneously, and given the perceived high risks of operative intervention, they are often first approached endoscopically with reported re-recurrence rates approaching 63%.[23,28–31] Surgical techniques to address rec/acqTEFs include placing autologous tissue (pleural or muscle flaps) or prosthetic material (mesh) between the repair. Re-recurrence rates for these cases, although better than endoscopic interventions, still range from 11% to 22%.[23,28,29] At our institution, posterior tracheopexy and rotational esophagoplasty is the backbone of surgical repair of rec/acqTEFs in order to completely separate suture lines without the need for interposing tissue.[32,33] Our published experience involving 62 patients who underwent rec-TEF repair reports 0 re-recurrences during a median follow-up of 2.5 years.[33] We prefer an upfront surgical approach as we think repeated endoscopies can be futile and/or harmful and surgery allows for addressing coexisting TBM, strictures, or other intrathoracic pathologic conditions.

TRACHEOBRONCHOMALACIA

Tracheomalacia is the most common congenital tracheobronchial anomaly (incidence 1/2100 children).[34] It refers to excessive compliance of the trachea, predisposing it to static or dynamic collapse. If the mainstem bronchi are also involved, TBM results. Tracheomalacia is common among EA/TEF patients (incidence of 10%–75%) due to shared embryologic origins of the trachea and esophagus.[35–38] Signs suggesting tracheomalacia include chronic barky cough, noisy breathing, exercise intolerance, expiratory stridor, frequent or more severe respiratory illnesses, feeding difficulties, development of bronchiectasis, or acute life-threatening events (ALTEs), including brief resolving unexplained events.

A detailed endoscopic airway assessment is essential to diagnosing TBM. The normal trachea and bronchi consist of C-shaped cartilages with a narrow posterior membrane that intrudes during cough without compromising overall airway patency. In TBM, malformed cartilages are often U or bow-shaped with a wider more pliable membrane that lends itself to significant posterior intrusion, thereby collapsing the airway lumen. This leads to impaired clearance of pulmonary secretions, ineffective cough, and insufficient air movement.

We perform rigid dynamic 3-phase tracheobronchoscopy to assess structure and function of the visible airways.[39] The first phase of assessment involves a spontaneously breathing patient. Anatomy is characterized with respect to tracheobronchial tree branching pattern, cartilage shape, posterior membrane intrusion at rest, and any fixed airway compression. Next, sedation is titrated to allow more vigorous breathing and cough. The degree of dynamic airway compression, particularly the extent of posterior membrane intrusion or anterior intrusion, is gauged at each portion of the visible airway, if possible. Finally, anesthesia provides additional sedation, and the airway is distended to inspect for tracheal diverticulums, occult TEFs, aberrant bronchi, and other abnormalities. Lesions suspicious for TEFs are probed with a catheter for passage into a tract or contrast is instilled to delineate communication with the esophagus. This assessment can also be performed with flexible bronchoscopy to evaluate small airway collapse in premature infants, those with bronchopulmonary dysplasia, or older patients for whom the rigid bronchoscopes are not long enough.

The combination of symptoms with abnormal tracheobronchoscopy supports further intervention. In our experience, children with symptomatic TBM often demonstrate greater than 75% narrowing of the airway during forced exhalation or coughing.[38,40] However, bronchoscopic findings must correlate with concerning symptoms to warrant the risks of any proposed interventions.

MANAGEMENT OF TRACHEOBRONCHOMALACIA

Many think that children with TBM will outgrow their symptoms but this is a common misconception. Although milder cases may become less symptomatic because the airway diameter enlarges with the child's growth, TBM will not simply resolve on its own and, in fact, can exacerbate with age. A graduated approach to management is therefore essential. We begin with medical management. Optimizing mucociliary clearance involves decreasing quantity of secretions without thickening them (using ipratropium bromide [atrovent]) and loosening secretions (with normal saline or hypertonic saline nebulizers). Chest physiotherapy enhances clearance. Low-dose inhaled corticosteroids help reduce mucosal inflammation but should be used cautiously to minimize any negative effects on cartilage development. Early initiation of antibiotics during an active infection is also part of our strategy to decrease severity and length of symptoms. Patients with documented severe collapse on tracheobronchoscopy and failure of maximal medical management are considered operative candidates.

Surgical management of TBM depends on the type and location of disease and the airway's relationship to major blood vessels and the esophagus. For this reason, preoperative evaluation also includes multidetector CT (MDCT) with 3-dimensional reconstruction.

Historically, TBM was addressed with anterior aortopexy. This entails sternotomy for thymectomy, after which the innominate artery and ascending aorta or aortic arch are pulled anteriorly by suturing it to the posterior aspect of the sternum, thereby relieving anterior airway compression. Because the vessels remain attached to the airway through areolar tissue, pulling the vessels anteriorly effectively opens the airway as well. This strategy, however, does not address posterior membranous tracheal intrusion, which is the more common finding seen in patients with a history of EA/TEF.

In this patient population, we begin with posterior tracheopexy. This involves a right thoracotomy for esophageal mobilization, being mindful of the vagus nerves, the RLNs, and the thoracic duct. The aorta is mobilized if a descending aortopexy is anticipated. If a recTEF or tracheal diverticulum from prior TEF repair is noted, it is corrected by dividing and repairing the TEF or resecting the tracheal diverticulum flush with the tracheal wall under bronchoscopic visualization. The resultant tracheal defect is primarily closed using interrupted absorbable monofilament suture. An air-leak test is performed in coordination with our anesthesiologists.

After this, posterior tracheopexy is performed by passing autologous-pledgeted polypropylene sutures into, but not through, the posterior membrane of the trachea using bronchoscopic guidance to assure no bite is full thickness. These bites are mattress fashion and taken to the anterior longitudinal spinal ligament, thus securing the posterior membrane there. All stitches are placed first and then sequentially tied with no retractors in place. A negative-pressure suction test is typically performed after the completion of tracheopexy to assess for residual posterior intrusion and airway patency. The end result is opening of the airway and rotation of the esophagus laterally such that variations in luminal size with feeding no longer cause intrusion into the posterior tracheal membrane.

If a descending aortopexy is indicated, it is performed before posterior tracheopexy. We do this procedure if the descending aorta is located too far anteriorly on cross-sectional imaging such that the midportion of the left mainstem bronchus is trapped between the descending aorta and the pulmonary artery, resulting in narrowing of the bronchus.[41,42] Identification of the Artery of Adamkiewicz during the MDCT guides the surgeon in avoiding injury to this artery during the case.

Long-term results of posterior tracheopexy (**Fig. 6**) for severe TBM were evaluated for 98 consecutive patients at our institution; with a 5-month follow-up period, we reported improvements in clinical symptoms, including chronic cough, noisy breathing, prolonged and recurrent respiratory infections, transient respiratory distress requiring

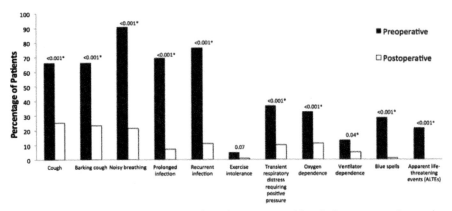

Fig. 6. Preoperative and postoperative clinical symptoms with relation to posterior tracheopexy. There were statistically significant improvements in clinical symptoms after posterior tracheopexy, including report of barking cough, noisy breathing, prolonged and recurrent respiratory infections, need for positive pressure, oxygen dependence, blue spells, and ALTEs. *statistical significance. (*From* Shieh HF, Smithers CJ, Hamilton TE, Zurakowski D, Rhein LM, Manfredi MA, Baird CW, Jennings RW. Posterior tracheopexy for severe tracheomalacia. J Pediatr Surg. 2017 Jun;52(6):951-955.)

positive pressure, oxygen dependence, blue spells, ALTEs, and ventilator dependence (**Fig. 7**).[37] Only 9% of patients had persistent symptomatic tracheomalacia requiring reoperation (in the form of anterior aortopexy).[37]

Most patients with EA/TEF will likely not need surgical management for tracheomalacia but if such interventions are being considered, patients should be referred to institutions with experience performing the procedures described above.

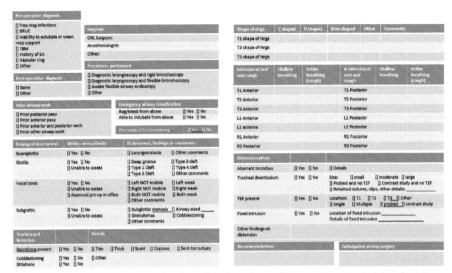

Fig. 7. Standardized airway evaluation. This form is used in a systematic fashion for airway evaluation in our patients.

LONG-TERM MULTIDISCIPLINARY CARE AND MANAGEMENT

Of utmost importance in the care of patients with complex esophageal and airway disorders is a comprehensive and multidisciplinary team-based mentality. Patients treated by our institution are followed longitudinally across numerous disciplines, including but not limited to general surgery, gastroenterology, pulmonology, otolaryngology, speech language pathology, nutrition, social work, anesthesia, cardiac surgery, plastic surgery, and orthopedic surgery. It is the multidisciplinary team's tireless efforts that has yielded durable success in the surgical and nonsurgical management of this highly complicated subset of neonatal and pediatric patients.

REFERENCES

1. Sfeir R, Bonnard A, Khen-Dunlop N, et al. Esophageal atresia: data from a national cohort. J Pediatr Surg 2013;48(8):1664–9.
2. Pinheiro PF, Simoes e Silva AC, Pereira RM. Current knowledge on esophageal atresia. World J Gastroenterol 2012;18(28):3662–72.
3. Goyal A, Jones MO, Couriel JM, et al. Oesophageal atresia and tracheo-oesophageal fistula. Arch Dis Child Fetal Neonatal 2006;91(5):F381–4.
4. Gupta DK, Sharma S. Esophageal atresia: the total care in a high-risk population. Semin Pediatr Surg 2008;17(4):236–43.
5. Bradshaw CJ, Thakkar H, Knutzen L, et al. Accuracy of prenatal detection of tracheoesophageal fistula and oesophageal atresia. J Pediatr Surg 2016;51(8): 1268–72.
6. Fallon SC, Ethun CG, Olutoye OO, et al. Comparing characteristics and outcomes in infants with prenatal and postnatal diagnosis of esophageal atresia. J Surg Res 2014;190(1):242–5.
7. Kunisaki SM, Bruch SW, Hirschl RB, et al. The diagnosis of fetal esophageal atresia and its implications on perinatal outcome. Pediatr Surg Int 2014;30(10): 971–7.
8. Garabedian CSR, Langlois C, Bonnard A, et al. Does prenatal diagnosis modify neonatal treatment and early outcome of children with esophageal atresia? Am J Obstet Gynecol 2015;212(3):340–7.
9. Ethun CG, Fallon SC, Cassady CI, et al. Fetal MRI improves diagnostic accuracy in patients referred to a fetal center for suspected esophageal atresia. J Pediatr Surg 2014;49(5):712–5.
10. Tracy S, Buchmiller TL, Ben-Ishay O, et al. The distended fetal hypopharynx: a Sensitive and Novel sign for the prenatal diagnosis of esophageal atresia. J Pediatr Surg 2018;53(6):1137–41.
11. van der Zee DCBP, Faure C. Position paper of INoEA working group on long-gap esophageal atresia: for better care. Front Pediatr 2017;5:1–3.
12. Svetanoff WJ, Zendejas B, Hernandez K, et al. Contemporary outcomes of the Foker process and evolution of treatment algorithms for long-gap esophageal atresia. J Pediatr Surg 2021;56(12):2180–91.
13. Foust AM, Zendejas B, Mohammed S, et al. Radiographic assessment of traction-induced esophageal growth and traction-related complications of the Foker process for treatment of long-gap esophageal atresia. Pediatr Radiol 2021. https://doi.org/10.1007/s00247-021-05228-z.
14. Yasuda JL, Taslitsky GN, Staffa SJ, et al. Utility of repeated therapeutic endoscopies for pediatric esophageal anastomotic strictures. Dis Esophagus 2020; 33(12). https://doi.org/10.1093/dote/doaa031.

15. Baghdadi O, Clark S, Ngo P, et al. Initial esophageal anastomosis diameter predicts treatment outcomes in esophageal atresia patients with a high risk for stricture development. Front Pediatr 2021;9:710363.

16. Liu J, Yang Y, Zheng C, et al. Surgical outcomes of different approaches to esophageal replacement in long-gap esophageal atresia: a systematic review. Medicine (Baltimore) 2017;96(21):e6942.

17. Lal DR, Gadepalli SK, Downard CD, et al. Perioperative management and outcomes of esophageal atresia and tracheoesophageal fistula. J Pediatr Surg 2017;52(8):1245–51.

18. Manfredi MA, Clark SJ, Staffa SJ, et al. Endoscopic esophageal vacuum therapy: a Novel therapy for esophageal Perforations in pediatric patients. J Pediatr Gastroenterol Nutr 2018;67(6):706–12.

19. Yasuda JL, Svetanoff WJ, Staffa SJ, et al. Prophylactic negative vacuum therapy of high-risk esophageal anastomoses in pediatric patients. J Pediatr Surg 2021; 56(5):944–50.

20. Heits N, Stapel L, Reichert B, et al. Endoscopic endoluminal vacuum therapy in esophageal perforation. Ann Thorac Surg 2014;97(3):1029–35.

21. Loske G, Schorsch T, Muller C. Intraluminal and intracavitary vacuum therapy for esophageal leakage: a new endoscopic minimally invasive approach. Endoscopy 2011;43(6):540–4.

22. Schorsch T, Muller C, Loske G. Endoscopic vacuum therapy of anastomotic leakage and iatrogenic perforation in the esophagus. Surg Endosc 2013;27(6): 2040–5.

23. Lal DR, Oldham KT. Recurrent tracheoesophageal fistula. Eur J Pediatr Surg 2013;23(3):214–8.

24. Coran AG. Redo esophageal surgery: the diagnosis and management of recurrent tracheoesophageal fistula. Pediatr Surg Int 2013;29(10):995–9.

25. Koivusalo AI, Pakarinen MP, Lindahl HG, et al. Revisional surgery for recurrent tracheoesophageal fistula and anastomotic complications after repair of esophageal atresia in 258 infants. J Pediatr Surg 2015;50(2):250–4.

26. Kovesi T, Rubin S. Long-term complications of congenital esophageal atresia and/or tracheoesophageal fistula. Chest 2004;126(3):915–25.

27. Ein SH, Stringer DA, Stephens CA, et al. Recurrent tracheoesophageal fistulas seventeen-year review. J Pediatr Surg 1983;18(4):436–41.

28. Aworanti O, Awadalla S. Management of recurrent tracheoesophageal fistulas: a systematic review. Eur J Pediatr Surg 2014;24(5):365–75.

29. Daniel SJ, Smith MM. Tracheoesophageal fistula: open versus endoscopic repair. Curr Opin Otolaryngol Head Neck Surg 2016;24(6):510–5.

30. Meier JD, Sulman CG, Almond PS, et al. Endoscopic management of recurrent congenital tracheoesophageal fistula: a review of techniques and results. Int J Pediatr Otorhinolaryngol 2007;71(5):691–7.

31. Richter GT, Ryckman F, Brown RL, et al. Endoscopic management of recurrent tracheoesophageal fistula. J Pediatr Surg 2008;43(1):238–45.

32. Smithers CJ, Hamilton TE, Manfredi MA, et al. Categorization and repair of recurrent and acquired tracheoesophageal fistulae occurring after esophageal atresia repair. J Pediatr Surg 2017;52(3):424–30.

33. Kamran A, Zendejas B, Meisner J, et al. Effect of posterior tracheopexy on risk of recurrence in children after recurrent tracheo-esophageal fistula repair. J Am Coll Surg 2021;232(5):690–8.

34. Boogaard R, Huijsmans SH, Pijnenburg MW, et al. Tracheomalacia and broncho-malacia in children: incidence and patient characteristics. Chest 2005;128(5): 3391–7.
35. Spitz L, Kiely E, Brereton RJ. Esophageal atresia: five year experience with 148 cases. J Pediatr Surg 1987;22(2):103–8.
36. Filler RM, Messineo A, Vinograd I. Severe tracheomalacia associated with esoph-ageal atresia: results of surgical treatment. J Pediatr Surg 1992;27(8):1136–40 [discussion: 40–1].
37. Shieh HF, Smithers CJ, Hamilton TE, et al. Posterior tracheopexy for severe tra-cheomalacia. J Pediatr Surg 2017;52(6):951–5.
38. Fraga JC, Jennings RW, Kim PC. Pediatric tracheomalacia. Semin Pediatr Surg 2016;25(3):156–64.
39. Kamran A, Jennings RW. Tracheomalacia and tracheobronchomalacia in pediat-rics: an Overview of evaluation, medical management, and surgical treatment. Front Pediatr 2019;7:512.
40. Choi S, Lawlor C, Rahbar R, et al. Diagnosis, classification, and management of pediatric tracheobronchomalacia: a review. JAMA Otolaryngol Head Neck Surg 2019;145(3):265–75.
41. Shieh HF, Smithers CJ, Hamilton TE, et al. Descending aortopexy and posterior tracheopexy for severe tracheomalacia and left mainstem bronchomalacia. Semin Thorac Cardiovasc Surg 2019;31(3):479–85.
42. Svetanoff WJ, Zendejas B, Frain L, et al. When to consider a posterolateral de-scending aortopexy in addition to a posterior tracheopexy for the surgical treat-ment of symptomatic tracheobronchomalacia. J Pediatr Surg 2020;55(12): 2682–9.

Abdominal Wall Defects
A Review of Current Practice Guidelines

Alyssa R. Mowrer, MD[a,*], Daniel A. DeUgarte, MD[b],
Amy J. Wagner, MD[a]

KEYWORDS

• Abdominal wall defect • Gastroschisis • Omphalocele

KEY POINTS

• Congenital abdominal wall defects can be diagnosed prenatally and are best managed at a perinatal center to improve clinical outcomes.
• Gastroschisis has a low mortality rate but can be complicated by intestinal abnormalities and a prolonged hospital stay.
• Omphalocele is frequently associated with chromosomal anomalies and other birth defects, which can lead to worse prognosis and complicate abdominal wall closure.

INTRODUCTION

The 2 most common abdominal wall defects are gastroschisis and omphalocele (**Table 1**). These 2 entities are common, creating a need for multidisciplinary collaboration and thorough understanding of the intricate disease processes by all members of the treatment team.

Gastroschisis has an incidence of 4.7 per 10,000 live births and has been demonstrated to be increasing in the western population of the past several decades. Omphalocele occurs more rarely, with an incidence of 1.9 per 10,000 live births, yet has a higher mortality rate due to associated anomalies.[1] Clinical outcomes vary between these 2 disease processes as well as within the spectrum of patients with each diagnosis. As abdominal wall defects can be challenging to manage in all aspects of clinical care, the emphasis on prenatal diagnosis, family counseling, and coordinated perinatal care cannot be underappreciated.

[a] Division of Pediatric Surgery, Department of Surgery, Medical College of Wisconsin, Children's Wisconsin, Administration Office, 999 North 92nd Street Suite 320, Milwaukee, WI 53226, USA;
[b] UCLA Division of Pediatric Surgery, Westwood Clinic Location, 200 UCLA Medical Plaza, Suite 265, Los Angeles, CA 90095, USA
* Corresponding author.
E-mail address: amowrer@chw.org

Clin Perinatol 49 (2022) 943–953
https://doi.org/10.1016/j.clp.2022.07.004
0095-5108/22/© 2022 Elsevier Inc. All rights reserved.

Table 1
Gastroschisis and omphalocele comparison

	Gastroschisis	Omphalocele
Defect location	Abdominal wall, typically right of umbilical cord	Umbilical Cord
Incidence	4.7 per 10,000 live births	1.9 per 10,000 live births
Associations	Young mothers	Chromosomal anomalies and other birth defects
Mortality	<5%	13%–40%
Method of delivery	Vaginal unless obstetric contraindication	Cesarean section if giant or liver herniation

GASTROSCHISIS
Background

Gastroschisis is defined as an abdominal wall defect to the right of the umbilicus with exposed abdominal contents lacking an overlying covering (**Fig. 1**). Although the specific pathogenesis of gastroschisis is not fully understood, the current understanding revolves around a multifactorial cause during embryologic development. The exact cause of this disease process remains unknown but there have been some risk factors identified, both environmental and genetic. Age of the mother, drug and tobacco use during pregnancy, maternal infection, and some medications have been demonstrated to influence the development of the disease process. The diagnosis is often made prenatally by ultrasound early in pregnancy.

On postnatal evaluation, gastroschisis is often divided into 2 categories: simple and complicated. Complicated gastroschisis is defined as an association with intestinal perforation, stenosis, volvulus, atresia, or necrotizing enterocolitis.[2] Patients with complicated gastroschisis have longer lengths of stay, increased mortality, and increased long-term morbidity with feeding difficulty, need for parenteral nutrition, and risk of intestinal failure.

Prenatal Considerations for Gastroschisis

There are several crucial components of prenatal care for patients with gastroschisis. Many of these topics remain in debate without an overall standard of care, such as

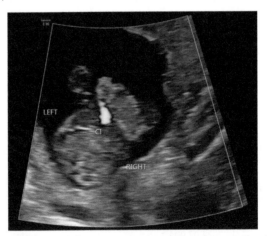

Fig. 1. Gastroschisis—Ultrasound demonstrating herniation through the abdominal wall, on the right, lateral to the umbilical cord insertion (CI).

imaging guidelines, method of monitoring, and delivery timing. Current practices regarding the frequency and method of several maternal–fetal specialists surveyed nationally suggest surveillance with a combination of nonstress tests, biophysical profile, and amniotic fluid index be implemented weekly at 32 weeks gestation.[3] Serial ultrasound imaging has largely been used to assess for the development of in utero growth restriction (IUGR) as well as oligohydramnios to anticipate the development of subsequent problems.

Fetal intervention is not currently indicated in gastroschisis. Due to the caustic effects of amniotic fluid on the abdominal contents, amniotic fluid exchange was proposed as a possible method to remove harmful substances and limit this damage. A study from Italy examined amniotic fluid exchange bimonthly throughout the third trimester for patients with gastroschisis.[4] No significant benefit was identified with this intervention, and due to the potential associated risks, this method fell largely out of favor.

Predicting outcomes prenatally is largely due to ultrasound findings. Several factors, such as intra-abdominal bowel dilation, polyhydramnios, and gastric distention, may be identified in the prenatal period and have been found to predict a higher risk of complications postnatally.[5] Specifically, it was demonstrated that intra-abdominal bowel dilation and polyhydramnios were associated with a higher risk of bowel atresia, and gastric distention was associated with a higher risk of neonatal death.

Liver herniation from the abdominal defect is often associated with omphalocele but has been identified in rare cases of gastroschisis. The identification of a normal umbilical cord adjacent to the abdominal wall defect and the absence of a remnant omphalocele sac can differentiate gastroschisis from a ruptured omphalocele. Giant gastroschisis with liver herniation is associated with worse outcomes including a high mortality rate likely due to associated pulmonary hypoplasia, other comorbidities, and severe visceroabdominal disproportion complicating closure.[6]

The prolapse of organs other than the liver (eg, stomach, bladder, and reproductive organs) does not seem to have an adverse impact on prognosis and may indeed have a positive impact. Organ prolapse may indicate a larger abdominal defect and a decreased risk of mesenteric compression and bowel ischemia. This concept was reinforced by the association of prolapsed organs with simple rather than complicated gastroschisis and suggests a positive correlation with several other outcomes.[2]

The method of delivery is one aspect of care that has reached a consensus. Vaginal delivery has been demonstrated widely as a safe option for delivery of infants with gastroschisis with no other indication for cesarean delivery. In addition, most authors advocate for delivery at a perinatal center when feasible to avoid the need for transfer, which has been associated with increased time to closure, increased length of stay, and higher complication rates.

The optimal timing of delivery for patients with gastroschisis is a topic that is frequently debated. There are several theories regarding potential benefits and consequences to delivery timing among experts in the field. Those in favor of early delivery often focus on the exposure of the abdominal contents to the caustic amniotic fluid environment. It has also been previously demonstrated that the risk of fetal demise is 7 times greater in patients with gastroschisis suggesting an earlier elective delivery may mitigate this risk.[7,8] Furthermore, concerns remain about the small but real risk of closing gastroschisis in which the fascial defect contracts and strangulates the eviscerated bowel resulting in vanishing bowel syndrome and short gut.[9] For these reasons, many centers advocate for delivery no later than 38 weeks estimated gestational age.

Elective preterm delivery remains controversial. In a recent retrospective meta-analysis, elective preterm delivery had a positive impact on feeding and sepsis.[10]

One prior randomized study of elective preterm delivery at 34 weeks was conducted with the goal of addressing this issue. Unfortunately, due to high rates of neonatal sepsis in the early delivery group, the study was aborted.[11] Another randomized study in the United Kingdom evaluated elective delivery at 36 weeks. Although this was a single-institution study with small sample size, no significant difference was observed by early delivery. Early gestation age at delivery (<35 weeks EGA) was identified as a significant predictor of adverse outcomes in a study from the University of California Fetal Consortium.[12] A large multicenter, randomized, prospective study evaluating the timing of delivery is currently underway. This trial, The Gastroschisis Outcomes of Delivery, or GOOD Study, randomizes patients to deliver at either 35 weeks or 38 weeks gestation. The primary outcomes include stillbirth, neonatal death, sepsis, respiratory morbidity, and gastrointestinal morbidity. There are currently 26 centers participating nationally, and the study is scheduled to be completed in 2026 (Clinical trial identifier NCT02774746).

Postnatal Considerations for Gastroschisis

After delivery, the initial treatment consists of addressing acute issues with examination of the protruding abdominal contents for signs of ischemia. On visual inspection, an important patient factor to observe is the presence and severity of bowel matting. This clinical component is one of the components of the Gastroschisis Prognostic Score, and it has been demonstrated that a more severe degree of bowel matting is associated with a higher risk of mortality.[13] After timely visual inspection, priority should be placed on warming the infant as well as covering the exposed contents. The management strategy following delivery includes several possible options including universal silo placement or immediate surgical intervention.

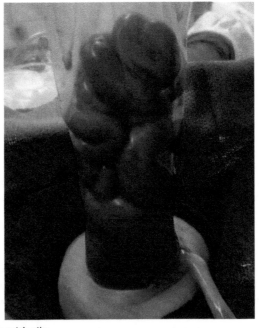

Fig. 2. Gastroschisis with silo.

In a recent multicenter retrospective analysis, the universal utilization of silo as a reasonable management strategy was explored (**Fig. 2**). This study examined outcomes of patients with immediate closure compared with those placed in a silo with closure within 5 days.[14] The results demonstrated no significant difference in the outcomes between these 2 groups, suggesting that universal silo utilization is a safe management strategy for gastroschisis patients. This strategy has proposed benefits of gradual reduction of abdominal contents, which some have suggested may lead to earlier tolerance of enteral feeding and shorter time to full feeds as well as a higher incidence of ventral hernia in patients who received immediate closure.[14,15]

Although the intricate components of patient care for gastroschisis patients remain multifactorial and varied, there have been some efforts to standardize the overall care plan. With common practice guidelines for aspects of care such as intubation, antibiotic choices, pain management regimens, and feeding protocols, it has been suggested that reductions in utilization of resources is both necessary and practical for implementation.[16] A major factor in this overall strategy incorporates multidisciplinary care teams with common goals with a major factor including the possibility of bedside surgical care rather than the traditional operating room setting.

Specific surgical management of the abdominal wall defect has 2 most common approaches, primary surgical closure of the fascia and the more recently proposed sutureless repair, using the umbilical cord as a biologic covering of the defect. In patients with sutureless closure, it has been demonstrated that patients may have less antibiotic use, less exposure to anesthetic due to bedside performance, less infectious complications, and decreased ventilator time compared with patients with primary surgical closure.[17] This literature suggests a sutureless closure for gastroschisis patients proposes significant clinical benefits.

One major limiting factor in the progression toward discharge for gastroschisis patients is the timing of initiation of and progression to full enteral feeds due to prolonged bowel dysmotility. Several institutions have implored efforts to standardize feeding practice guidelines with implementation of a protocol. Studies have demonstrated that the use of such protocols can result in shorter length of stay due to a faster progression to full feeding of gastroschisis patients.[18] This finding was specific to patients with uncomplicated gastroschisis that underwent primary surgical closure. However, when viewed in combination with the data regarding the newer method of sutureless closure, the standardized feeding protocol approach may have a significant benefit in gastroschisis patients of that population as well.

A major concern immediately following the delivery of an infant with gastroschisis is the prevention of temperature and fluid losses due to the exposed abdominal contents. The overall rate of hypothermia in gastroschisis patients has been identified as high as 42%, with significant variability in this number across institutions.[19] Perioperative hypothermia has the potential to increase the infectious complications in the adult population and may have similar effect on the pediatric gastroschisis patient.[10] As infectious complications can have a significant effect on the morbidity and mortality of gastroschisis patients, efforts have been implemented to decrease the frequency of these events. Further research in this setting is necessary as a potential modifiable risk factor for overall clinical outcomes in this population.

Growth failure is a common and significant clinical outcome in the gastroschisis population with as many as 28% of patients meeting criteria for this diagnosis at the time of hospital discharge.[20] As discussed previously, the intestinal dysmotility observed in gastroschisis patients may play a role in the growth failure observed. This highlights the need for further multidisciplinary collaboration to develop a method of intervention to prevent growth failure before hospital discharge.

After discharge, gastroschisis patients have a high rate of hospital readmission.[21] Patients have a risk of adhesive bowel obstruction. Additionally, gastroschisis patients inherently all have some form of intestinal rotational abnormality. The mesenteric base in gastroschisis patients may be narrow, promoting the development of possible midgut volvulus. However, most likely due to the bowel inflammation and adhesion formation, volvulus in gastroschisis patients is rare. Midgut volvulus was identified in 1% of patients with gastroschisis.[22]

OMPHALOCELE
Background

Omphalocele occurs when the intestines fail to return to the abdominal cavity after herniation into the umbilical cord, resulting in a folding defect in the midline of the abdominal wall.[23] The presence of an overlying sac composed of 3 layers, peritoneum, Wharton's jelly, and amnion, is one of the significant differences from gastroschisis patients (**Fig. 3**).[24] In cases of ruptured omphalocele when an overlying sac is not present, the diagnosis can be made by evaluating the location of bowel herniation relative to the umbilical cord insertion (**Fig. 4**). The bowel herniates through the umbilical cord insertion in omphalocele and laterally through the abdominal wall in gastroschisis.[25]

Subsequent clinical outcomes in omphalocele patients are largely dependent on associated anomalies. Chromosomal defects, most commonly Trisomy 18, 13, and 21, occur in approximately 30% to 70% of patients with omphalocele.[26] Other genetic associations occur with syndromes such as Beckwith-Wiedemann, Pentalogy of Cantrell, and cloacal exstrophy. Nonintestinal anomalies, such as cardiac, occur in up to 24% of omphalocele patients.[27] Due to the significant relationship of omphalocele and associated disorders, genetic testing via amniocentesis should be offered to all prenatally diagnosed cases of omphalocele.[26]

Several risk factors for the development of omphalocele have been identified. Maternal age has been associated with increased risk of omphalocele with the highest prevalence in the age range of 35 to 39 years.[28] Women with prepregnancy obesity have also been identified as having a higher risk of omphalocele when compared with mothers at a healthy weight before pregnancy.[29]

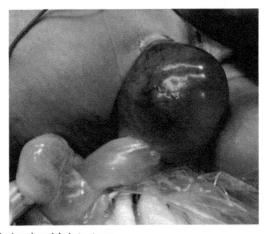

Fig. 3. Small omphalocele with intact sac.

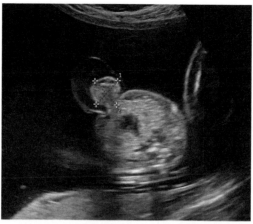

Fig. 4. Omphalocele– Ultrasound demonstrating herniation through the umbilical cord insertion.

Prenatal Considerations for Omphalocele

Prenatal diagnosis of omphalocele is often achieved with routine ultrasound surveillance. Physiologic herniation of the bowel may be observed on early ultrasound; however, the presence of herniated liver or stomach at any point in pregnancy is likely to be an omphalocele.[30] Once identified, it is recommended these patients proceed with fetal cardiac investigation through fetal echocardiogram.[31]

The omphalocele size can vary substantially, leading to the classification of small and giant omphaloceles. Although the definition of a giant omphalocele can vary, many consider a patient with a defect of 5 cm or greater, the presence of herniated liver, or a ruptured sac to have a giant omphalocele.[32] The significance of a giant omphalocele lies mainly in delivery planning and concern for pulmonary hypoplasia. A giant omphalocele is thought to cause an abnormally narrow chest, leading to poor chest expansion in utero, and therefore inadequate lung growth.[33]

Some prenatal tests have been used for large omphaloceles to predict poor prognosis. Fetal MRI can be used to calculate lung volumes and identify patients at risk for pulmonary hypoplasia. Observed to expected lung volumes less than 50% have been associated with higher rates of death and prolonged hospital stay.[34] Ultrasound can be used to calculate an omphalocele ratio (omphalocele diameter/abdominal circumference), which has been shown to help predict respiratory insufficiency and feeding intolerance (**Fig. 5**).[22]

Due to the associated anomalies, patients with omphalocele are also recommended to undergo serial ultrasound surveillance due to the increased risk of IUGR and polyhydramnios. Around the time of 32 weeks, it is also suggested to obtain weekly nonstress tests and biophysical profiles for this patient population.[30] The timing of delivery for omphalocele patients should be dictated mainly by standard obstetric guidelines, with no clear evidence to suggest a specific time or method of delivery as superior. However, in the case of a giant omphalocele, a Cesarean section should be considered to avoid injury to the herniated contents.[35]

Postnatal Considerations for Omphalocele

Immediate postnatal management of omphalocele should include investigation for associated anomalies. Contrary to gastroschisis, if the sac remains intact, the

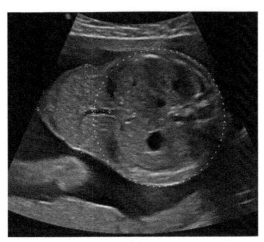

Fig. 5. Omphalocele ratio (omphalocele diameter/abdominal circumference), which has been shown to help predict respiratory insufficiency and feeding intolerance.

potential for heat and fluid losses is significantly lower. The next surgical steps are often dictated by the size of the defect and associated anomalies whether to perform immediate surgical repair or delayed closure.

Although small defects are more likely to undergo immediate primary surgical repair, larger defects or giant omphaloceles may be best managed with a delayed closure (**Fig. 6**). The evolution of the method often referred to as "paint and wait" developed as a combination of 2 prior methods: cicatrization and delayed operative reconstruction (**Fig. 7**).[36] This approach is recommended for large defects, patients at high risk of abdominal compartment syndrome, or patients in whom comorbidities pose excessive risk for primary surgical reconstruction. Although some patients may close the

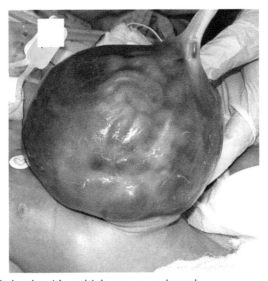

Fig. 6. Giant omphalocele with multiple organs prolapsed.

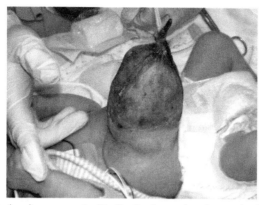

Fig. 7. Large omphalocele managed with the "paint and wait" method for delayed repair.

abdominal wall defect over time, many will have a remaining ventral hernia requiring surgical repair between ages 1 and 5 years.[37]

The risk of early complications following surgical repair of omphalocele is significant, with a frequency of up to 12% related to increased abdominal pressure and 25% related to wound complications.[38] Similar to gastroschisis, these patients have inherent rotational abnormalities leading to a rare occurrence of midgut volvulus. One study demonstrated a low but significant risk of volvulus at a rate of 4.4%, which is 4 times more frequent than seen in gastroschisis patients and 67 times more frequent than the general population.[22] Although data is insufficient to mandate routine performance of a Ladd's procedure in this population, it is imperative to remain aware of this rare but potentially devastating complication.

Although survival rates for omphalocele are reported between 20% and 50%, they are likely higher when including only live births.[37] There remains a close association in overall morbidity and mortality for omphalocele patients with chromosomal or other anomalies. Despite the associated increased morbidity and mortality with giant omphaloceles, those who survive to young adulthood have been shown to reach a similar quality of life and overall state of health when compared with their peers.[39]

CLINICS CARE POINTS

- The prenatal diagnosis of gastroschisis may include assessment of growth restriction, intra-abdominal bowel dilation, amniotic fluid levels, and rarely liver herniation because they are relevant to outcomes.

- Gastroschisis requires emergent surgical care after delivery to maintain normothermia and provide coverage with either closure or silo placement.

- Omphalocele is often associated with chromosomal, cardiac, or other anomalies that should be investigated both prenatally and postnatally.

- Closure of the omphalocele defect is not emergent, and a thorough workup and assessment of size should dictate primary closure versus desiccation of the sac.

DISCLOSURE

The authors have nothing to disclose.

REFERENCES

1. Parker SE, Mai CT, Canfield MA, et al. Updated National Birth Prevalence estimates for selected birth defects in the United States, 2004-2006. Birth Defects Res A Clin Mol Teratol 2010;88(12):1008–16.
2. Koehler SM, Szabo A, Loichinger M, et al. The significance of organ prolapse in gastroschisis. J Pediatr Surg 2017;52(12):1972–6.
3. Amin R, Domack A, Bartoletti J, et al. National practice patterns for prenatal monitoring in gastroschisis: gastroschisis outcomes of delivery (GOOD) provider survey. Fetal Diagn Ther 2019;45(2):125–30.
4. Midrio P, Stefanutti G, Mussap M, et al. Amnioexchange for fetuses with gastroschisis: is it effective? J Pediatr Surg 2007;42(5):777–82.
5. D'Antonio F, Virgone C, Rizzo G, et al. Prenatal risk factors and outcomes in gastroschisis: a meta-analysis. Pediatrics 2015;136(1):e159–69.
6. McClellan EB, Shew SB, Lee SS, et al. Liver herniation in gastroschisis: incidence and prognosis. J Pediatr Surg 2011;46(11):2115–8.
7. South AP, Stutey KM, Meinzen-Derr J. Metaanalysis of the prevalence of intrauterine fetal death in gastroschisis. Am J Obstet Gynecol 2013;209(2).
8. Sparks TN, Shaffer BL, Page J, et al. Gastroschisis: mortality risks with each additional week of expectant management. Am J Obstet Gynecol 2017;216(1): 66.e1-7.
9. Dennison FA. Closed gastroschisis, vanishing midgut and extreme short bowel syndrome: case report and review of the literature. Ultrasound 2016;24(3):170–4.
10. Landisch RM, Yin Z, Christensen M, et al. Outcomes of gastroschisis early delivery: a systematic review and meta-analysis. J Pediatr Surg 2017;52(12):1962–71.
11. Shamshirsaz AA, Lee TC, Hair AB, et al. Elective delivery at 34 weeks vs routine obstetric care in fetal gastroschisis: randomized controlled trial. Ultrasound Obstet Gynecol 2020;55(1):15–9.
12. Overcash RT, DeUgarte DA, Stephenson ML, et al. Factors associated with gastroschisis outcomes. Obstet Gynecol 2014;124(3):551–7.
13. Cowan KN, Puligandla PS, Laberge JM, et al. The gastroschisis prognostic score: reliable outcome prediction in gastroschisis. J Pediatr Surg 2012;47(6):1111–7.
14. Hawkins RB, Raymond SL, St Peter SD, et al. Immediate versus silo closure for gastroschisis: results of a large multicenter study. J Pediatr Surg 2020;55(7): 1280–5.
15. Harris J, Poirier J, Selip D, et al. Early closure of gastroschisis after silo placement correlates with earlier enteral feeding. J Neonatal Surg 2015;4(3):28.
16. DeUgarte DA, Calkins KL, Guner Y, et al. Adherence to and outcomes of a University-Consortium gastroschisis pathway. J Pediatr Surg 2020;55(1):45–8.
17. Fraser JD, Deans KJ, Fallat ME, et al. Sutureless vs sutured abdominal wall closure for gastroschisis: operative characteristics and early outcomes from the Midwest Pediatric Surgery Consortium. J Pediatr Surg 2020;55(11):2284–8.
18. Utria AF, Wong M, Faino A, et al. The role of feeding advancement strategy on length of stay and hospital costs in newborns with gastroschisis. J Pediatr Surg 2021. https://doi.org/10.1016/j.jpedsurg.2021.04.011. S0022-3468(21)00313-4.
19. Bence CM, Landisch RM, Wu R, et al. Risk factors for perioperative hypothermia and infectious outcomes in gastroschisis patients. J Pediatr Surg 2021;56(7): 1107–12.
20. Strobel KM, Romero T, Kramer K, et al. Growth failure prevalence in neonates with gastroschisis : a statewide cohort study. J Pediatr 2021;233:112–8.e3.

21. South AP, Wessel JJ, Sberna A, et al. Hospital readmission among infants with gastroschisis. J Perinatol 2011;31(8):546–50.
22. Fawley JA, Abdelhafeez AH, Schultz JA, et al. The risk of midgut volvulus in patients with abdominal wall defects: a multi-institutional study. J Pediatr Surg 2017; 52(1):26–9.
23. Christison-Lagay ER, Kelleher CM, Langer JC. Neonatal abdominal wall defects. Semin Fetal Neonatal Med 2011;16(3):164–72.
24. Bence CM, Wagner AJ. Abdominal wall defects. Transl Pediatr 2021;10(5): 1461–9.
25. Ledbetter DJ. Congenital abdominal wall defects and reconstruction in pediatric surgery: gastroschisis and omphalocele. Surg Clin North Am 2012;92(3):713–x.
26. Schindewolf E, Moldenhauer JS. Genetic counseling for fetal gastrointestinal anomalies. Curr Opin Obstet Gynecol 2020;32(2):134–9.
27. Corey KM, Hornik CP, Laughon MM, et al. Frequency of anomalies and hospital outcomes in infants with gastroschisis and omphalocele. Early Hum Dev 2014; 90(8):421–4.
28. Rankin J, Dillon E, Wright C. Congenital anterior abdominal wall defects in the north of England, 1986-1996: occurrence and outcome. Prenat Diagn 1999; 19(7):662–8.
29. Watkins ML, Rasmussen SA, Honein MA, et al. Maternal obesity and risk for birth defects. Pediatrics 2003;111(5 Pt 2):1152–8.
30. Mann S, Blinman TA, Douglas Wilson R. Prenatal and postnatal management of omphalocele. Prenat Diagn 2008;28(7):626–32.
31. Adams AD, Stover S, Rac MW. Omphalocele-What should we tell the prospective parents? Prenat Diagn 2021;41(4):486–96.
32. Barrios Sanjuanelo A, Abelló Munarriz C, Cardona-Arias JA. Systematic review of mortality associated with neonatal primary staged closure of giant omphalocele. J Pediatr Surg 2021;56(4):678–85.
33. Victoria T, Andronikou S, Bowen D, et al. Fetal anterior abdominal wall defects: prenatal imaging by magnetic resonance imaging. Pediatr Radiol 2018;48(4): 499–512.
34. Chock VY, Davis AS, Cho SH, et al. Prenatally diagnosed omphalocele: characteristics associated with adverse neonatal outcomes. J Perinatol 2019;39(8): 1111–7.
35. Lurie S, Sherman D, Bukovsky I. Omphalocele delivery enigma: the best mode of delivery still remains dubious. Eur J Obstet Gynecol Reprod Biol 1999;82(1): 19–22.
36. Wagner JP, Cusick RA. Paint and wait management of giant omphaloceles. Semin Pediatr Surg 2019;28(2):95–100.
37. Islam S. Advances in surgery for abdominal wall defects: gastroschisis and omphalocele. Clin Perinatol 2012;39(2):375–86.
38. Maksoud-Filho JG, Tannuri U, da Silva MM, et al. The outcome of newborns with abdominal wall defects according to the method of abdominal closure: the experience of a single center. Pediatr Surg Int 2006;22(6):503–7.
39. Van Eijck FC, Hoogeveen YL, van Weel C, et al. Minor and giant omphalocele: long-term outcomes and quality of life. J Pediatr Surg 2009;44(7):1355–9.

Review of Necrotizing Enterocolitis and Spontaneous Intestinal Perforation Clinical Presentation, Treatment, and Outcomes

Laura A. Rausch, MD, MPH, MA[a,b,c], David N. Hanna, MD[a],
Anuradha Patel, MD[d], Martin L. Blakely, MD, MS[d],*

KEYWORDS

- Necrotizing enterocolitis • Spontaneous intestinal perforation • Toll-like receptor 4
- Nitric oxide synthase • Cerebral palsy

KEY POINTS

- Surgeons should make deliberate attempts to distinguish NEC and SIP when considering surgical treatment options.
- Use of ultrasound to inform surgical treatment requires further study.
- With presumed NEC, initial laparotomy likely leads to lower rates of death and neurodevelopmental impairment.

INTRODUCTION

Necrotizing enterocolitis (NEC) and spontaneous intestinal perforation (SIP) are 2 neonatal conditions that have been widely investigated but continue to have frequent morbidity and high mortality. In this review, we will discuss the differences and similarities in clinical presentation, pathophysiology, treatment, and outcomes for NEC and SIP. NEC effects 2% to 9% of preterm neonates, and nearly 10% of preterm infants with very low birthweight (VLBW, <1500 grams).[1,2] The mortality rate of extremely low birth weight (ELBW, <1000 grams) neonates is 30% to 50% and for VLBW neonates ranges from 10% to 30%. There is variation in incidence of disease based on gestational age (GA), birthweight, country of origin, with the lowest reported

[a] Vanderbilt University Medical Center, 2200 Children's Way, Suite 7100, Nashville, TN 37232, USA; [b] Vanderbilt University Master of Public Health School, 2200 Children's Way, Suite 7100, Nashville, TN 37232, USA; [c] Geriatric Research Education and Clinical Center, 2200 Children's Way, Suite 7100, Nashville, TN 37232, USA; [d] Monroe Carell Jr. Children's Hospital at Vanderbilt, 2200 Children's Way, Suite 7100, Nashville, TN 37232, USA
* Corresponding author.
E-mail address: martin.blakely@vumc.org

Clin Perinatol 49 (2022) 955–964
https://doi.org/10.1016/j.clp.2022.07.005
0095-5108/22/© 2022 Elsevier Inc. All rights reserved.

incidence in Japan (2%) and the highest in Australia, Canada, and Italy ranging from 7% to 9% of preterm infants. This variation in incidence rates among countries[1,2] suggests that there are various factors influencing the development of NEC including environment, diet, and genetic predisposition.[1]

Over the years, there have been increasing reports of SIP in VLBW and ELBW neonates. For neonates with a GA less than 32 weeks, the reported incidence rate was 1.6% based on National Inpatient Sample dataset from 2002 to 2017. This cohort demonstrated increased incidence of SIP with decreasing GA. In the cohort, 90% of cases were less than or equal to 28-week GA, with 82% of the neonates being ELBW and more prevalent in male versus female neonates.[3] The incidence rates of NEC and SIP change over time, and ongoing study is important.

CLINICAL PRESENTATION

NEC and SIP are 2 intra-abdominal conditions that have significant overlap in clinical presentation. The optimal treatment modality of these 2 distinct disorders likely differs; therefore it is important for clinicians to distinguish between NEC and SIP before initiating the surgical treatment. NEC is thought to be primarily driven by ischemia and initiation of enteral feeds resulting in full-thickness hemorrhagic necrosis. SIP is localized to the area of perforation and is characterized as isolated mucosal ulceration with submucosal thinning.[4,5] Thus, SIP can occur before the initiation of enteral feeds in LBW and ELBW infants.[6,7] In SIP, operative findings typically involve a single subcentimeter perforation, usually on the antimesenteric border of the small intestine with minimal peritoneal contamination and healthy appearing surrounding intestine.[5] Although a perforation is often present in NEC, the surrounding bowel is not typically healthy-appearing and requires a small bowel resection with or without stoma creation.

A particular challenge in differentiating NEC from SIP is that the definition of NEC has evolved during the last several decades. Scoring systems, such as Bell's criteria and the modified Bell's criteria, have primarily served to communicate severity of disease, rather than specifically diagnose NEC from other forms of gastrointestinal illness.[8] More recent attempts to standardize the definition of NEC, including the Stanford NEC score, the International Neonatal Consortium NEC workgroup definition, and the Centers for Disease Control and Prevention definition, incorporate laboratory and radiographic signs that help limit and objectify the definition of NEC.[9-11] However, such definitions and scoring systems are seldom used by clinicians at the bedside when evaluating a neonate with symptoms typical of NEC or SIP. Thus, clinicians should consider risk factors, physical examination findings, radiographic findings, and specific laboratory markers that are specific to NEC or SIP.

No maternal characteristics, such as age, parity, multiple gestations, or mode of delivery, have been implicated in NEC or SIP, and there is significant overlap in the clinical presentation of infants with NEC and SIP.[4,6] Infants with either disorder may develop bloody stools, abdominal distension, and may have an accompanying bilious output from a nasogastric decompression tube. However, infants with SIP consistently develop a bluish discoloration of the abdomen, which is a hallmark differentiator from NEC.[5,12-15]

There are multiple risk factors that are associated with the development of NEC. The following are consistently described: formula feeding, intestinal dysbiosis, low birthweight, and prematurity.[1,16] It has also been reported with acid-suppressing medications, acute hypoxia, antibiotic exposure, blood transfusions, cardiac anomalies, neonatal anemia, and mechanical ventilation.[2,17] Prematurity is the only well-established risk factor for SIP, although there are other antenatal and prenatal risk factors based on limited data from case series, for which a conclusive association has not been established.[10]

IMAGING

The diagnosis of NEC or SIP is supported by standard imaging modalities, such as abdominal X-rays and ultrasound. Abdominal X-rays (supine and lateral) may provide findings that can help the clinician differentiate between NEC and SIP. Although pneumoperitoneum occurs in both entities, neonates with NEC may demonstrate significant bowel distension or fixed bowel loops, whereas neonates with SIP are likely to demonstrate a paucity of bowel gas or a gasless abdomen.[18] Abdominal ultrasound may provide other specific signs of NEC, such as thickened intestinal walls, pneumatosis intestinalis, and portal venous gas. Ultrasound has been shown to be a valuable tool in differentiating NEC from SIP. Several early studies demonstrated portal venous gas to be a highly sensitive and specific sign of NEC, and more recent studies have demonstrated its high specificity.[19–23] Additionally, ultrasound may demonstrate a localized area of peritoneal contamination that may direct peritoneal drain placement should the clinician elect to place one, although this is not used commonly. There are no large, multicenter studies clearly documenting the added value of ultrasound in the diagnostic distinction of NEC and SIP or in the management of these conditions, and this is an important area where further study is needed. It likely can play an important role but reliable supporting evidence is in the early phases.

PATHOPHYSIOLOGY

The pathophysiology of NEC is multifactorial, and there is active ongoing research to determine factors and processes that lead to this devastating disease. The time from birth to the onset of NEC is inversely proportional to GA,[10] with the more premature infants developing NEC at a later postnatal age and less preterm infant developing it sooner after birth. The development of NEC seems to reach a peak around 29 to 32 weeks postmenstrual age.[16] The classic pathophysiology understanding is that intraluminal bacteria disrupt and invade intestinal epithelium at the tip of the intestinal villi. This then leads to the endotoxin from the bacteria to bind to the toll-like receptor 4 (TLR4) on intestinal epithelial cells, leading to the activation of the pathogen-associated molecular pattern receptors. This ultimately leads to break down of gut barrier and allows bacteria to translocate inciting an inflammatory response in lamina propria led by TNF-alpha, IL-1beta, and other cytokines. The activation of complement and coagulation systems causes leukocytes and platelets adherence to the endothelium, thereby decreasing blood flow in microvasculature and causing tissue injury leading to coagulative necrosis and sepsis.[1] Currently, there are multiple potential mechanisms that have been extensively researched and currently investigated, including the role of TLR4 and nitric oxide, disruption of microvascular blood flow (intestinal ischemia), the effect of dysbiosis, and the reduced activity of intestinal stem cells.[1,4–7]

The cause of SIP largely remains unknown, with several cases reporting thinning or absence of muscularis propria at the site of perforation.[5] One mechanism regarding the role for abnormal or delayed nitric oxide synthase (NOS) has been hypothesized, this is based on single study of NOS knock out mouse model that demonstrated ileal perforation with exposure to indomethacin and/or dexamethasone.[24] The following processes have been demonstrated to be upregulated in SIP but milder in samples taken from patients with SIP compared with those with NEC: changes in immunoregulatory pathways regarding angiogenesis, arginine metabolism, cell adhesion and chemotaxis, extracellular matrix remodeling, hypoxia and oxidative stress, inflammation, and muscle contraction.[25,26]

TREATMENT OF SURGICAL NECROTIZING ENTEROCOLITIS AND SPONTANEOUS INTESTINAL PERFORATION

There are promising signs that the incidence of NEC is decreasing over time but until this devastating disease of prematurity can be reliably prevented, it is incumbent on pediatric surgeons and neonatologists to study outcomes with currently available surgical treatments with the goal of optimizing outcomes.[27] Unlike many other neonatal surgical therapies, which typically are "understudied," there have now been 3 randomized clinical trials (RCT) comparing laparotomy versus peritoneal drainage at disease onset. Questions remain but there is reliable evidence for pediatric surgeons and neonatologists to now use in their clinical decision-making and to use in discussions with parents of infants with these conditions.

The first 2 RCTs compared initial laparotomy versus peritoneal drainage in different populations of infants with surgical NEC or SIP and each of these primarily evaluated mortality rates.[28,29] The NEC Steps trial was an important RCT within pediatric surgery, being one of the very few multicenter RCTs supported by National Institutes of Health (NIH) funding. This trial enrolled 117 infants up to 1500 grams birthweight and found that there was no difference in mortality at 90 days with initial peritoneal drainage (34.5%) compared with initial laparotomy (35.5%). This trial strongly discouraged subsequent laparotomy after initial drainage and can be viewed as laparotomy versus "definitive" drainage rather than initial "temporizing" drainage. The second RCT comparing initial laparotomy versus peritoneal drainage enrolled 69 ELBW infants at 31 centers in 13 countries.[29] This trial was more permissive of subsequent laparotomy after initial drainage, which 74% of initial drainage patients had. Six-month survival with the initial drainage was 51.4% versus 63.6% with laparotomy ($P = .3$; risk difference 12% [95% CI: $-11, 34\%$]). As discussed later in this section, the conclusion that there was "no significant difference" in this finding meets the traditional dichotomous views centered around a P value of less than or greater than .05 but possibly also showed clinically relevant differences in mortality rates. Importantly, neither of these early RCTs comparing laparotomy versus peritoneal drainage attempted to measure the possible impact of the preoperative diagnosis of NEC versus SIP on the treatment effect. These trials were a very important start in the investigation of our 2 current "standard" therapies but without delving into differences between NEC and SIP, it is likely that the true story is more complicated than presented.

The Necrotizing Enterocolitis Surgery Trial (NEST) is the third RCT comparing initial laparotomy versus peritoneal drainage and advances our understanding of outcomes of these therapies in infants with surgical NEC or SIP in several important ways. This trial was conducted within the robust infrastructure of the National Institute of Child Health and Human Development- Neonatal Research Network and was the first trial to meet its designated sample size, randomizing 310 ELBW infants.[30] The primary outcome was death or neurodevelopmental impairment (NDI) at 18 to 22 months corrected age, which was based on a prior observational study showing that mortality was not different in laparotomy versus drainage groups but later NDI possibly was.[31] This trial also formally assessed the possibility that the preoperative diagnosis of NEC or SIP affected the treatment effect of laparotomy versus drainage, which had not been tested previously. The NEST reported that infants with NEC do have many differences from those with a preoperative diagnosis of SIP, although some do present

Table 1
Necrotizing enterocolitis surgery trial patient characteristics by preoperative diagnosis[30]

Variable	Preop NEC (n = 95)	Preop IP (n = 213)	P Value
Age at initial surgery, mean (SD), d	20.93 (11.90)	7.84 (5.19)	<.001
Pneumatosis, No. (%)	34 (35.79)	11 (5.16)	<.001
Pneumoperitoneum, No. (%)	48 (50.53)	198 (92.96)	<.001
Portal vein air, No. (%)	18 (18.95)	5 (2.35)	<.001
Gasless abdomen, No. (%)	9 (9.47)	8 (3.76)	.04
Vasopressors at time of randomization, No. (%)	43 (45.26)	57 (26.76)	.001
Ventilatory support			
Conventional vent, No. (%)	56 (58.95)	151 (70.89)	.04
High frequency ventilation, No. (%)	36 (37.89)	44 (20.66)	.001
Fio_2, mean (SD)	57.71 (27.90)	39.87 (21.73)	<.001
pH, mean (SD)	7.21 (0.15)	7.25 (0.11)	.007
Birthweight, mean (SD), g	728.34 (147.05)	710.58 (132.17)	.29
Gestational Age, mean (SD), wk	25.15 (1.95)	24.88 (1.61)	.21
Weigh at initial surgery, mean (SD), g	900.37 (314.64)	706.56 (157.83)	<.001
Bluish discoloration, No. (%)	40 (42.11)	80 (37.56)	.45
Measures Prior to Randomization			
Received indomethacin before randomization, No. (%)	40 (45.45)	116 (54.98)	.13
Received postnatal steroids before randomization, No. (%)	34 (35.79)	40 (18.78)	.001
Received enteral feedings before randomization, No. (%)	65 (92.86)	120 (71.86)	<.001

Abbreviation: SD, standard deviation.

with similar features (**Table 1**). Although this distinction is challenging and imperfect, many pediatric surgeons use this distinction in surgical decision-making in clinical practice, typically preferring drainage for cases of SIP and laparotomy for those with NEC.[32–34] The NEST found that the preoperative diagnosis of NEC versus SIP was indeed important and significantly affected the overall treatment effect (P = .03). In infants with a preoperative diagnosis of NEC (n = 94), the rate of death or NDI (primary outcome) at 18 to 22 months with initial drainage was 85% compared with 69% with initial laparotomy (adjusted relative risk = 0.81 [95% CI: 0.64–1.04). The Bayesian posterior probability that laparotomy reduced the rate of death or NDI in this diagnostic group was 97%. However, in infants with a preoperative diagnosis of SIP (n = 201), the treatment effect was in the opposite direction, finding that the rate of death/NDI after initial drainage was 63% compared with 69% with laparotomy (Bayesian posterior probability with laparotomy of 18%). Stated a different way, in infants with a preoperative diagnosis of NEC, the rate of survival without impairment with laparotomy was twice that with initial drainage (31% vs 15%). The final recommendations of the NEST were that a robust effort should be made at the time of consult to distinguish NEC from SIP and that initial laparotomy is the optimal therapy for infants diagnosed with NEC. Further studies are being developed to investigate the adoption of these recommendations into practice and to elicit attitudes of pediatric surgeons, neonatologists, and parents of affected infants regarding implementation of these findings and the ethical considerations involved.

SHORT-TERM OUTCOMES

Most of the focus of larger studies evaluating outcomes with surgical NEC and SIP has appropriately been on mortality and later NDI, although other early outcomes are also important in surgical decision-making. A fairly recent systematic review reported that the overall mortality rate with surgical NEC was 34.5% and was 40.5% for ELBW infants with surgical NEC.[35] The incidence of intestinal failure, in a limited number of studies (n = 1370 infants), was between 15% and 35%. In NEST, which had a predominance of SIP infants (n = 213) compared with NEC (n = 95), the overall mortality was 29% at 18 to 22 months corrected age. The mortality with a preoperative diagnosis of NEC was 46%, consistent with prior studies and with SIP was 21%. In infants with a preoperative diagnosis of NEC, initial laparotomy resulted in a mortality rate of 40% compared with 51% with drainage. With SIP, the initial laparotomy had a mortality rate of 23% compared with 19% with initial drainage.

In NEST, infants with a preoperative diagnosis of NEC and initial laparotomy had similar duration of mechanical ventilation but shorter duration of parenteral nutrition, time to full feeds, and length of hospital stay.[30] This advantage with laparotomy was not seen with SIP infants. An important finding in NEST was that the intraoperative complication rate was higher with initial laparotomy (20%) compared with initial drainage (13%), and the most common intraoperative complication was liver hemorrhage (5% of laparotomy patients). There is likely some degree of ascertainment bias involved in intraoperative complication measurement because complications during drainage are likely more occult compared with laparotomy, nevertheless this is an important finding to consider in surgical decision-making. An outcome favoring laparotomy in NEST was that 7% of infants with a preoperative diagnosis of NEC or SIP actually had neither condition at laparotomy (2 cases of intestinal volvulus, 2 gastric perforations, and 6 other diagnoses). Also influential is the finding that 50% of initial drainage infants had a subsequent laparotomy compared with 24% after initial laparotomy (this excludes ostomy closure).

NEURODEVELOPMENTAL OUTCOMES

NDI continues to be a major problem in infants treated for surgical NEC and SIP. In the recently reported NEST, the overall rate of NDI in survivors at 18 to 22 months corrected age was 56%, which is consistent with other publications during the past decade.[30,36] NDI in this study was defined as having any of the following: moderate-to-severe cerebral palsy (CP) with Gross Motor Function Classification System level 2 or greater, Bayley-III cognitive composite score less than 85, severe bilateral visual impairment consistent with vision less than 20/200, or permanent hearing loss despite amplification that prevents communication or understanding the examiner. For infants with a preoperative diagnosis of NEC, initial laparotomy resulted in a lower rate of NDI in survivors (48%) compared with initial peritoneal drainage (68%), with a Bayesian posterior probability that laparotomy was beneficial of 89%. The rates of any NDI in infants with a preoperative diagnosis of SIP did not differ much with initial laparotomy (59%) compared with drainage (53%). Interestingly, the rate of moderate-to-severe CP did seem to be somewhat lower with initial laparotomy (16%) compared with initial drainage (24%) in infants with presumed SIP (Bayesian posterior probability of benefit with lap 89%). In infants with a preoperative diagnosis of NEC, the benefit of initial laparotomy in reducing moderate to severe CP was larger (20% with lap vs 44% with drain; Bayesian posterior probability of benefit with initial laparotomy of 94%). This protection against CP with initial laparotomy deserves further investigation to verify and determine possible mechanisms.

Although the incidence of NDI in infants with surgical NEC and SIP has not improved, the mechanisms involved are becoming clearer. A recent investigation involving an NEC mouse model and also brain tissues from infants that died with NEC (and controls) found that an underlying mechanism of NEC-related brain injury were because of gut-derived CD4+ T lymphocytes that mediated neuroinflammation, and these authors concluded that early management of intestinal inflammation in cases of NEC may improve neurologic outcomes.[37] This is a possible underlying mechanism for the lower rate of NDI in surgical NEC infants after laparotomy versus drainage reported in NEST. Other mechanisms shown to be involved include proinflammatory cytokines secondary to intestinal damage, increased growth hormone during an acute illness leading to decreased insulin-like growth factor (IGF-1) levels, changes in gut microbiome and malnutrition.[38,39]

SUMMARY

The distinction of NEC and SIP before laparotomy does need much improvement and deserves the focus of high-quality research efforts. When there is discrepancy between the preoperative and the intraoperative diagnosis of NEC or SIP, it is usually assumed that the preoperative diagnosis was incorrect. However, there has never been a study, to our knowledge, investigating the validity and consistency of the intraoperative distinction of NEC and SIP and it is likely that there is important variability in this measure. Prospective studies investigating the distinction of NEC and SIP as the primary study focus are needed but currently not available. The definitions of these conditions are also being questioned and refined over time.[40]

An interesting and unanswered question, after the publication of the 3 RCTs reviewed, is what is the level of evidence that pediatric surgeons and neonatologists should require to potentially change their practice. This question applies especially to neonatal surgery, wherein RCTs are few and far between and those that are done are typically small. For surgeons that prefer initial laparotomy for infants with a preoperative diagnosis of NEC and reserve initial drainage for those with SIP, these trial findings may serve to reinforce their practice. However, do the NEST findings warrant a change in practice for surgeons or neonatologists that may prefer initial drainage for presumed NEC infants or for those that chose between laparotomy and drainage based on patient weight or measures of acuity of illness? There is a growing call from the scientific community to avoid dichotomous conclusions based on a P value of less than or greater than .05 (or any other statistical metric) and the recommendation is to evaluate the point estimate of the treatment effect, the confidence interval, the quality of the conduct of the study including data integrity, the costs and risks of the therapies, and the likelihood of other trials producing more high-quality evidence.[41,42] However, many surgeons still have the dichotomous world view around the P value, despite often not understanding the true meaning of the P value. The facts that 2 of the 3 RCTs did not reach their designed sample size and that the NEST required 10 years to complete, indicate that there will not be other RCTs addressing these therapies any time soon and possibly ever. Therefore, pediatric surgeons and neonatologists will need to carefully review these data and decide for themselves how to use this in their clinical practice.

Best practices

- Make deliberate effort to distinguish NEC from SIP prior to initial operation and use the presumed preoperative diagnosis in surgical decision making.

DISCLOSURE

The authors have nothing to disclose.

REFERENCES

1. Alganabi M, Lee C, Bindi E, et al. Recent advances in understanding necrotizing enterocolitis. F1000Res 2019;8.
2. Rose AT, Patel RM. A critical analysis of risk factors for necrotizing enterocolitis. Semin Fetal Neonatal Med 2018;23(6):374–9.
3. Elgendy MM, Othman HF, Heis F, et al. Spontaneous intestinal perforation in premature infants: a national study. J Perinatol 2021;41(5):1122–8.
4. Hwang H, Murphy JJ, Gow KW, et al. Are localized intestinal perforations distinct from necrotizing enterocolitis? J Pediatr Surg 2003;38(5):763–7.
5. Pumberger W, Mayr M, Kohlhauser C, et al. Spontaneous localized intestinal perforation in very-low-birth-weight infants: a distinct clinical entity different from necrotizing enterocolitis. J Am Coll Surg 2002;195(6):796–803.
6. Fatemizadeh R, Mandal S, Gollins L, et al. Incidence of spontaneous intestinal perforations exceeds necrotizing enterocolitis in extremely low birth weight infants fed an exclusive human milk-based diet: a single center experience. J Pediatr Surg 2021;56(5):1051–6.
7. Neu J. Necrotizing enterocolitis: the mystery goes on. Neonatology 2014;106(4): 289–95.
8. Patel RM, Ferguson J, McElroy SJ, et al. Defining necrotizing enterocolitis: current difficulties and future opportunities. Pediatr Res 2020;88(Suppl 1):10–5.
9. Battersby C, Santhalingam T, Costeloe K, et al. Incidence of neonatal necrotising enterocolitis in high-income countries: a systematic review. Arch Dis Child Fetal Neonatal Ed 2018;103(2):F182–9.
10. Caplan MS, Underwood MA, Modi N, et al. Necrotizing enterocolitis: Using Regulatory science and Drug development to improve outcomes. J Pediatr 2019;212: 208–215 e1.
11. Torrazza RM, Li N, Neu J. Decoding the enigma of necrotizing enterocolitis in premature infants. Pathophysiology 2014;21(1):21–7.
12. Aschner JL, Deluga KS, Metlay LA, et al. Spontaneous focal gastrointestinal perforation in very low birth weight infants. J Pediatr 1988;113(2):364–7.
13. Meyer CL, Payne NR, Roback SA. Spontaneous, isolated intestinal perforations in neonates with birth weight less than 1,000 g not associated with necrotizing enterocolitis. J Pediatr Surg 1991;26(6):714–7.
14. Mintz AC, Applebaum H. Focal gastrointestinal perforations not associated with necrotizing enterocolitis in very low birth weight neonates. J Pediatr Surg 1993; 28(6):857–60.
15. Buchheit JQ, Stewart DL. Clinical comparison of localized intestinal perforation and necrotizing enterocolitis in neonates. Pediatrics 1994;93(1):32–6.
16. Bazacliu C, Neu J. Pathophysiology of necrotizing enterocolitis: an Update. Curr Pediatr Rev 2019;15(2):68–87.
17. Meister AL, Doheny KK, Travagli RA. Necrotizing enterocolitis: It's not all in the gut. Exp Biol Med (Maywood) 2020;245(2):85–95.
18. Ahle M, Ringertz HG, Rubesova E. The role of imaging in the management of necrotising enterocolitis: a multispecialist survey and a review of the literature. Eur Radiol 2018;28(9):3621–31.

19. Merritt CR, Goldsmith JP, Sharp MJ. Sonographic detection of portal venous gas in infants with necrotizing enterocolitis. AJR Am J Roentgenol 1984;143(5): 1059–62.
20. Robberecht EA, Afschrift M, De Bel CE, et al. Sonographic demonstration of portal venous gas in necrotizing enterocolitis. Eur J Pediatr 1988;147(2):192–4.
21. Lindley S, Mollitt DL, Seibert JJ, et al. Portal vein ultrasonography in the early diagnosis of necrotizing enterocolitis. J Pediatr Surg 1986;21(6):530–2.
22. Dordelmann M, Rau GA, Bartels D, et al. Evaluation of portal venous gas detected by ultrasound examination for diagnosis of necrotising enterocolitis. Arch Dis Child Fetal Neonatal Ed 2009;94(3):F183–7.
23. Dilli D, Suna Oguz S, Erol R, et al. Does abdominal sonography provide additional information over abdominal plain radiography for diagnosis of necrotizing enterocolitis in neonates? Pediatr Surg Int 2011;27(3):321–7.
24. Gordon PV, Herman AC, Marcinkiewicz M, et al. A neonatal mouse model of intestinal perforation: investigating the harmful synergism between glucocorticoids and indomethacin. J Pediatr Gastroenterol Nutr 2007;45(5):509–19.
25. Chan KY, Leung FW, Lam HS, et al. Immunoregulatory protein profiles of necrotizing enterocolitis versus spontaneous intestinal perforation in preterm infants. PLoS One 2012;7(5):e36977.
26. Chan KY, Leung KT, Tam YH, et al. Genome-wide expression profiles of necrotizing enterocolitis versus spontaneous intestinal perforation in human intestinal tissues: dysregulation of functional pathways. Ann Surg 2014;260(6):1128–37.
27. Ellsbury DL, Clark RH, Ursprung R, et al. A Multifaceted Approach to improving outcomes in the NICU: the Pediatrix 100 000 Babies Campaign. Pediatrics 2016; 137(4).
28. Moss RL, Dimmitt RA, Barnhart DC, et al. Laparotomy versus peritoneal drainage for necrotizing enterocolitis and perforation. N Engl J Med 2006;354(21):2225–34.
29. Rees CM, Eaton S, Kiely EM, et al. Peritoneal drainage or laparotomy for neonatal bowel perforation? A randomized controlled trial. Ann Surg 2008;248(1):44–51.
30. Blakely ML, Tyson JE, Lally KP, et al. Initial laparotomy versus peritoneal drainage in extremely low birthweight infants with surgical necrotizing enterocolitis or isolated intestinal perforation: a multicenter randomized clinical trial. Ann Surg 2021;274(4):e370–80.
31. Blakely ML, Tyson JE, Lally KP, et al. Laparotomy versus peritoneal drainage for necrotizing enterocolitis or isolated intestinal perforation in extremely low birth weight infants: outcomes through 18 months adjusted age. Pediatrics 2006; 117(4):e680–7.
32. Cass DL, Brandt ML, Patel DL, et al. Peritoneal drainage as definitive treatment for neonates with isolated intestinal perforation. J Pediatr Surg 2000;35(11): 1531–6.
33. Jakaitis BM, Bhatia AM. Definitive peritoneal drainage in the extremely low birth weight infant with spontaneous intestinal perforation: predictors and hospital outcomes. J Perinatol 2015;35(8):607–11.
34. Quiroz HJ, Rao K, Brady AC, et al. Protocol-driven surgical Care of necrotizing enterocolitis and spontaneous intestinal perforation. J Surg Res 2020;255: 396–404.
35. Jones IH, Hall NJ. Contemporary outcomes for infants with necrotizing enterocolitis-A systematic review. J Pediatr 2020;220:86–92 e3.
36. Hintz SR, Kendrick DE, Stoll BJ, et al. Neurodevelopmental and growth outcomes of extremely low birth weight infants after necrotizing enterocolitis. Pediatrics 2005;115(3):696–703.

37. Zhou Q, Nino DF, Yamaguchi Y, et al. Necrotizing enterocolitis induces T lymphocyte-mediated injury in the developing mammalian brain. Sci Transl Med 2021;13(575). https://doi.org/10.1126/scitranslmed.aay6621.
38. Hickey M, Georgieff M, Ramel S. Neurodevelopmental outcomes following necrotizing enterocolitis. Semin Fetal Neonatal Med 2018;23(6):426–32.
39. Vlug LE, Verloop MW, Dierckx B, et al. Cognitive outcomes in Children with conditions affecting the small intestine: a systematic review and Meta-analysis. J Pediatr Gastroenterol Nutr 2022;74(3):368–76.
40. Swanson JR, Hair A, Clark RH, et al. Spontaneous intestinal perforation (SIP) will soon become the most common form of surgical bowel disease in the extremely low birth weight (ELBW) infant. J Perinatol 2022. https://doi.org/10.1038/s41372-022-01347-z.
41. Ronald L, Wasserstein A. Moving to a world beyond "p < 0.05". Am Statistician 2019;73:1–19.
42. Amrhein V, Greenland S, McShane B. Scientists rise up against statistical significance. Nature 2019;567(7748):305–7.

Advances in the Management of the Neonate Born with an Anorectal Malformation

Sebastian K. King, PhD, FRACS[a,b,c],*, Marc A. Levitt, MD[d,e]

KEYWORDS

- Anorectal malformations • Newborn • Pediatric • Anorectoplasty

KEY POINTS

- The management of infants with anorectal malformations requires a systematic approach to diagnosis and treatment.
- Careful physical examination of the newborn will determine the operative or nonoperative management for the first 24 to 48 h in most of the patients.
- Investigation for associated anomalies requires specialized radiological testing and an excellent relationship with radiological colleagues.

INTRODUCTION

The management of the neonate born with an anorectal malformation (ARM) has matured and dramatically improved over the last two decades. Advances in antenatal diagnosis have led to an increased number of patients being born with a presumptive diagnosis of an ARM, though the numbers remain small. More accurate assessment of the malformation type in the first few days of life, and an improvement in decision-making regarding the need for colostomy formation, has led to decreased morbidity in affected neonates. The long-term needs of the patients, including into adulthood, have been recognized. The outlook for a neonate born with an ARM has never been better, but there remains much to do.

[a] Colorectal and Pelvic Reconstruction Service, Department of Paediatric Surgery, The Royal Children's Hospital, Melbourne 3052, Australia; [b] Department of Paediatrics, University of Melbourne, Australia; [c] F. Douglas Stephens Surgical Research Group, Murdoch Children's Research Institute, Melbourne, Australia; [d] Division of Colorectal and Pelvic Reconstruction, Children's National Hospital, Washington, DC, USA; [e] The George Washington School of Medicine, Washington, DC, USA
* Corresponding author. Colorectal and Pelvic Reconstruction Service, Department of Paediatric Surgery, The Royal Children's Hospital, Melbourne 3052, Australia.
E-mail address: sebastian.king@rch.org.au

Clin Perinatol 49 (2022) 965–979
https://doi.org/10.1016/j.clp.2022.08.002   perinatology.theclinics.com
0095-5108/22/Crown Copyright © 2022 Published by Elsevier Inc. All rights reserved.

ANTENATAL DIAGNOSIS

The diagnosis of an ARM on antenatal imaging remains a rare event, except in the situation of a cloacal anomaly. Although the absence of the perianal musculature may be diagnosed on 3D ultrasonography, and standard 2D ultrasonography may identify dilatation of the distal bowel and intraluminal calcified meconium, neither of these findings typically lead to recognition of the ARM. However, the presence of a large cystic mass arising from the pelvis may lead to a presumptive diagnosis of cloaca, with the fluid-filled vagina (hydrocolpos) being responsible for the abnormal finding.[1] (**Fig. 1**).

More often, the presence of an ARM is suggested by the findings of potential associated anomalies (vertebral, cardiac, tracheoesophageal, renal, limb) and/or syndromes (trisomy 21). In these cases, a fetal MRI after 20 weeks' gestation may be used to delineate the musculature of the external anal sphincter complex and the presence of the *levator ani* complex. Additional abnormalities of the urinary tract, Mullerian anomalies, limb anomalies, an absent sacrum, and a presacral mass may also be detected on MRI.

HOW TO DIAGNOSE THE DIFFERENT TYPES OF ANORECTAL MALFORMATION

Careful physical examination and inspection of the perineum of the neonate should lead to the initial diagnosis of the ARM. However, more subtle or rare malformation types (rectoperineal fistula, anal stenosis, rectal atresia) may be missed initially, as passage of meconium does not necessarily exclude abnormal anatomy. In many neonates with an ARM, the clinical examination will be sufficient to determine the correct diagnosis. Those patients with more complex malformations will need additional studies and imaging.

The two key determinants of whether a neonate has an ARM are as follows:

1. an inadequately sized anal opening

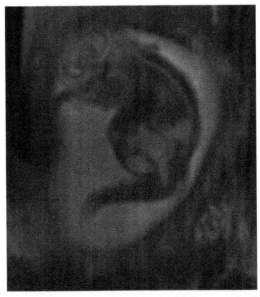

Fig. 1. Antenatal MRI. Antenatal MRI in 20-week-old fetus with cloacal anomaly and hydrocolpos.

2. an anal opening that is atypically located and, thus, not completely within the sphincter complex

A typical term neonate should be able to have a size 12 Hegar dilator placed into the anus without difficulty. Initial assessment of the sphincter complex may be performed at the bedside, but definitive assessment requires an examination under anesthesia and muscle stimulation. It is important to note that the length of the perineal body (the so-called anteriorly displaced anus) is not a determining factor for ARM. If the anal opening fulfills the size and sphincter requirements, then the child does not have an ARM.

A method of accurate physical examination of the neonate with a suspected ARM includes having the clinician:

1. Place neonate in a comfortable supine position with legs pulled up to the abdomen
2. Inspect the shape and contour of the buttocks' gluteal groove (ie, is there a "flat bottom"?)
3. Identify the presumed muscle complex, typically as an area with pigmented or pinkish color
4. In males, look for a fistula, meconium or mucous beads, or a "bucket handle"
5. In females, lift the labia up and out, and flatten the perineal to body to inspect and determine the presence or absence of the three perineal openings (urethra, vagina, and anus/fistula)
6. Gently lift the labia toward you in cases where you cannot identify the three openings to obtain a better view of the tibule. Spreading carefully with two cotton-tip applicators may help in identifying the presence of a separate urethra and vagina
7. Palpate for the tip of the coccyx to identify a possible sacral anomaly

MALFORMATIONS IN MALES
Perineal Fistula

In male patients with a fistulous tract to the perineum, the opening is placed anterior to the actual center of the normal anal dimple (**Fig. 2**). In some neonates, there may be meconium (black and/or white) or mucous beads on the perineum, or these may be deposited up to the midline raphe of the scrotum. The fistulous tract starts anterior to the correct location of the anus and, importantly, there is no communication with the urinary tract. The "bucket-handle" deformity occurs in the setting of a perineal

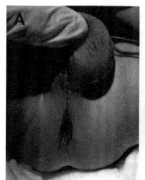 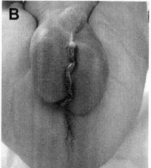 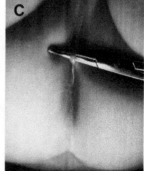

Fig. 2. Perineal fistula—male. (*A*) Perineal fistula with meconium indicating the orifice 24 h after birth. (*B*) Perineal fistula with mucus beads along the midline raphe of the scrotum. (*C*) "Bucket handle" deformity.

fistula. In many of these males, the fistulous opening lies just beneath the exuberant skin of the "bucket handle" and may be shown with a lacrimal probe.

In those neonates where a clearly visible fistula (or mucous beads or meconium) is not initially shown, it is important to wait at least 24 h after birth and repeat the clinical examination. This delay may allow the significant intraluminal pressure that is required for the meconium to be forced through the fistula to develop. If there is no obvious perineal fistula during that time period, the neonate may require the formation of a colostomy.

No Perineal Fistula

In those male patients with no fistulous opening on the perineum, there are several different possibilities (**Fig. 3**). The two most likely malformation types in this clinical setting are a rectobulbar fistula and a rectoprostatic fistula. Indeed, these are the most common ARM types seen in males.

Alternative diagnoses include rectobladder neck fistula (rare) and ARM without fistula (almost exclusively associated with trisomy 21; see below). Only an ARM without fistula may be excluded when meconium is passed via the urethra. Otherwise, it is not possible to differentiate between the three remaining malformation types without further radiological assessment. These patients require the formation of a colostomy to divert the stool, for access to the distal colostogram study, and to protect the ultimate anorectal repair.

MALFORMATIONS IN FEMALES
Perineal Fistula

One of the two most common types of malformation in female patients, the perineal fistula is characterized by a fistulous opening that is separated from the vagina and the urethra by a very short perineal body (**Fig. 4**). In some cases, even though the perineal body is short, the anus may still lie within the muscular complex. In these cases, the caliber of the anal opening must be determined. If a true perineal fistula is present, the opening is narrow and requires intervention. It is important to spread the perineum to correctly identify the anatomy. In unclear cases, the patient may need an examination under anesthesia and electric stimulation to rule out a perineal fistula, by confirming regular anatomy and muscular contractions within a centered anal opening.

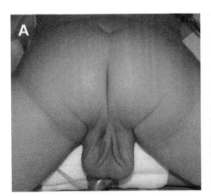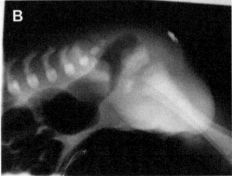

Fig. 3. No perineal fistula in male. (*A*) Perineum of male (in prone position), with no perineal fistula. (*B*) Lateral radiograph (in prone position) of the same patient showing a dysplastic sacrum. The patient was subsequently found to have a rectoprostatic fistula.

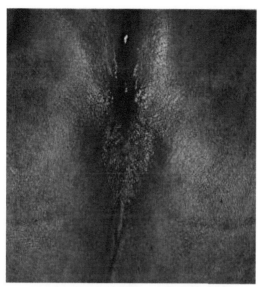

Fig. 4. Perineal fistula—female. Perineal fistula in a female patient. The fistula is located posterior to the fourchette. The muscle complex is most likely located in the pinkish area posterior to the fistula.

Rectovestibular Fistula

The other most common type of malformation in female patients is the rectovestibular fistula (**Fig. 5**). In this setting, the fistula appears directly posterior to the vagina, within the confines of the tibule, with three openings (urethra, vagina, fistula) seen on clinical examination. It may help to lift the labia on both sides to enhance the view of the posterior aspect of the tibule to visualize the fistulous opening. When examining a patient with a rectovestibular fistula, the presence and patency of the vagina needs to be considered, as up to 5% of affected females have an associated vaginal septum. In rare circumstances, there may even be agenesis of the vagina.

Cloacal Anomaly

The presence of a single opening on the perineum in a female neonate establishes the diagnosis of a cloacal anomaly, one of the most complex of all congenital malformations diagnosed in children (**Fig. 6**). It is impossible to determine the length of the common channel, the associated genitourinary anomalies, or the location of the rectal fistulous opening, without further imaging and intraoperative assessments. These patients require the formation of a colostomy.

Anteriorly Displaced Anus

This common congenital abnormality of the anorectal region leads to a variety of presumptive diagnoses, including perineal fistula (**Fig. 7**). The diagnosis should be able to made easily, with simple physical examination and assessment of the perianal and anorectal region. The female has a normal urethra and vagina, and an anal opening that appears slightly anterior. If the anal opening is of normal caliber (Hegar 11 or 12 in a neonate), lies within the sphincter, is supple (not fistulous tissue), even if a small perineal body is present then this is a normal variant and no operative intervention is required. It is important to recognize that females with an anteriorly displaced anus

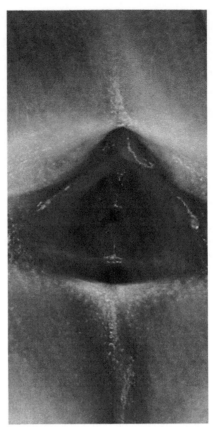

Fig. 5. Rectovestibular fistula. The fistula may be identified directly posterior to the introitus with mild distraction of the labia.

may show an increased frequency of constipation symptoms throughout their childhood.

Perineal Groove

Another common referral for assessment of the perineum in females is a perineal groove (**Fig. 8**). In this condition, there is a mucosa-lined tract of variable length that passes along the perineal body from the anus toward the posterior fourchette. These females have an anus that is normal and require no operative intervention.

Rectovaginal Fistula

In this malformation, there is no visible anus and there are two perineal openings, a normal urethra and the introitus, with the fistula visible deep in the back wall of the posterior aspect of the vagina above the hymen (**Fig. 9**). The urethra and vagina are identified separately, but the fistulous opening may be difficult to show on clinical examination alone. The most likely clinical presentation for affected females is of meconium discharging from the vagina. Most of the patients initially diagnosed with a rectovaginal fistula are likely to actually have a misdiagnosed rectovestibular fistula. These patients require the formation of a colostomy.

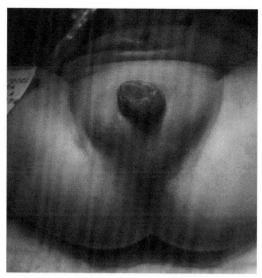

Fig. 6. Cloaca. A single perineal opening may be identified upon clinical examination.

H-type Anovestibular Fistula

This very rare malformation may be difficult to diagnose, and typically presents outside the neonatal period with the passage of stool from the vagina and tibule (**Fig. 10**). The female has a normal appearing perineum and anus, with the fistulous openings located just distal to the hymen and at the level of the dentate line.[2]

MALFORMATIONS IN MALES AND FEMALES
Anorectal Malformation Without Fistula

This malformation occurs in both males and females, and almost exclusively in children with trisomy 21. The perineal examination reveals a normal urethra, a normal introitus in a female, and no anal opening. There is no passage of meconium onto the perineum due to the lack of an associated rectourinary fistula. These patients require the formation of a colostomy within 24–36 h of birth, as they are at an increased risk of colonic perforation due to the lack of a decompressing fistula.[3]

Anal Stenosis/Rectal Atresia

These are both rare malformations, which affect males and females (**Fig. 11**).[4] The patients are born with a normal anal canal (which is sometimes skin-lined, also known as a funnel anus). However, there is a stricture or complete atresia located a few centimeters proximal to the dentate line, which typically leads to a delay in diagnosis. The strong association of these types of malformations, particularly that of anal stenosis, with a sacral anomaly, mandates accurate assessment. The diagnosis of Currarino triad (ARM, presacral mass, abnormal sacrum) must be considered and excluded.[5] Patients with anal stenosis will not necessarily require colostomy formation. However, patients with rectal atresia will require colostomy formation within 24–36 h of life. For the definitive operative repair of rectal atresia, a modified posterior sagittal anorectoplasty (PSARP) technique may be used, which allows the sparing of the anterior dentate line.[6]

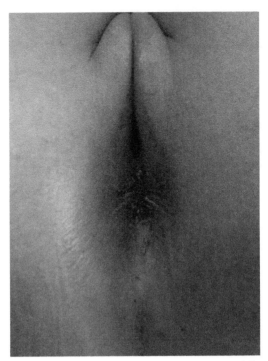

Fig. 7. Anteriorly displaced anus. The opening on the perineum, while anterior in its position, is surrounded by the sphincter mechanism and is able to be calibrated to the appropriate size for the patient's age.

THE ROLE OF INVESTIGATIONS IN THE ASSESSMENT OF ASSOCIATED ANOMALIES

Associated anomalies are shown in most of the neonates born with an ARM. In general, the more severe the type of ARM that is diagnosed, the more likely it is that there will be associated anomalies. Genitourinary anomalies are the most common. Neonates may also have musculoskeletal, cardiovascular, and gastrointestinal anomalies.[6] All neonates must be assessed for the VACTERL (Vertebral, Anal, Cardiac, Tracheo-Esophageal, Renal, and Limb) associations.[7] Despite their prevalence, these anomalies are often under-intigated, particularly in those patients with seemingly less complex malformations.[8]

As stated above, the likelihood of an associated anomaly is influenced by the complexity of the ARM. For example, in males with the rare malformation type of rectobladder neck fistula, the incidence of an associated genitourinary anomaly is significantly higher than in males with a rectobulbar fistula. All patients must undergo an abdominal and renal ultrasound to exclude the presence of hydronephrosis (most likely due to icoureteric reflux), as well as other anomalies (eg, duplex system, renal agenesis, multi-cystic dysplastic kidney) or hydrocolpos in female patients with a cloacal anomaly.

In addition, all neonates should have a focused ultrasound of the spine, as this will aid in the identification of abnormalities in sacral segments and the presence or absence of a tethered spinal cord. The ability of the ultrasound to diagnose occult spinal dysraphism is, however, less certain. It is ideal to perform the ultrasound within the first 1-2 weeks of life; however, the investigation may be useful up to 3 months of life

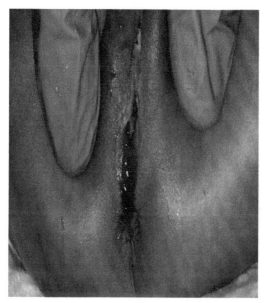

Fig. 8. Perineal groove. The mucosa-lined tract is visible passing from the anus to the posterior fourchette.

before the sacrum has ossified. In those patients in whom significant spinal anomalies are detected on ultrasound, it is likely that they will require further imaging with a spinal MRI. This may be performed in the neonatal period, using a "feed and wrap"

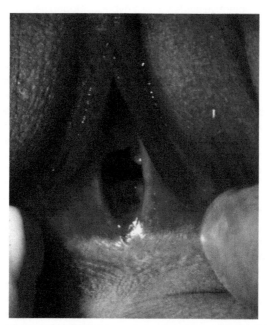

Fig. 9. Rectovaginal fistula. This patient has a normal urethra, with the fistula visible deep in the back wall of the posterior aspect of the vagina, above the hymen.

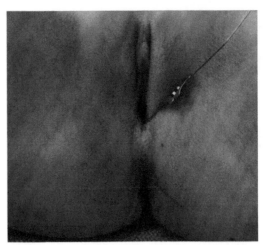

Fig. 10. Anovestibular fistula. This patient has a normally positioned anus, with the fistulous connection lying between the tibule and the anus.

approach, hence avoiding the need for a general anesthetic. However, the investigation is rarely required in the neonatal period, and the quality of spinal imaging impro when the child is older, between 6 and 12 months. The indications for assessment and intervention should be discussed with a pediatric neurosurgeon.

Further spinal imaging, beyond the neonatal period, may include a spinal radiograph (both anteroposterior and lateral) to identify the presence or absence of hemivertebrae and sacral segments. The relevance of these findings is that they may have negative prognostic implications for both fecal and urinary control. A sacral ratio may be calculated which, if low, is objective evidence of a hypodeveloped sacrum, which correlates with poor development of the perineal ner and muscles.

The final component of the VACTERL screen is the echocardiogram. Depending upon the antenatal imaging that was performed, the echocardiogram may need to be completed before any operative intervention to exclude cardiac lesions, including tetralogy of Fallot and a significant ventricular septal defect. This part of the screening for associated anomalies must not be missed in patients with an ARM.[8]

A small proportion of patients with an ARM will be diagnosed outside the neonatal period. This most typically occurs in girls with a perineal fistula or an H-type fistula, and occasionally in boys with a perineal fistula, or those with anal stenosis. In this setting, it remains important to exclude associated anomalies, so consultation with a pediatric nephrologist, cardiologist, and neurosurgeon is recommended.

A Structured Approach to the Initial Operative Management

Following a focused clinical examination of the neonate, and their perineal region, the decision must be made as to whether the neonate requires the formation of a colostomy. The colostomy is ideally formed at the junction of the descending and sigmoid colon (**Fig. 12**). By placing the colostomy at this more proximal site the surgeon may ensure that the distal colonic segment will be sufficient in length to facilitate a tension-free anorectoplasty. In addition, a colostomy that is formed at the proximal sigmoid colon junction will be less likely to prolapse because the colon is tethered by the lateral attachments. Narrowing of the opening of the mucous fistula should reduce the risk of prolapse of the more redundant and dilated distal colonic segment. Both a divided

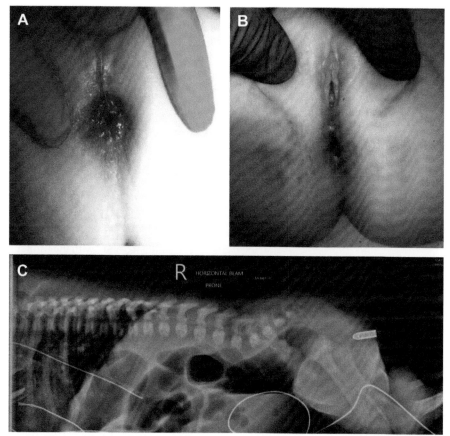

Fig. 11. Anal stenosis and rectal atresia. (*A*) Anal stenosis in a male. (*B*) Anal stenosis in a female. (*C*) Rectal atresia, shown by rectal thermometer probe in a patent anus, with distension of rectum.

stoma and a loop stoma are good choices.[9] In addition, a laparoscopic approach provides excellent visualization.

The formation of a transverse colostomy is not recommended, for serveral important reasons. First, it makes it very difficult to clear inspissated meconium from the distal colonic segment. Second, it makes performing an adequate distal colostogram very challenging as obtaining sufficient pressure is difficult. Finally, the presence of a fistula to the urinary tract may result in the resorption of urine, which predisposes to acidosis.

However, not all neonates born with an ARM will require immediate operative intervention.[10] Colostomy formation may be deferred in the following situations, after waiting 24 h:

1. Perineal fistula in a male or female: if the neonate is passing meconium without difficulty, and/or the fistula is able to be dilated easily, then the anoplasty may be deferred. It is recommended that the anoplasty be performed within the first three months of life, with or without a covering colostomy depending upon the experience of the surgeon and the local circumstances. Delaying the anoplasty may be indicated in those neonates who are initially unstable with associated anomalies (particularly cardiac), and/or premature.

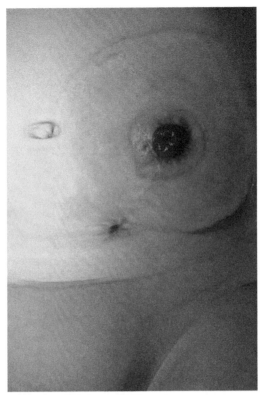

Fig. 12. Colostomy formation. Divided colostomy, with the proximal limb positioned laterally and the mucous fistula positioned medially.

2. Rectovestibular fistula: if the neonate is passing meconium without difficulty, and/ or the fistula is able to be dilated easily, then the anorectoplasty may be deferred. Again, it is recommended that the anoplasty be performed within the first three months of life, with or without a covering colostomy depending upon the experience of the surgeon and the local circumstances.

3. Anal stenosis: if the stenosis is easily dilated, then an operative intervention may be deferred. Rarely, the stenosis may be amenable to dilatations only and no further intervention is required. However, if the stenosis is refractory to dilations, then repair is indicated. It is important that a presacral mass is definitively excluded in all of these patients.

The Need for Additional Interventions in the Neonate with an Anorectal Malformation

There are several clinical situations in which additional operative interventions may be required during the same anesthetic for the colostomy formation. In females with a cloacal anomaly it may be necessary, in those in whom catheterization via the perineum has been unsuccessful, to perform a vaginostomy (tube or cutaneous) to relieve urinary obstruction.[11] Formation of a icostomy is rarely required to relieve urinary obstruction, but may be needed in those patients with significant bilateral icoureteric reflux or if the common channel is atretic. The ideal time to perform a cystoscopy to assess the common channel and urethral lengths is after a few months of life. There is superior visualization when the baby is older.

A significant proportion of neonates with an ARM will have at least one associated anomaly. For some of these neonates, the associated anomalies may represent a major comorbidity that will influence their immediate clinical care. Esophageal atresia (EA), which occurs in 5-9% of neonates with an ARM, has significant implications for the immediate clinical management and timing of operative intervention.[12] (**Fig. 13**) As most EA patients will have an associated tracheoesophageal fistula (TEF), the preferential passage of air through the TEF to the gastrointestinal tract, and onto the rectum, may lead to the need for an earlier formation of colostomy.

EA is not the only gastrointestinal atresia that must be considered in a neonate with an ARM. Duodenal atresia (DA), though less frequent than EA, does impact the operative approach to the ARM, and is seen more commonly in patients with co-existing trisomy 21. Owing to the proximal obstruction in DA, enteric content flow has been significantly minimized during the fetal period. This often leads to a reduction of meconium present in the rectum and a distal colon that is typically less distended. Although this may lead to an easier formation of a colostomy, it is critical to identify the correct section of bowel and appropriately orientate the divided colostomy. An operative technique that has been previously used by the authors to help facilitate choosing the correct section of colon is to use the vision afforded by the transverse laparotomy incision for the DA repair to mark the proximal and distal sigmoid colon with sutures. This

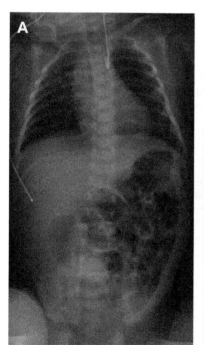
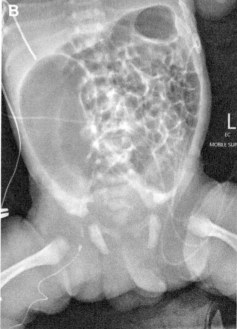

Fig. 13. Esophageal atresia, with distal tracheoesophageal fistula, and anorectal malformation. (*A*) Esophageal atresia with distal tracheoesophageal fistula, and an associated anorectal malformation. (*B*) Same patient, 12 h later, with significant distension of the sigmoid colon and rectum.

will then facilitate the delivery of the correctly oriented colonic loops through a smaller incision in the left lower quadrant.

In ARM patients with associated EA/TEF and DA, the authors recommend the "top-down" approach to operative repair. This invol division of the TEF, esophageal anastomosis, formation of a duodenoduodenostomy, and then colostomy formation. These may be all undertaken under the one anesthetic, as long as the patient remains hemodynamically stable.[13] In those patients who are unstable, it may be necessary to stage the separate procedures, with preference for early division of the TEF.

As stated previously, cardiac anomalies are relatively common in ARM patients. The cardiac lesion most commonly requiring operative intervention is a ventricular septal defect. This defect rarely impacts physiologically upon the patient undergoing the formation of a colostomy, so should not be a cause for delay in the operative course. In most patients, the echocardiogram may be delayed until after colostomy formation, unless the patient shows early signs of central cyanosis.

A very rare association with ARM is the presence of an abdominal wall defect. The omphalocele–exstrophy–imperforate anus–spinal defects (OEIS) complex, first described in 1978, includes cloacal extrophy.[14] Marked improvements in antenatal ultrasonography have led to increased fetal diagnosis, and have shown a greater incidence of this complex than previously documented. In addition, the association between prune belly syndrome and congenital pouch colon has been described by several authors, but appears to be mostly limited to Asia.[15]

The association between colonic atresia and ARM is exceedingly rare, as documented in a very small series.[16] The key clinical findings that may aid in the diagnosis include the markedly reduced caliber of the distal colon and rectum, as well as the character of its contents, namely white mucus rather than normal meconium. The relationship between colonic atresia and Hirschsprung disease must also be borne in mind, though it is a rare finding.

An even rarer situation is the neonate with both Hirschsprung disease and an ARM. There are very few published case reports, and the coexistence of trisomy 21 (and, therefore ARM without fistula) is common.[17] We recommend a formal rectal biopsy in those patients in whom a distal bowel obstruction persists following colostomy closure.

CLINICS CARE POINTS

- Antenatal diagnosis of anorectal malformations is rare. In the presence of a cystic structure in the pelvis of a female fetus, the diagnosis of a cloacal malformation must be considered.
- The key components of a diagnosis of an anorectal malformation are an inadequately sized anal opening and an anal opening that is located in the incorrect position.

ACKNOWLEDGEMENT

Professor Sebastian King's position as an Academic Paediatric Surgeon is generously supported by The Royal Children's Hospital Foundation and the Australian Government.

DISCLOSURE

The authors have no commercial or financial conflicts of interest or any funding sources to disclose.

REFERENCES

1. Calvo-Garcia M, Kline-Fath B, Levitt MA, et al. Fetal MRI clues to diagnose cloacal malformations. Pediatr Radiol 2011;41:1117.
2. Lawal T, Chatoorgoon K, Bischoff A, et al. Management of H-type rectovestibular and rectovaginal fistulas. J Pediatr Surg 2011;46(6):1226–30.
3. King SK, Cooksey R, Atkinson J, et al. Colonic performation in a neonate with an anorectal malformation. ANZ J Surg 2016;86(5):418–9.
4. Hamrick M, Eradi B, Bischoff A, et al. Rectal atresia and stenosis: unique anorectal malformations. J Pediatr Surg 2012;47(6):1280–4.
5. AbouZeid A, Mohannad S, Abolfotoh M, et al. The Currarino triad: what pediatric surgeons need to know. J Pediatr Surg 2017;52(8):1260–8.
6. Levitt MA, Pena A. Anorectal malformations. Orphanet J Rare Dis 2007;2:33.
7. Rittler M, Paz JE, Castilla EE. VACTERL association, epidemiologic definition and delineation. Am J Med Genet 1996;63:529–36.
8. Kruger P, Teague WJ, Khanal R, et al. Screening for associated anomalies in anorectal malformations: the need for a standardized approach. ANZ J Surg 2019;89:1250–2.
9. Youssef F, Arbash G, Puligandla PS, et al. Loop versus divided colostomy for the management of anorectal malformations: a systematic review and meta-analysis. J Pediatr Surg 2017;52(5):783–90.
10. van der Steeg HJ, Schmiedeke E, Bagolan P, et al. European consensus meeting of ARM-Net members concerning diagnosis and early management of newborns with anorectal malformations. Tech Coloproctol 2015;19(3):181–5.
11. Levitt MA, Bischoff A, Pena A. Pitfalls and challenges of cloaca repair: how to reduce the need for reoperations. J Pediatr Surg 2011;46(6):1250–5.
12. Lautz TB, Mandelia A, Radhakrishnan J. VACTERL associations in children undergoing surgery for esophageal atresia and anorectal malformations: implications for pediatric surgeons. J Pediatr Surg 2015;50:1245–50.
13. Ceccanti S, Midrio P, Messina M, et al. The date association: a separate entity or a further extension of the VACTERL association? J Surg Res 2019;241:128–34.
14. Carey JC, Greenbaum B, Hall BD. The OEIS complex (omphalocele, exstrophy, imperforate anus, spinal defects). Birth Defects Orig Artic Ser 1978;14:253–63.
15. Bangroo AK, Tiwari S, Khetri R, et al. Congenital pouch colon with prune belly syndrome and megalouretha. Pediatr Surg Int 2005;21:474–7.
16. Goodwin S, Schlatter M, Connors R. Imperforate anus and colon atresia in a newborn. J Pediatr Surg 2006;41:583–5.
17. Raboei EH. Patients with anorectal malformation and Hirschsprung's disease. Eurj Pediatr Surg 2009;19:1–3.

Advances in the Treatment of Neonatal Biliary Disease

Sarah Mohamedaly, MD, MPH[a], Amar Nijagal, MD[a,b,c],*

KEYWORDS

- Neonatal biliary disease • Biliary atresia • Choledochal cyst

KEY POINTS

- Advances in management of neonatal biliary disease.
- Surgical management of biliary atresia.
- Surgical management of choledochal cyst.

Abbreviations	
BA	Biliary Atresia
CC	Choledochal Cyst
ERCP	Endoscopic Retrograde Cholangiopancreatography
GCSF	Granulocyte Colony-Stimulating Factor
HD	Hepaticoduodenostomy
HSC	Hematopoeitic Stem Cell
IBAT	Ileal Bile Acid Transporter
KPE	Kasai Portoenterostomy
MMP-7	Matrix Metalloproteinase-7
PTX	Pentoxifylline
RYHJ	Roux-en-Y hepaticojejunostomy
SDVS	SpyGlass Direct Visualization System

INTRODUCTION

Neonatal biliary diseases are rare in occurrence. However, when present, they can be associated with severe morbidities including cholangitis, pancreatitis, and liver cirrhosis. In this article, we review the two most common surgical neonatal biliary diseases: biliary atresia (BA) and choledochal cyst (CC). In addition to discussing current standard of care for surgical treatment, this review will emphasize advances in the field

[a] Division of Pediatric Surgery, Department of Surgery, University of California, San Francisco, 513 Parnassus Avenue, HSW 1652, Campus Box 0570, San Francisco, CA 94143-0570, USA; [b] The Liver Center, University of California, San Francisco, CA, USA; [c] The Pediatric Liver Center at UCSF Benioff Childrens' Hospitals, San Francisco, CA, USA
* Corresponding author. Division of Pediatric Surgery, University of California, San Francisco, 513 Parnassus Avenue, HSW 1652, Campus Box 0570, San Francisco, CA 94143-0570.
E-mail address: Amar.Nijagal@ucsf.edu

Clin Perinatol 49 (2022) 981–993
https://doi.org/10.1016/j.clp.2022.07.006
0095-5108/22/© 2022 Elsevier Inc. All rights reserved.
perinatology.theclinics.com

for each condition and will cover promising avenues of inquiry that may improve our understanding of disease pathogenesis and therapy.

BILIARY ATRESIA

BA is a progressive inflammatory liver disease that results in rapid obliteration of the bile ducts, leading to liver failure and cirrhosis. Accounting for approximately 75% of liver transplants in children aged younger than 2 years, BA is the most common indication for pediatric liver transplant.[1,2] The cause of BA is not fully understood; however, it is thought to be attributed to multiple factors including genetic predisposition, immune dysregulation, and toxic and infectious causes.[2] Timing of such injury is also unclear, although our current understanding supports the idea that an insult during fetal development triggers an inflammatory cascade in the liver that persists postnatally.[3]

Given the multifactorial etiology and demographic differences between patients, clinical characterization of BA has been variable. However, there are 3 generally accepted broad categories of BA: (1) BA without other anomalies or malformations, (2) BA in association with laterality malformation, also known as BA splenic malformation (BASM), and (3) BA in association with other congenital malformations.[4] Additional subgroups include cystic BA, cytomegalovirus (CMV)-associated BA, and cardiac-associated BA.[5–8]

Clinical diagnosis of BA remains difficult because other neonatal cholestatic conditions such as Alagille Syndrome and progressive familial intrahepatic cholestasis can have similar presentations. Laboratory testing with liver enzymes is also nonspecific, thereby necessitating liver biopsy to aid in the diagnosis of BA. Recently, however, matrix metalloproteinase-7 (MMP-7) has been described as a less invasive diagnostic biomarker in BA that can potentially alleviate the need for an invasive diagnostic procedure (biopsy or cholangiogram).[9] Although the role by which MMP-7 alters the pathogenesis of BA is not fully understood, several studies have shown high MMP-7 levels in livers of BA patients, particularly those with advanced fibrosis.[10–12] Further research is needed, however, in order to investigate the relationship between BA and MMP-7 and support its use as a diagnostic and prognostic biomarker.

Kasai Portoenterostomy

Although there have been major advancements in understanding the variables that contribute to BA, improvement in long-term outcomes and cessation of disease progression have been largely unsuccessful. Current standard of care includes sequential surgical management with initial Kasai portoenterostomy (KPE) followed by liver transplantation for those patients who progress to end-stage liver disease.[13] The goal of KPE is to restore bile flow into the small intestine by removing the obliterated extrahepatic biliary tree and diverting bile flow using a Roux-en-Y hepaticojejunostomy (RYHJ). Although the KPE can temporarily relieve the biliary obstruction, most patients will continue to experience progressive liver disease with at least 50% of patients requiring liver transplantation by 2 years of age.[14]

Early restoration of bile flow is associated with improved outcomes after KPE. In patients who undergo KPE within the first 30 days of life, there is a 50% chance of native liver survival at 4 years of age and 40% at 15 years.[13–15] However, among those who undergo KPE between 31 to 90 days of life, the chance of native liver survival at 4 years of age diminishes to 36%.[13] In addition to the age at diagnosis, other factors contribute to the efficacy of KPE. In particular, the presence of liver fibrosis portends poor prognosis.[14] These studies indicate the importance of making an expeditious diagnosis of BA before potentially irreversible sequelae of liver inflammation (eg, fibrosis) set in.

Surgical Approach

Open KPE is considered the standard of care at most centers who treat patients with BA. Early experience with laparoscopic KPE has been associated with worse clearance of jaundice and shorter native liver survival at 2-year and 5-year follow-ups compared with open KPE.[16–19] Additionally, the need for reoperation and revision after laparoscopic KPE is significantly higher than with open surgery.[16,20] However, several recent studies have examined outcomes between open and laparoscopic KPE demonstrating similar rates of postoperative cholangitis and native liver survival between the two groups.[21,22] Furthermore, a comparative study of both approaches in children who subsequently underwent liver transplantation demonstrated that laparoscopic KPE is associated with a lower risk of reoperation and portal vein complications at the time of transplant.[23]

This shift in outcomes is most likely associated with the learning curve that is seen with the introduction of any new laparoscopic surgical technique.[24,25] Because case volume has increased, pediatric surgeons have become more experienced in laparoscopic KPEs and thus surgical outcomes improved.[16,24] Despite the encouraging outcomes achieved with laparoscopic KPE, an open approach should be used except in select centers who have extensive experience in minimally invasive approaches for BA.

Role of Liver Transplantation

The use of sequential surgical treatment is currently the standard of care for patients with BA. KPE performed during infancy followed by selective liver transplantation as clinically indicated for children with progressive hepatic deterioration is used to treat patients with BA.[13,26] Indication for liver transplant in patients after KPE include liver cirrhosis, liver failure, gastrointestinal bleeding secondary to portal hypertension, growth retardation, pruritis, progressive intrapulmonary shunting, hepatopulmonary syndrome, and repeated cholangitis.[26,27] Current recommendations support prompt liver transplant evaluation if the total bilirubin is greater than 6 mg/dL 3 months after KPE or if total bilirubin persistently remains between 2 and 6 mg/dL.[27] Primary liver transplantation should be considered in patients with late presentation (beyond 100 days) and overt cirrhosis.[27,28]

Current Adjuvant Therapies

The use of adjuvant therapies to improve bile drainage after KPE has been described; however, evidence to support these therapies is largely inconclusive. Post-KPE regimens to promote bile flow, such as ursodeoxycholic acid, are based on analogous adult conditions such as sclerosing cholangitis and primary biliary cirrhosis.[29] However, there are no current recommendations that support bile acid analogs in children, despite its common use after KPE.[27] Corticosteroids have also been proposed to improve post-KPE biliary drainage without success. A recent trial investigating the use of high-dose corticosteroid therapy within 72 hours after KPE demonstrated no benefit in bile drainage at 6 months after KPE and no improvement in native liver survival at 2 years of age.[14] Other therapies such as intravenous immunoglobulin (IVIG) have also been shown to be equivocal in a phase I/IIa trial following KPE.[30,31] Although IVIG infusions in infants with BA after KPE were feasible and safe, there was no evidence of lower bilirubin levels or improved 1 year survival with the native liver.[31]

High-quality evidence to support the use of prophylactic antibiotics to reduce recurrent rates of cholangitis and improve survival is also lacking. A recent systematic review supports the use of prophylactic antibiotics in BA patients after KPE although these conclusions were based on one randomized control trial.[32,33] The trial investigated the efficacy of trimethoprim–sulfamethoxazole or oral neomycin in BA patients who had one episode of cholangitis.[32] Rates of recurrent cholangitis were significantly lower in both antibiotic groups and thus support the use of prophylactic antibiotics in BA patients after KPE.[32]

Aggressive nutritional support after KPE is recommended to ensure adequate growth and prevent fat-soluble vitamin deficiency.[27,34] Malnutrition after KPE is associated with poor neurologic development and worse transplant outcomes. Thus, close surveillance of the child's nutritional status and a tiered approach for interventions is highly recommended.[27,35] Infants with BA may require up to 150% of the recommended calories/energy for age to maintain or restore growth.[34] In order to meet such requirements, oral intake with a high content of medium chain triglycerides to maximize intestinal lipid absorption is recommended.[34] Protein intake should range from 3 to 4 g/kg/d and carbohydrates should make up 40% to 60% of the total energy intake.[34] If oral intake is insufficient to meet these nutritional requirements, supplemental nasogastric (NG) feeds should be initiated. Due to the potential complications associated with gastric varices in the setting of portal hypertension, gastrotomy tubes are not recommended for enteral feeds.[34] In children with enteral feeding intolerance or persistent growth retardation despite maximum NG feeds, parenteral nutrition is recommended.[34]

Prognosis

Long-term prognosis for BA remains variable; however, 90% of patients who undergo early KPE and, if indicated, liver transplantation after 2 years of age, survive into adulthood.[36,37] Variability in prognosis is thought to be associated with the various subtypes of BA, with BASM and CMV-associated BA associated with poorer overall outcomes and higher mortality.[5] Patients with cystic BA tend to have more favorable outcomes and better long-term survival.[5]

Future Directions

Understanding the underlying cause and pathogenesis of BA is essential for the development of future therapeutic agents. Several studies highlight the possible autoimmune contributions to the pathogenesis of BA.[38–41] A recent study, in particular, highlighted the tolerance defects in hepatic B cells that promote IgG-autoantibody accumulation in BA.[42] In a well-established murine model of BA, depleting B cells or blocking antigen presentation alleviated liver damage.[42] Furthermore, in a small pilot study (n = 4), anti-CD20 treatment with rituximab in infants with BA resulted in B cell depletion and halted the accumulation of IgG-autoantibodies.[42] Further long-term studies are needed to assess whether this promising finding is associated with halting disease progression in the clinical setting.

Several other groups have studied the contribution of immune cells to disease pathogenesis.[43–45] Studies in our laboratory support the contribution of the innate immune system to the pathogenesis of BA. We previously demonstrated that the physiologic abundance of Ly6C^{Lo} nonclassic monocytes during perinatal life is associated with susceptibility to liver injury in an infectious model of BA.[46] Furthermore, experimental manipulation of Ly6C^{Lo} nonclassic monocytes in neonatal pups rendered animals to be resistant to liver injury.[46]

Current trials are predominately focused on investigating therapies to mitigate disease progression after KPE. A recent phase I trial examined the safety of granulocyte colony-stimulating factor (GCSF) in patients with BA, with the hypothesis that GCSF therapy attenuates biliary fibrosis and progression to cirrhosis after KPE.[47] GCSF is known to enhance hematopoietic stem cell (HSC) mobilization and engraftment in the liver with attenuated hepatic necrosis and fibrosis.[47] This phase I trial demonstrated that infants after KPE can mount an effective neutrophil and CD34+ HSC response to GCSF within a week of surgery.[47] Additionally, a 3-day dose of 10 μg/kg/d of GCSF within 3 days of surgery was shown to be well tolerated and enhanced HSC mobilization.[47] A preliminary comparison of patients who received GCSF to those who underwent KPE without receiving GCSF demonstrated reduced cholestasis at one month with a trend toward lower complications after KPE including lower rates of cholangitis at 6 months.[47] A phase II trial is currently underway to investigate GCSF response on bile flow by measuring the percentage of subjects with total bilirubin less than 2 mg/dL at 3 months after KPE (**Table 1**).[48] Primary outcomes also include GCSF response on transplant-free survival in patients who do not undergo KPE.[48]

Another phase II trial is investigating a phosphodiesterase inhibitor, pentoxifylline (PTX), in BA with the hypothesis that PTX can improve bile flow after KPE.[49] PTX has been shown to prevent liver fibrosis, improve liver regeneration, and reduce cirrhosis-related complications in adults.[49] Subjects will receive PTX orally for 90 days as an adjunct to standard therapy, and the primary outcome will measure the change in conjugated bilirubin levels after 90 days.[49] Secondary outcomes include changes in body weight, serum markers, liver imaging, and time to liver transplant in infants with BA.[49] In a similar phase II trial, N-acetylcysteine (NAC) will be investigated as a therapeutic agent to improve bile flow after KPE.[50] NAC is a precursor for glutathione, and is a choleretic molecule that creates an osmotic gradient in the bile duct lumen to allow for biliary flow.[50] Glutathione is also an antioxidant that could scavenge free radicals contributing to cirrhosis.[50] Subjects will receive intravenous NAC for 7 days after KPE with the primary outcome being normal levels of total serum bile acids within 24 weeks of surgery.[50] Markers of BA progression, such as bilirubin levels, failure-to-thrive, and cirrhosis-related complications, will also be evaluated during the first 2 years of life.[50]

Two additional studies are investigating the role of ileal bile acid transporter (IBAT) inhibitors in BA.[51,52] IBAT inhibitors decrease the reabsorption of bile acids from the terminal ileum and thus may potentially lessen or delay liver damage associated with the hepatotoxicity and cholangiopathy of bile acid accumulation.[51,52] In a phase II trial investigating maralixibat, subjects will receive maralixibat oral solution twice daily for 26 weeks after KPE with the primary outcome of mean changes to total bilirubin level from baseline to 26 weeks.[51] Additional outcomes such as time to liver transplantation or death, and the proportion of subjects with total bilirubin less than 2 mg/dL will also be measured.[51] A similar trial, currently in phase III, will investigate odevixibat, with patients receiving the medication orally once daily for 104 weeks after KPE.[52] The proportion of patients who are alive and have not undergone a liver transplantation after 104 weeks will be the primary outcome.[52]

CHOLEDOCHAL CYSTS

CCs are congenital dilations of the intrahepatic and extrahepatic biliary tree and can be associated with complications such as cholangitis, perforation, liver failure, and malignancy. CCs are more common among Asian populations with an incidence of

Table 1
Adjunct therapy for management of biliary atresia

Clinicaltrials.gov Identifier	Study Name	Status	Hypothesis/Objective
NCT04373941	GCSF Adjunct Therapy for BA	Phase I completed, phase 2 pending	Post-KPE GCSF therapy attenuates biliary fibrosis and progression to cirrhosis
NCT01774487	Pentoxifylline Therapy in BA	Phase 2	PTX can improve bile flow after KPE
NCT03499249	N-Acetylcysteine (NAC) in BA After Kasai Portoenterostomy	Phase 2	IV NAC can improve bile flow after KPE
NCT04524390	Efficacy and Safety of Maralixibat in the Treatment of Subjects With BA After HPE	Phase 2	Maralixibat can reduce reabsorption of bile acids from the terminal ileum and delay the liver damage associated with the hepatotoxicity and cholangiopathy of bile acid accumulation
NCT04336722	Efficacy and Safety of Odevixibat in Children With BA Who Have Undergone a Kasai HPE	Phase 3	Investigate the efficacy and safety of Odevixibat compared with placebo in children with BA who have undergone a KPE

1 in 13,000 versus 1 in 100,000 in Western populations.[53] Although the cause of CCs is not fully understood, the predominant theory is that an anomalous pancreaticobiliary union results in increased reflux of pancreatic enzymes with ductal wall injury and subsequent ductal dilation.[54,55]

The most commonly used classification system is the updated Todani classification, which describes five different types of CC.[54,56,57] **(Table 2)**

Management

The approach to management of CCs largely depends on the cyst type and potential for associated malignancy. Gallbladder carcinoma or cholangiocarcinoma occurs in 6% to 30% in adults with CCs, with a life-long malignancy risk of up to 4% even after excision.[54] Patients with type I, II, or IV usually undergo surgical resection of the cysts due to a high risk of malignancy.[53,54] Type III cysts are typically not associated with neoplasia and can be managed with sphincterotomy or endoscopic resection if patients are symptomatic.[58] Type V cysts are typically difficult to treat due to their intrahepatic nature and can ultimately require liver transplantation.[53,54] In the acute setting, patients with ascending cholangitis require antibiotics and drainage regardless of the cyst type with definitive surgical management of the cyst after resolution of the infection if indicated.

Table 2
Types and incidence of choledochal cysts

Type I	80%–90%	Cystic, saccular, or fusiform dilation of the common bile duct (CBD)
Type II	2%	True diverticulum of the extrahepatic bile ducts
Type III	4%–5%	Choledochocele—cystic dilation of the intraduodenal portion of the CBD
Type IV	10%–15%	Both intrahepatic and extrahepatic cysts or multiple extrahepatic cysts
Type V	<1%	Intrahepatic cysts only, without extrahepatic disease

Surgical Approach

Due to high risk of recurrence and malignant transformation associated with CCs, cystenterostomy is an inadequate surgical option for definitive management.[53,59] Currently, the standard of care consists of cyst excision and biliary-enteric reconstruction with either a RYHJ or hepaticoduodenostomy (HD).[53,59,60] RYHJ reconstruction is the more commonly used approach and is favored due to the higher rates of bile reflux and cholangitis associated with HD.[53,59,61,62] However, in recent years, HD has been gaining popularity due to the simplicity of a single anastomosis in the setting of laparoscopic cyst excision.[61,63] Additionally, HD allows for easier postoperative endoscopic access if further interventions are necessary.[61,63] Due to the lack of concrete evidence supporting either of the reconstruction options, the decision between RYHJ and HD depends on surgeon preference. Similarly, although there is sufficient evidence supporting minimally invasive cyst excision, the decision for open versus laparoscopic surgery is based on surgeon experience and comfort with laparoscopic biliary surgery. Benefits of laparoscopic cyst excision include lower rates of intraoperative blood transfusions, shorter length of stay, and lower adhesive intestinal obstruction.[64–66]

Early surgical excision is recommended and is also associated with lower morbidity compared with late diagnosis and treatment.[59] For these reasons, prenatal diagnosis is imperative and has been shown to result in earlier definitive management.[67,68] A study comparing outcomes between patients diagnosed prenatally and postnatally found that prenatal diagnosis was associated with surgical cyst excision at 4.4 months versus 5.7 years in the postnatally diagnosed group.[68] Late diagnosis is associated with more complications such as pancreatitis, cholangitis, and liver fibrosis.[68,69]

Overall, complete cyst excision is associated with excellent prognosis, with the exception of a higher risk of biliary and pancreatic cancer compared with the general population.[53,70,71] The risk for malignancy after complete excision can be up to 4% and 18% in patients treated with cyst enterostomy.[53,71] There are no clear guidelines on surveillance strategies after surgical resection of CC; however, serial CA19-9, CEA, and imaging of the biliary tree are widely used. Current understanding of which factors are associated with malignant transformation is limited; however, recent studies have implicated de novo somatic mutations in TP53 and RBM10, and amplification of KRAS as potential contributors.[60,72]

Future Directions

Although management of CC has been largely unchanged in recent years, emerging endoscopic technology shows promise for advances in diagnostics and surveillance. The use of endoscopic retrograde cholangiopancreatography (ERCP) has transformed the field with improved diagnostics and less invasive therapeutic options for biliary drainage, however, it remains limited by several factors.[73] First, ERCP only offers indirect fluoroscopic visualization of the biliary tree, which limits the endoscopists' assessment of abnormal tissue.[73,74] Additionally, ERCP techniques such as brush cytology and biopsy have low sensitivity for the detection of malignant lesions.[74,75] In the pediatric population, ERCP is also exceptionally challenging due to the small size of the common bile duct.[76] Recent advances in peroral cholangioscopy, however, address some of these limitations. Although predominately described in adult patients, the use of the SpyGlass Direct Visualization System (SDVS) has offered multiple diagnostic and therapeutic benefits such as visually guided biopsies of abnormal tissue, improved evaluation of indeterminate strictures, visually guided ablation of ductal tumors and lithotripsy.[74,77,78] SVDS has also been associated with a 77% to 82% accuracy in the diagnosis of malignancy when ERCP-guided brush biopsies of biliary strictures were inconclusive.[76,79,80] Although limited in quantity, recent reports in pediatric patients demonstrate similar favorable benefits and promising potentials.[76,81] Additional investigation is warranted to compare complication rates of SVDS to ERCP in the pediatric population.

SUMMARY

The understanding of neonatal biliary diseases such as BA and choledochal cysts has improved tremendously during the past decade and has offered a multitude of advancements in diagnosis and management. However, some areas of controversy and research dilemmas persist to date. Further understanding of the pathophysiology of such diseases can highlight potential areas of continued investigation to improve treatment.

FUNDING

Funding was provided by the NIH FAVOR T32 training grant (5T32AI125222-05, SM), American Pediatric Surgical Association Foundation Jay Grosfeld, MD Scholar Award (AN), an American College of Surgeons Faculty Research Fellowship (AN), a UCSF Liver Center Pilot Award (NIH P30 DK026743, AN), the UCSF Parnassus Flow Cytometry Core (DRC Center Grant NIH P30 DK063720), and core resources of the UCSF Liver Center (P30 DK026743).

DISCLOSURE

The authors have no disclosures to declare.

REFERENCES

1. Verkade HJ, Bezerra JA, Davenport M, et al. Biliary atresia and other cholestatic childhood diseases: advances and future challenges. J Hepatol 2016;65(3): 631–42.
2. Hartley JL, Davenport M, Kelly DA. Biliary atresia. Lancet 2009;374(9702): 1704–13.
3. Harpavat S, Garcia-Prats JA, Shneider BL. Newborn bilirubin screening for biliary atresia. Available at: https://doi-org.ucsf.idm.oclc.org/101056/NEJMc1601230. Accessed August 10, 2016.
4. Schwarz KB, Haber BH, Rosenthal P, et al. Extra-hepatic anomalies in infants with biliary atresia: results of a large prospective North American multi-center study. Hepatology 2013;58(5):1724–31.
5. Lakshminarayanan B, Davenport M. Biliary atresia: a comprehensive review. J Autoimmun 2016;73:1–9.

6. Caponcelli E, Knisely AS, Davenport M. Cystic biliary atresia: an etiologic and prognostic subgroup. J Pediatr Surg 2008;43(9):1619–24.

7. De Tommaso AM, Andrade PD, Costa SC, et al. High frequency of Human Cytomegalovirus DNA in the liver of infants with extrahepatic neonatal cholestasis. BMC Infect Dis 2005;5:108.

8. Zani A, Quaglia A, Hadzić N, et al. Cytomegalovirus-associated biliary atresia: an aetiological and prognostic subgroup. J Pediatr Surg 2015;50(10):1739–45.

9. Thomas H. MMP7 — a diagnostic biomarker for biliary atresia. Nat Rev Gastroenterol Hepatol 2018;15(2):68.

10. Huang CC, Chuang JH, Chou MH, et al. Matrilysin (MMP-7) is a major matrix metalloproteinase upregulated in biliary atresia-associated liver fibrosis. Mod Pathol 2005;18(7):941–50.

11. Lertudomphonwanit C, Mourya R, Fei L, et al. Large-scale proteomics identifies MMP-7 as a sentinel of epithelial injury and of biliary atresia. Sci Translational Med 2017;9(417):eaan8462.

12. Kerola A, Lampela H, Lohi J, et al. Increased MMP-7 expression in biliary epithelium and serum underpins native liver fibrosis after successful portoenterostomy in biliary atresia. J Pathol Clin Res 2016;2(3):187–98.

13. Schreiber RA, Barker CC, Roberts EA, et al. Biliary atresia: the Canadian experience. The J Pediatr 2007;151(6):659–65.e1.

14. Bezerra JA, Wells RG, Mack CL, et al. Biliary atresia: clinical and research challenges for the Twenty-first Century. Hepatology 2018;68(3):1163–73.

15. Serinet MO, Wildhaber BE, Broué P, et al. Impact of age at Kasai operation on its results in late childhood and Adolescence: a Rational Basis for biliary atresia Screening. Pediatrics 2009;123(5):1280–6.

16. Kiblawi R, Zoeller C, Zanini A, et al. Laparoscopic versus open pediatric surgery: three decades of comparative studies. Eur J Pediatr Surg 2022;32(01):009–25.

17. Chan KWE, Lee KH, Wong HYV, et al. Ten-year native liver survival rate after laparoscopic and open Kasai portoenterostomy for biliary atresia. J Laparoendoscopic Adv Surg Tech 2019;29(1):121–5.

18. Chan KWE, Lee KH, Tsui SYB, et al. Laparoscopic versus open Kasai portoenterostomy in infant with biliary atresia: a retrospective review on the 5-year native liver survival. Pediatr Surg Int 2012;28(11):1109–13.

19. Hussain MH, Alizai N, Patel B. Outcomes of laparoscopic Kasai portoenterostomy for biliary atresia: a systematic review. J Pediatr Surg 2017;52(2):264–7.

20. Huang SY, Yeh CM, Chen HC, et al. Reconsideration of laparoscopic Kasai operation for biliary atresia. J Laparoendoscopic Adv Surg Tech 2018;28(2):229–34.

21. Hinojosa-Gonzalez DE, Bueno LC, Roblesgil-Medrano A, et al. Laparoscopic vs open portoenterostomy in biliary atresia: a systematic review and meta-analysis. Pediatr Surg Int 2021;37(11):1477–87.

22. Shirota C, Hinoki A, Tainaka T, et al. Laparoscopic Kasai portoenterostomy can be a standard surgical procedure for treatment of biliary atresia. World J Gastrointest Surg 2022;14(1):56–63.

23. Takeda M, Sakamoto S, Uchida H, et al. Comparative study of open and laparoscopic Kasai portoenterostomy in children undergoing living donor liver transplantation for biliary atresia. Pediatr Surg Int 2021;37(12):1683–91.

24. Ji Y, Yang K, Zhang X, et al. Learning curve of laparoscopic Kasai portoenterostomy for biliary atresia: report of 100 cases. BMC Surg 2018;18(1):107.

25. van der Poel MJ, Fichtinger RS, Bemelmans M, et al. Implementation and outcome of minor and major minimally invasive liver surgery in The Netherlands. HPB 2019;21(12):1734–43.

26. Kasahara M, Umeshita K, Sakamoto S, et al. Liver transplantation for biliary atresia: a systematic review. Pediatr Surg Int 2017;33(12):1289–95.

27. Squires RH, Ng V, Romero R, et al. Evaluation of the pediatric patient for liver transplantation: 2014 practice guideline by the american association for the study of liver diseases, american society of transplantation and the north american society for pediatric gastroenterology, hepatology and nutrition. Hepatology 2014; 60(1):362–98.

28. Davenport M, Puricelli V, Farrant P, et al. The outcome of the older (≥100 days) infant with biliary atresia. J Pediatr Surg 2004;39(4):575–81.

29. Davenport M. Adjuvant therapy in biliary atresia: hopelessly optimistic or potential for change? Pediatr Surg Int 2017;33(12):1263–73.

30. Nijagal A, Perito ER. Treating biliary atresia: the challenge continues. J Pediatr Gastroenterol Nutr 2019;68(4):464–5.

31. Mack CL, Spino C, Alonso EM, et al. A phase I/IIa trial of intravenous Immunoglobulin following portoenterostomy in biliary atresia. J Pediatr Gastroenterol Nutr 2019;68(4):495–501.

32. Bu LN, Chen HL, Chang CJ, et al. Prophylactic oral antibiotics in prevention of recurrent cholangitis after the Kasai portoenterostomy. J Pediatr Surg 2003; 38(4):590–3.

33. Decharun K, Leys CM, West KW, et al. Prophylactic antibiotics for prevention of cholangitis in patients with biliary atresia status post-Kasai portoenterostomy: a systematic review. Clin Pediatr (Phila) 2016;55(1):66–72.

34. Boster JM, Feldman AG, Mack CL, et al. Malnutrition in biliary atresia: assessment, management, and outcomes. Liver Transplant 2022;28(3):483–92.

35. Barshes NR, Chang IF, Karpen SJ, et al. Impact of Pretransplant growth retardation in pediatric liver transplantation. J Pediatr Gastroenterol Nutr 2006;43(1): 89–94.

36. Chardot C, Buet C, Serinet MO, et al. Improving outcomes of biliary atresia: French national series 1986-2009. J Hepatol 2013;58(6):1209–17.

37. Wildhaber BE, Majno P, Mayr J, et al. Biliary atresia: Swiss national study, 1994-2004. J Pediatr Gastroenterol Nutr 2008;46(3):299–307.

38. Mack CL, Tucker RM, Lu BR, et al. Cellular and Humoral autoimmunity Directed at bile duct Epithelia in murine biliary atresia. Hepatology 2006;44(5):1231–9.

39. Shivakumar P, Sabla G, Mohanty S, et al. Effector role of neonatal hepatic CD8+ lymphocytes in epithelial injury and autoimmunity in experimental biliary atresia. Gastroenterology 2007;133(1):268–77.

40. LU BR, BRINDLEY SM, TUCKER RM, et al. α-Enolase autoantibodies Cross-Reactive to Viral Proteins in a Mouse model of biliary atresia. Gastroenterology 2010;139(5):1753–61.

41. Pang SY, Dai YM, Zhang RZ, et al. Autoimmune liver disease-related autoantibodies in patients with biliary atresia. World J Gastroenterol 2018;24(3):387–96.

42. Wang J, Xu Y, Chen Z, et al. Liver immune profiling reveals pathogenesis and therapeutics for biliary atresia. Cell 2020;183(7):1867–83, e26.

43. Mohanty SK, Donnelly B, Temple H, et al. A rotavirus-induced mouse model to study biliary atresia and neonatal cholestasis. In: Vinken M, editor. Experimental cholestasis research. Methods in molecular biology. New York: Springer; 2019. p. 259–71.

44. Riepenhoff-talty M, Schaekel K, Clark HF, et al. Group A Rotaviruses Produce extrahepatic biliary obstruction in orally Inoculated Newborn Mice. Pediatr Res 1993;33(4):394–9.

45. Allen SR, Jafri M, Donnelly B, et al. Effect of rotavirus Strain on the murine model of biliary atresia. J Virol 2007;81(4):1671–9.

46. Alkhani A, Levy CS, Tsui M, et al. Ly6c Lo non-classical monocytes promote resolution of rhesus rotavirus-mediated perinatal hepatic inflammation. Scientific Rep 2020;10(1):7165.

47. Holterman A, Nguyen HPA, Nadler E, et al. Granulocyte-colony stimulating factor GCSF mobilizes hematopoietic stem cells in Kasai patients with biliary atresia in a phase 1 study and improves short term outcome. J Pediatr Surg 2021;56(7):1179–85.

48. Holterman A-X. Granulocyte-colony stimulating factor Adjunct therapy for biliary atresia: Part II of a prospective, randomized Controlled, multi-Institutional trial. clinicaltrials.gov. 2020. Available at: https://clinicaltrials.gov/ct2/show/NCT04373941.

49. Harpavat S. A phase II trial of pentoxifylline in Newly-diagnosed biliary atresia. clinicaltrials.gov. 2021. Available at: https://clinicaltrials.gov/ct2/show/NCT01774487.

50. Harpavat S. A phase 2 trial of N-acetylcysteine in biliary atresia after Kasai portoenterostomy. clinicaltrials.gov. 2021. Available at: https://clinicaltrials.gov/ct2/show/NCT03499249.

51. Mirum Pharmaceuticals. Inc. Randomized, Double-Blind, Placebo-Controlled phase 2 study to evaluate the efficacy and safety of Maralixibat in the treatment of subjects with biliary atresia after Hepatoportoenterostomy. clinicaltrials.gov. 2022. Available at: https://clinicaltrials.gov/ct2/show/NCT04524390.

52. Albireo A. Double-blind, randomized, Placebo-Controlled study to evaluate the efficacy and safety of Odevixibat (A4250) in children with biliary atresia who have undergone a Kasai Hepatoportoenterostomy. clinicaltrials.gov. 2022. Available at: https://clinicaltrials.gov/ct2/show/NCT04336722.

53. Soares KC, Goldstein SD, Ghaseb MA, et al. Pediatric choledochal cysts: diagnosis and current management. Pediatr Surg Int 2017;33(6):637–50.

54. Jones RE, Zagory JA, Clark RA, et al. A narrative review of the modern surgical management of pediatric choledochal cysts. Transl Gastroenterol Hepatol 2021;6:37.

55. Ashcraft KW, Holcomb GW, Murphy JP, et al. Ashcraft's pediatric surgery. Saunders/Elsevier; 2010.

56. Singham J, Yoshida EM, Scudamore CH. Choledochal cysts: Part 1 of 3: classification and pathogenesis. Can J Surg 2009;52(5):434–40.

57. Todani T, Watanabe Y, Toki A, et al. Classification of congenital biliary cystic disease: special reference to type Ic and IVA cysts with primary ductal stricture. J Hepato-Biliary-Pancreatic Surg 2003;10(5):340–4.

58. Law R, Topazian M. Diagnosis and treatment of Choledochoceles. Clin Gastroenterol Hepatol 2014;12(2):196–203.

59. Jabłońska B. Biliary cysts: etiology, diagnosis and management. World J Gastroenterol 2012;18(35):4801–10.

60. Schwab ME, Song H, Mattis A, et al. De novo somatic mutations and KRAS amplification are associated with cholangiocarcinoma in a patient with a history of choledochal cyst. J Pediatr Surg 2020;55(12):2657–61.

61. Yeung F, Fung ACH, Chung PHY, et al. Short-term and long-term outcomes after Roux-en-Y hepaticojejunostomy versus hepaticoduodenostomy following laparoscopic excision of choledochal cyst in children. Surg Endosc 2020;34(5):2172–7.

62. Liem NT, Pham HD, Dung LA, et al. Early and Intermediate outcomes of laparoscopic surgery for choledochal cysts with 400 patients. J Laparoendoscopic Adv Surg Tech 2012;22(6):599–603.

63. Santore MT, Deans KJ, Behar BJ, et al. Laparoscopic hepaticoduodenostomy versus open hepaticoduodenostomy for reconstruction after resection of choledochal cyst. J Laparoendoscopic Adv Surg Tech 2011;21(4):375–8.

64. Zhen C, Xia Z, Long L, et al. Laparoscopic excision versus open excision for the treatment of choledochal cysts: a systematic review and meta-analysis. Int Surg 2015;100(1):115–22.

65. Margonis GA, Spolverato G, Kim Y, et al. Minimally invasive resection of choledochal cyst: a feasible and safe surgical option. J Gastrointest Surg 2015;19(5): 858–65.

66. Qiao G, Li L, Li S, et al. Laparoscopic cyst excision and Roux-Y hepaticojejunostomy for children with choledochal cysts in China: a multicenter study. Surg Endosc 2015;29(1):140–4.

67. She WH, Chung HY, Lan LCL, et al. Management of choledochal cyst: 30 years of experience and results in a single center. J Pediatr Surg 2009;44(12):2307–11.

68. Foo DC, Wong KK, Lan LC, et al. Impact of prenatal diagnosis on choledochal cysts and the benefits of early excision. J Paediatrics Child Health 2009; 45(1–2):28–30.

69. Tsai MS, Lin WH, Hsu WM, et al. Clinicopathological Feature and surgical outcome of choledochal cyst in different age groups: the implication of surgical timing. J Gastrointest Surg 2008;12(12):2191.

70. Madadi-Sanjani O, Wirth TC, Kuebler JF, et al. Choledochal cyst and malignancy: a Plea for Lifelong follow-up. Eur J Pediatr Surg 2019;29(02):143–9.

71. ten Hove A, de Meijer VE, Hulscher JBF, et al. Meta-analysis of risk of developing malignancy in congenital choledochal malformation. Br J Surg 2018;105(5): 482–90.

72. Weinberg BA, Xiu J, Lindberg MR, et al. Molecular profiling of biliary cancers reveals distinct molecular alterations and potential therapeutic targets. J Gastrointest Oncol 2019;10(4):652–62.

73. Drabek J, Keil R, Stovicek J, et al. The role of endoscopic retrograde cholangiopancreatography in choledochal cysts and/or abnormal pancreatobiliary junction in children. Prz Gastroenterol 2017;12(4):303–9.

74. Yodice M, Choma J, Tadros M. The Expansion of cholangioscopy: established and investigational Uses of SpyGlass in biliary and pancreatic Disorders. Diagnostics (Basel) 2020;10(3):132.

75. Navaneethan U, Njei B, Lourdusamy V, et al. Comparative effectiveness of biliary brush cytology and intraductal biopsy for detection of malignant biliary strictures: a systematic review and meta-analysis. Gastrointest Endosc 2015;81(1):168–76.

76. Rowland KJ, Cunningham AJ, Jazrawi SF, et al. Novel application of SpyGlass™ cholangioscopy in the diagnosis and treatment of extrahepatic biliary obstruction in infants. J Pediatr Surg Case Rep 2018;38:19–22.

77. Mou S, Waxman I, Chennat J. Peroral cholangioscopy in roux-en-Y hepaticojejunostomy anatomy by using the SpyGlass Direct visualization system (with video). Gastrointest Endosc 2010;72(2):458–60.

78. Hülagü S, Şirin G, Duman AE, et al. Use of SpyGlass for peroral cholangioscopy in the diagnosis and treatment of hepatobiliary diseases in over five years follow-up: a single centre experience. Turk J Gastroenterol 2019;30(12):1044–54.

79. Siddiqui AA, Mehendiratta V, Jackson W, et al. Identification of cholangiocarcinoma by using the Spyglass Spyscope system for peroral cholangioscopy and biopsy Collection. Clin Gastroenterol Hepatol 2012;10(5):466–71.

80. Ramchandani M, Reddy DN, Gupta R, et al. Role of single-operator peroral cholangioscopy in the diagnosis of indeterminate biliary lesions: a single-center, prospective study. Gastrointest Endosc 2011;74(3):511–9.

81. Harpavat S, Raijman I, Hernandez JA, et al. Single-center experience of choledochoscopy in pediatric patients. Gastrointestinal Endoscopy 2012;76(3):685–8.

UNITED STATES POSTAL SERVICE ® Statement of Ownership, Management, and Circulation
(All Periodicals Publications Except Requester Publications)

1. Publication Title	2. Publication Number	3. Filing Date
CLINICS IN PERINATOLOGY	001 – 744	9/18/2022

4. Issue Frequency	5. Number of Issues Published Annually	6. Annual Subscription Price
MAR, JUN, SEP, DEC	4	$331.00

7. Complete Mailing Address of Known Office of Publication (Not printer) (Street, city, county, state, and ZIP+4®)

ELSEVIER INC.
230 Park Avenue, Suite 800
New York, NY 10169

Contact Person
Malathi Samayan
Telephone (Include area code)
91-44-4299-4507

8. Complete Mailing Address of Headquarters or General Business Office of Publisher (Not printer)

ELSEVIER INC.
230 Park Avenue, Suite 800
New York, NY 10169

9. Full Names and Complete Mailing Addresses of Publisher, Editor, and Managing Editor (Do not leave blank)

Publisher (Name and complete mailing address)
DOLORES MELONI, ELSEVIER INC.
1600 JOHN F KENNEDY BLVD. SUITE 1800
PHILADELPHIA, PA 19103-2899

Editor (Name and complete mailing address)
KERRY HOLLAND, ELSEVIER INC.
1600 JOHN F KENNEDY BLVD. SUITE 1800
PHILADELPHIA, PA 19103-2899

Managing Editor (Name and complete mailing address)
PATRICK MANLEY, ELSEVIER INC.
1600 JOHN F KENNEDY BLVD. SUITE 1800
PHILADELPHIA, PA 19103-2899

10. Owner (Do not leave blank. If the publication is owned by a corporation, give the name and address of the corporation immediately followed by the names and addresses of all stockholders owning or holding 1 percent or more of the total amount of stock. If not owned by a corporation, give the names and addresses of the individual owners. If owned by a partnership or other unincorporated firm, give its name and address as well as those of each individual owner. If the publication is published by a nonprofit organization, give its name and address.)

Full Name	Complete Mailing Address
WHOLLY OWNED SUBSIDIARY OF REED/ELSEVIER, US HOLDINGS	1600 JOHN F KENNEDY BLVD. SUITE 1800 PHILADELPHIA, PA 19103-2899

11. Known Bondholders, Mortgagees, and Other Security Holders Owning or Holding 1 Percent or More of Total Amount of Bonds, Mortgages, or Other Securities. If none, check box → ☐ None

Full Name	Complete Mailing Address
N/A	

12. Tax Status (For completion by nonprofit organizations authorized to mail at nonprofit rates) (Check one)
The purpose, function, and nonprofit status of this organization and the exempt status for federal income tax purposes:
☒ Has Not Changed During Preceding 12 Months
☐ Has Changed During Preceding 12 Months (Publisher must submit explanation of change with this statement)

PS Form **3526**, July 2014 (Page 1 of 4 (see instructions page 4)) PSN: 7530-01-000-9931   PRIVACY NOTICE: See our privacy policy on www.usps.com.

---

13. Publication Title	14. Issue Date for Circulation Data Below
CLINICS IN PERINATOLOGY	JUNE 2022

15. Extent and Nature of Circulation		Average No. Copies Each Issue During Preceding 12 Months	No. Copies of Single Issue Published Nearest to Filing Date
a. Total Number of Copies (Net press run)		564	492
b. Paid Circulation (By Mail and Outside the Mail)	(1) Mailed Outside-County Paid Subscriptions Stated on PS Form 3541 (Include paid distribution above nominal rate, advertiser's proof copies, and exchange copies)	427	378
	(2) Mailed In-County Paid Subscriptions Stated on PS Form 3541 (Include paid distribution above nominal rate, advertiser's proof copies, and exchange copies)	0	0
	(3) Paid Distribution Outside the Mails Including Sales Through Dealers and Carriers, Street Vendors, Counter Sales, and Other Paid Distribution Outside USPS®	103	77
	(4) Paid Distribution by Other Classes of Mail Through the USPS (e.g., First-Class Mail®)	0	0
c. Total Paid Distribution (Sum of 15b (1), (2), (3), and (4)) ►		530	455
d. Free or Nominal Rate Distribution (By Mail and Outside the Mail)	(1) Free or Nominal Rate Outside-County Copies Included on PS Form 3541	16	19
	(2) Free or Nominal Rate In-County Copies Included on PS Form 3541	0	0
	(3) Free or Nominal Rate Copies Mailed at Other Classes Through the USPS (e.g., First-Class Mail)	0	0
	(4) Free or Nominal Rate Distribution Outside the Mail (Carriers or other means)	0	0
e. Total Free or Nominal Rate Distribution (Sum of 15d (1), (2), (3) and (4)) ►		16	19
f. Total Distribution (Sum of 15c and 15e) ►		546	474
g. Copies not Distributed (See Instructions to Publishers #4 (page #3)) ►		18	18
h. Total (Sum of 15f and g) ►		564	492
i. Percent Paid (15c divided by 15f times 100) ►		97.06%	95.99%

* If you are claiming electronic copies, go to line 16 on page 3. If you are not claiming electronic copies, skip to line 17 on page 3.

16. Electronic Copy Circulation		Average No. Copies Each Issue During Preceding 12 Months	No. Copies of Single Issue Published Nearest to Filing Date
a. Paid Electronic Copies ►			
b. Total Paid Print Copies (Line 15c) + Paid Electronic Copies (Line 16a) ►			
c. Total Print Distribution (Line 15f) + Paid Electronic Copies (Line 16a) ►			
d. Percent Paid (Both Print & Electronic Copies) (16b divided by 16c × 100) ►			

☒ I certify that 50% of all my distributed copies (electronic and print) are paid above a nominal price.

17. Publication of Statement of Ownership
☒ If the publication is a general publication, publication of this statement is required. Will be printed ☐ Publication not required.
in the DECEMBER 2022 issue of this publication.

18. Signature and Title of Editor, Publisher, Business Manager, or Owner

Malathi Samayan   Date 9/18/2022

Malathi Samayan - Distribution Controller

I certify that all information furnished on this form is true and complete. I understand that anyone who furnishes false or misleading information on this form or who omits material or information requested on the form may be subject to criminal sanctions (including fines and imprisonment) and/or civil sanctions (including civil penalties).

PS Form **3526**, July 2014 (Page 3 of 4)   PRIVACY NOTICE: See our privacy policy on www.usps.com

Moving?

Make sure your subscription moves with you!

To notify us of your new address, find your **Clinics Account Number** (located on your mailing label above your name), and contact customer service at:

Email: journalscustomerservice-usa@elsevier.com

800-654-2452 (subscribers in the U.S. & Canada)
314-447-8871 (subscribers outside of the U.S. & Canada)

Fax number: 314-447-8029

Elsevier Health Sciences Division
Subscription Customer Service
3251 Riverport Lane
Maryland Heights, MO 63043

*To ensure uninterrupted delivery of your subscription, please notify us at least 4 weeks in advance of move.

Printed and bound by CPI Group (UK) Ltd, Croydon, CR0 4YY

08/06/2025

01896870-0002